01. 05. 1987.

ADVANCES IN HOST DEFENSE MECHANISMS
Volume 4

MUCOSAL IMMUNITY

Advances in Host Defense Mechanisms
Volume 4

Mucosal Immunity

Editors

John I. Gallin, M.D.

Chief, Bacterial Diseases Section
Laboratory of Clinical Investigation
National Institute of Allergy and
Infectious Diseases
National Institutes of Health
Bethesda, Maryland

Anthony S. Fauci, M.D.

Director
National Institute of Allergy and
Infectious Diseases
National Institutes of Health
Bethesda, Maryland

Raven Press ■ New York

Raven Press, 1140 Avenue of the Americas, New York, New York 10036

Made in the United States of America

Library of Congress Cataloging in Publication Data
Main entry under title:

Mucosal immunity.

(Advances in host defense mechanisms ; v. 4)
Includes bibliographies and index.
1. Mucous membrane.   2. Immunity.   I. Gallin,
John I.   II. Fauci, Anthony S., 1940–   .
III. Series.   [DNLM: 1. Mucous Membrane—immunology.
W1 AD636 v.4 / QS 532.5.M8 M942]
QR185.9.M83M83   1985   616.07'9   83-48671
ISBN 0-88167-067-7

The material contained in this volume was submitted as previously unpublished material, except in the instances in which credit has been given to the source from which some of the illustrative material was derived.

Great care has been taken to maintain the accuracy of the information contained in the volume. However, Raven Press cannot be held responsible for errors or for any consequences arising from the use of the information contained herein.

Materials appearing in this book prepared by individuals as part of their official duties as U.S. Government employees are not covered by the above-mentioned copyright.

Preface

Mucosal immunity is an important subspecialty of the study of infectious diseases that has profound importance for both basic and clinical scientists as well as for clinicians. Yet, until recently it had received relatively little attention in terms of clinical investigation, largely because of the complexity of the systems involved.

This volume contains chapters covering major areas in the field. The first three chapters provide state-of-the-art reviews of the cellular and humoral components of mucosal immunity. The reviews by Strober and Jacobs and Tomasi and Plaut address the cellular and humoral defenses, and the review by Abraham and Beachey considers mechanisms of bacterial attachment to mucosal surfaces and host reactions to bacteria. The next three chapters focus on pulmonary host defenses. The chapters on specific cellular factors, by Hunninghake and colleagues, and humoral factors, by Rankin and Reynolds, provide background information, whereas Pennington's review on the effects of immunosuppression on pulmonary defenses is particularly relevant for clinicians. The final chapter, by Panosian and Gorbach, provides a comprehensive review of the general principles of the host defenses of the gastrointestinal tract and of the infectious diseases of this organ system.

The reviews in this volume clearly portray the enormous challenges awaiting investigators of mucosal immunity. The story that is told is timely and will be of interest to immunologists, pharmacologists, cell biologists, and clinicians.

John I. Gallin
Anthony S. Fauci

Contents

Contributors

Soman N. Abraham, M.D.: *Veterans Administration Medical Center, 1030 Jefferson Avenue, Memphis, Tennessee 38104*

Edwin H. Beachey, M.D.: *Veterans Administration Medical Center, 1030 Jefferson Avenue, Memphis, Tennessee 38104*

Robert B. Fick, M.D.: *Department of Medicine, University of Iowa College of Medicine, Iowa City, Iowa 52242*

Sherwood L. Gorbach, M.D.: *Chief, Division of Infectious Diseases, Tufts University School of Medicine, Tufts–New England Medical Center Hospital, Boston, Massachusetts 02111*

Gary W. Hunninghake, M.D.: *Director, Pulmonary Division, Department of Medicine, Room E325-1 GH, University of Iowa Hospitals and Clinics, Iowa City, Iowa 52242*

David Jacobs, M.D.: *Medical Staff Fellow, Department of Health and Human Services, Public Health Service, National Institutes of Health, Building 10, Room 11N244, Bethesda, Maryland 20205*

Kenneth M. Nugent, M.D.: *Department of Medicine, University of Iowa College of Medicine, Iowa City, Iowa 52242*

Claire B. Panosian, M.D.: *Chief, Division of Infectious Diseases, UCLA–Olive View Memorial Medical Center, Van Nuys, California 91405, and Assistant Professor of Medicine, UCLA School of Medicine, University of California at Los Angeles, Los Angeles, California 90024*

James E. Pennington, M.D.: *Associate Professor of Medicine, Harvard Medical School, and Associate Chief, Infectious Disease Division, Brigham and Women's Hospital, 75 Francis Street, Boston, Massachusetts 02115*

Andrew G. Plaut, M.D.: *Professor of Medicine, Tufts–New England Medical Center, 171 Harrison Avenue, Boston, Massachusetts 02111*

John A. Rankin, M.D.: *Assistant Professor of Medicine, Pulmonary Section, Department of Internal Medicine, Yale University School of Medicine, 333 Cedar Street, P. O. Box 3333, New Haven, Connecticut 06510*

Herbert Y. Reynolds, M.D.: *Professor of Medicine, Head, Pulmonary Section, Department of Internal Medicine, Yale University School of Medicine, 333 Cedar Street, P. O. Box 3333, New Haven, Connecticut 06510*

Warren Strober, M.D.: *Chief, Mucosal Immunity Section, Department of Health and Human Services, Public Health Service, National Institutes of Health, Building 10, Room 11N244, Bethesda, Maryland 20205*

Thomas B. Tomasi, M.D.: *Director, Cancer Center and Chairman, Department of Cell Biology, University of New Mexico School of Medicine, 900 Camino de Salud, Northeast, Albuquerque, New Mexico 81713*

ADVANCES IN HOST DEFENSE MECHANISMS
Volume 4

MUCOSAL IMMUNITY

Advances in Host Defense Mechanisms, Vol. 4,
edited by J. I. Gallin and A. S. Fauci.
Raven Press, New York © 1985.

Cellular Differentiation, Migration, and Function in the Mucosal Immune System

Warren Strober and David Jacobs

Mucosal Immunity Section, Laboratory of Clinical Investigation, National Institute of Allergy and Infectious Diseases, National Institutes of Health, Bethesda, Maryland 20205

Well over a decade ago Craig and Cebra (1) showed that cells obtained from Peyer's patches (PP) of donor rabbits could be used to repopulate the lymphoid tissues of irradiated recipient rabbits. However, the pattern of repopulation obtained with such cells was quite different from that obtained with peripheral node cells: PP cells led to a spleen B-cell population consisting mostly of IgA-containing cells and to abundant repletion of intestinal tissues, again mainly with IgA cells; in contrast, peripheral node cells led to a spleen B-cell population dominated by IgG-containing cells and to only marginal repletion of intestinal tissues, in this case largely by IgG cells (1). These studies established two important features of the mucosal immune system: First, PP provide a preferential site for IgA B-cell development; second, PP cells are the source of IgA B cells that are found in the mucosal areas generally. In the discussion to follow we shall examine these two concepts in light of recent studies of cell genesis and movement in the mucosal immune system. More specifically, we shall address the question why IgA B cells develop in mucosal lymphoid follicles and not in other lymphoid tissues, as well as the question why cells in mucosal lymphoid follicles tend to migrate out of these lymphoid tissues only to localize in the diffuse sites underlying the various mucosal epithelial layers.

IgA B-CELL DEVELOPMENT

Overview of B-Cell Differentiation

IgA B-cell development in PP is best discussed within the context of our current understanding of the major steps involved in general B-cell development. To begin with, B cells have their origin in pluripotential stem cells that give rise to cells destined for B-cell development in the bone marrow (or, during fetal life, in the liver). The earliest cells of the B-cell series are recognizable by the fact that they bear certain B-cell-specific surface determinants detected by monoclonal antibodies (2). These early B cells develop into "pre-B cells," which are cells that contain cytoplasmic μ-chain but not whole IgM molecules; such cells bear neither surface

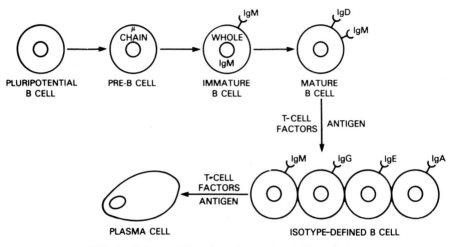

FIG. 1. Schema of B-cell development and differentiation.

immunoglobulins nor other mature B-cell markers (3). Pre-B cells develop into "immature B cells," cells that are capable of synthesizing whole IgM molecules and that bear surface IgM (sIgM) (4). Immature B cells, in turn, become "mature B cells," which synthesize both IgM and IgD and bear these immunoglobulins on their surfaces. Further development of the B cell involves interactions of the cell with antigen as well as several antigen-nonspecific factors derived from T cells (5,6). Such interactions initiate isotype differentiation, a process during which the B cell becomes a definitive IgM, IgG, IgE, or IgA B cell (7). Finally, B cells differentiate into Ig-secreting plasma cells, again under the influence of T-cell factors. An overview of B-cell development is shown in Fig. 1.

In the last few years it has become clear that these cellular transformations reflect genomic events that result in massive rearrangements of the DNA segments (the genes) encoding the heavy and light chains of the immunoglobulin molecule (8). Initially (prior to differentiation), the region of the genome dedicated to the Ig molecule consists of many structural genes on a relatively long stretch of DNA. In the case of the variable region of the heavy chain, these structural genes consist of several hundred variable-region (V-region) genes followed by approximately 20 diversity-region (D-region) genes, and four joining-region (J-region) genes. These V-region genes are followed by constant-region (C-region) genes arrayed on the DNA strand in a fixed order. In the mouse this consists first of μ and δ C-region genes, then the various γ-subclass C-region genes, and finally the ϵ and α C-region genes (9). In the human, this basic arrangement seems to have undergone gene-group duplication, in that we find the μ and δ C-region genes followed by two tandem segments each containing γ, ϵ, and α genes. The first segment is composed of γ_3 and γ_1 genes, followed by a nonexpressed ϵ gene and the α_1 genes. The second segment is composed of γ_2 and γ_4 genes, followed by an expressed ϵ gene and the α_2 gene (10).

The earliest step in the process leading to a functionally active immunoglobulin gene involves rearrangement of the DNA segment that controls the V region of the Ig molecule. During this step, one of the V-region genes is brought together with one of the D-region genes and one of the J-region genes by a molecular mechanism that involves the looping out and excision of DNA intervening between the retained genes (11). Variability in the sequencing of resultant V, D, and J genes and the occurrence of somatic mutations lead to diversity in the assembled V-region gene and explain why each cell is virtually unique with respect to antigenic specificity (8). Genes controlling the light-chain V region undergo similar rearrangements, but, as mentioned, in this case there are no D genes on the relevant DNA strand.

Following V-region DNA rearrangement, the heavy-chain Ig gene is composed of rearranged V-region DNA (a joined VDJ gene) juxtaposed to heavy-chain C-region-encoding genes. At this point the cell is at the pre-B-cell stage of development, and mRNA pairing with V-region and adjacent μ C-region genes can be synthesized. Such mRNA necessarily contains bases pairing with DNA intervening between the rearranged and joined V-region genes and the μ C-region gene; however, these bases are excised during post-transcriptional processing (12). At a later stage of B-cell development, a stage characteristic of the immature B cell, a longer mRNA transcript is formed that includes bases pairing with the δ C-region gene as well as the μ C-region gene. Following transcription, this mRNA is broken down into separate mRNAs that encode for either IgM or IgD molecules; thus, the cell can produce both immunoglobulins during this stage of its development (13).

In the next phase of B-cell differentiation, during the time cells bearing the individual immunoglobulin classes and subclasses arise (i.e., during isotype differentiation), further changes in the B-cell genome occur. In general, these changes involve additional DNA deletions that result in the juxtaposition of progressively more 3' C-region genes next to the VDJ gene (14,15). Thus, in cells differentiating into IgG B cells, μ and δ C-region DNA is deleted and γ C-region-encoding DNA comes to lie adjacent to the V-region DNA. Alternatively, in cells differentiating into IgA B cells, μ as well as γ C-region DNA is deleted and α C-region-encoding DNA lie next to the V-region DNA. The molecular processes governing the deletion of heavy-chain C-region-encoding DNA segments (and thus B-cell "switching") are not fully understood. Recently, however, some light was shed on the matter by Davis et al. (16), who described DNA regions located 5' to each heavy-chain C-region gene (except the δ heavy-chain C-region gene) that are involved in the C-region gene deletional process. These segments (called "switch sites") contain repeating base sequences and appear to be Ig-class-specific. It is postulated that during the deletional process certain of these switch sites become paired, and the loop of DNA that is formed is excised. For example, during deletion of IgM and IgG C-region genes (i.e., during transformation of an IgM B cell to an IgE B cell), a switch site 5' to the IgM gene pairs with a switch site 5' to the IgE gene, and the resultant DNA loop is deleted. On the basis of this information it can tentatively be proposed that the factors that determine switch-site interactions also determine

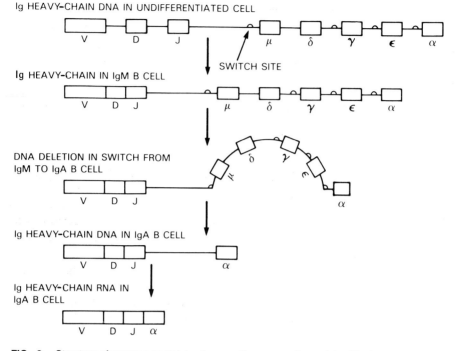

Ig HEAVY-CHAIN DNA IN UNDIFFERENTIATED CELL

SWITCH SITE

Ig HEAVY-CHAIN IN IgM B CELL

DNA DELETION IN SWITCH FROM
IgM TO IgA B CELL

Ig HEAVY-CHAIN DNA IN IgA B CELL

Ig HEAVY-CHAIN RNA IN
IgA B CELL

FIG. 2. Structure of genome containing Ig-encoding genes. As explained in the text, the rearranged VDJ region encodes for the V region of the Ig molecule. Genes encoding for various heavy-chain C regions are arranged in sequence and undergo deletion during isotype differentiation. Such deletion involves pairing of switch sites 5′ to C-region genes and deletion of the resulting loop. It is seen that the IgA C-region-encoding gene is the most-3′ of the various C-region genes.

the pathway of B-cell isotype differentiation. A diagrammatic representation of the molecular events of isotype differentiation is shown in Fig. 2.

The foregoing model of isotype switching is irreversible in the sense that once a DNA segment is deleted, the cell can no longer make the Igs encoded by the deleted genes. Recently, however, Honjo and associates presented evidence that B cells may sometimes pass through a stage in which the μ C-region gene and one downstream C-region gene are transcribed prior to any C-region gene deletion (17). In the studies supporting this concept, in a particular inbred mouse strain (SJA) preimmunized with a particular parasite, these investigators identified a stable population of cells that express both IgM and sIgE, but that have not undergone heavy-chain gene rearrangement and deletion. They proposed that in such cells an ultralong RNA transcript is synthesized that undergoes post-transcriptional processing to yield mRNA for IgM and IgE. If such a process can also occur in relation to other heavy-chain C-region genes, it is possible that all B cells may first express any given isotype (along with IgM) prior to the deletion of heavy-chain genes emplaced 5′ to it on the DNA strand. B cells in this state may revert

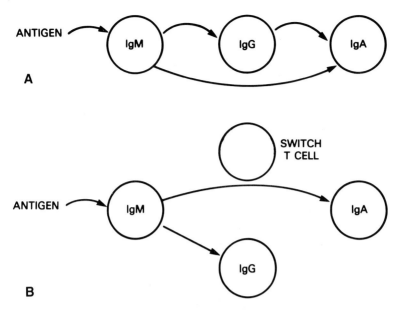

FIG. 3. Two theories of IgA B-cell differentiation. **A:** The B-cell-centered theory, which promotes the concept of an antigen-driven, sequential, random switch. **B:** The T-cell-centered theory, which suggests the presence of regulating T cells involved in isotype switching.

back to exclusive IgM expression or, alternatively, may proceed to gene deletion and irreversible commitment to the downstream heavy-chain gene already expressed.

Theories of IgA B-Cell Differentiation

With this knowledge of the cellular and molecular events of B-cell differentiation, we are in a position to discuss the factors that contribute to the differentiation of IgA B cells at mucosal sites. In one theory, events going on entirely within B cells subjected to repeated antigen stimulation are considered paramount, and influences arising from other cells are considered unimportant and unnecessary (18). In another theory, intracellular events occurring in the antigen-stimulated B cell are recognized as essential; nevertheless, such events are assumed to require regulation by signals derived from other cells, particularly T cells (19). These two theories are diagrammatically represented in Fig. 3 and, for convenience, will be referred to as the B-cell-centered and T-cell-centered theories, respectively.

The B-cell-centered theory is based chiefly on studies conducted by Cebra and associates in which the splenic-focus assay, originally developed by Klinman (20), was the method used to determine the nature of the progeny of individual B cells. In this assay, B cells (usually along with T cells) are obtained from various organs of an immunized animal and are injected into a lethally irradiated mouse. After a period of time, the spleen of the recipient mouse is harvested and cut into small fragments that are cultured *in vitro* in wells along with the original immunizing antigen. Finally, the supernatants of the spleen-fragment cultures are assayed for the presence of antibodies having particular isotypes and antigenic specificities. An essential feature of this procedure is that the lethally irradiated mice are given a B-cell dose chosen in such a way that most of the spleen fragments ultimately obtained are not seeded by more than one B cell; thus, any antibody appearing in the fragment cultures is the product of the progeny of a single B cell.

In studies in which the splenic-focus assay was applied to investigation of the mucosal immune system, Cebra and associates found that administration of an antigen by the oral route led to an increase in PP of precursor cells specific for the antigen and that such precursors consistently gave rise to progeny secreting some IgA or, more strikingly, progeny secreting only IgA (21,22). Furthermore, there appeared to be a gradient of B cells committed to IgA expression, in that precursors giving rise to progeny secreting only IgA were more numerous in PP than in mesenteric nodes and more numerous in the nodes than in the spleen. In other studies, the Cebra group tied the occurrence of IgA-only clones to antigen exposure by demonstrating that B cells committed to only IgA expression were increased in conventional animals as compared with germ-free animals, particularly when the antigen used to immunize animals was one that is naturally present in the mucosal environment. In addition, they established that following antigenic challenge via the gastrointestinal tract with environmental antigens, the frequency of clones making at least some IgA was remarkably high.

Cebra and associates used these data, as well as newly emerging information on the gene rearrangements that accompany B-cell development *(vide supra)*, to construct a theory of IgA B-cell differentiation (23,24). In particular, these investigators postulated that the intense antigenic drive encountered by B cells in PP leads to recurrent cell divisions and thus to progressive loss of heavy-chain C-region-encoding genes. Such cell-division-dependent deletion is assumed to occur in a manner that results in stepwise loss of a single C-region gene (stepwise deletion), or loss of several C-region genes at once. In either case, the process is "vectorial" and inevitably results (after a sufficient number of divisions) in a B-cell population that has arrived at the ultimate level of heavy-chain C-region gene deletion, that characteristic of IgA B cells.

This core conception was amplified by a number of corollary assertions. First, recognizing that terminal differentiation of B cells into IgM or IgG plasma cells would have the effect of depleting the total B-cell pool of cells potentially able to express IgA, the Cebra group postulated that such terminal differentiation was prohibited in PP (23). Second, the view was adopted that there is nothing intrinsically unique about PP B cells as far as IgA potential is concerned: Any B-cell population subject to an equivalent antigenic drive would move toward IgA expression; it is on this basis that we encounter some IgA B cells in clonal outgrowths obtained from spleen-cell populations. Third, the position was taken that regulatory T cells play little or no role in IgA B-cell development, because the factors essential for IgA expression are inherent in the potential of B cells to undergo DNA rearrangements and the antigenic drive present in the environment. The only possible effect of T cells is on B cells that have already become IgA B cells, in which case the effect is to play a minor role in the expansion of the already differentiated IgA B-cell population (24).

Although this B-cell-centered theory is logical and offers a comprehensive explanation for the emergence of IgA B cells, it is at odds with certain observations relative to B-cell differentiation generally and IgA B-cell differentiation specifically.

The first problem is based on the molecular biology of Ig genes reviewed earlier. In particular, whereas the gene encoding the α heavy-chain C region is the ultimate gene in the Ig DNA region of the mouse, in humans one α heavy-chain C-region gene (the α gene) appears in the middle of the C-region gene sequence, and one at the end of the sequence (the α_2 gene). Thus, in the case of the α_1 gene, progressive gene deletion in humans would not lead inevitably to IgA expression, because the α_1 gene is followed by several other non-α genes, including two γ genes and one ϵ gene.

The second problem with the theory is that it predicts, indeed requires, that IgG B cells can give rise to IgA B cells. This follows from the fact that the theory views DNA rearrangements as an unregulated accompaniment of B-cell division and places no restriction whatever on the kinds of rearrangements that occur; in particular, rearrangements involving stepwise deletion of C-region-encoding genes, such as those presumably involved in IgG-to-IgA transitions, are considered eminently feasible. Because the Cebra group found clonal outgrowths (in the splenic-focus assay) that produce IgG and IgA (but not other immunoglobulins), they postulated that IgG-to-IgA transitions are possible and that, in fact, observation does coincide with theory. However, various other data speak against IgG-to-IgA B-cell transitions. Thus, in studies of the nature of the Ig found on the surfaces of B cells performed with the use of fluoresceinated anti-Ig antibodies, it was found that whereas cells bearing both sIgM and sIgG or cells bearing both sIgM and sIgA (with or without accompaning sIgD) are frequently observed, cells bearing both sIgG and sIgA are never observed (7). In addition, in studies in which mitogen-induced Ig synthesis was inhibited with class- and subclass-specific antibodies, it was found that anti-Ig specific for a given class or subclass of IgG inhibited only that class or subclass, whereas anti-IgM inhibited all classes (26,27). Taken together, these data support the widely held view that sIgM B cells are the precursors of IgG B cells and that IgG B cells are not precursors of IgA B cells (or vice versa). In light of these data, one might want to explain the simultaneous occurrence of IgG and IgA B cells in clonal outgrowths of cells studied in the splenic-focus assay by saying that these B cells result from a common IgM B-cell precursor that rapidly disappears and therefore goes undetected, rather than by saying that these B cells result from transitions of IgG B cells to IgA B cells.

The third and perhaps most important problem with the B-cell-centered theory is its view of the role T cells play in B-cell differentiation. In addition to the fact that the theory simply has no need for T cells, Cebra and associates found (again using the splenic-focus assay) that whereas athymic mice have few precursors of IgA-expressing cells for naturally occurring environmental antigens, challenge of athymic mice with a new antigen such as cholera toxin leads to the appearance of IgA-expressing B cells, albeit at a substantially lower frequency than that observed in normal mice (24). Furthermore, they found that IgA-expressing cells occurred at approximately equal frequencies in splenic fragments developing after transfer of whole PP populations (containing both T cells and B cells) and after transfer of T-cell-depleted populations, although the IgA B cells developing in the absence of T cells made lesser amounts of antibody (24). These data would seem to further support the view that IgA B cells can arise in the absence of T cells and that the T cell is not normally a quantitatively important factor in IgA B-cell differentiation.

A far different picture of the role T cells play in B-cell differentiation has emerged from the work of Mongini et al. (29–31), using many of the same techniques as the Cebra group. In an initial series of studies these investigators determined the responses of athymic animals to TNP-Ficoll, a thymic-independent antigen (31). Of interest was the fact that whereas athymic animals had good *in vivo* IgM and IgG_3 anti-TNP responses, they had poor IgG_{2a} and IgG_{2b} anti-TNP responses; in addition, reconstitution of the athymic animals with T cells led to good IgG_{2a} responses. Because the positions of the genes on the DNA strands encoding for the C regions of the various IgG subclasses are in the order IgG_3, IgG_1, IgG_{2b}, and IgG_{2a} (moving in a 3' direction along the DNA strand), these results suggest that T cells somehow lead to the expression of genes located farther down the DNA strand.

In later studies these investigators studied responses to TNP-Ficoll at the clonal level by using the splenic-focus assay (30). Here they made the observation that addition of T cells to the inocula of cells given to irradiated recipients (whose spleen fragments were to be subsequently assayed *in vitro*) led to enhanced IgG_{2a} and IgG_{2b} responses, indicating that IgG_{2a} and IgG_{2b} expressions are dependent on the presence of T cells, as in the case of the *in vivo* responses of athymic animals. A further finding was that spleen fragments that produced IgG_{2a} also produced IgG_{2b}, whereas spleen fragments producing IgG_{2b} produced very little IgG_{2a}. Because IgG_{2a} is encoded by a gene located farther along the DNA strand than the gene encoding IgG_{2b}, these data (as well as related data) led to the view that a fragment producing a given IgG subclass would also produce all the IgG subclasses encoded by genes preceding its gene on the DNA strand, but not the IgG subclasses following its gene on the DNA strand. These findings relative to the T-cell effects on IgG isotype expression intermesh with those of Isakson and associates, who studied B-cell responses in polyclonal systems (32). In the relevant studies it was shown that a factor derived from a concanavalin-A-activated (Con-A-activated) alloreactive T-cell line, when added to lipopolysaccharide-stimulated (LPS-stimulated) B cells, resulted in cells secreting more IgG_1 and less IgG_3 as compared with LPS-stimulated B cells cultured without the factor. In all, the foregoing studies are consistent with the view that T cells are essential to the synthesis of a full range of IgG subclasses and that the role of T cells is to provide a signal that somehow facilitates the emergence of cells expressing IgG subclasses encoded for by ever-more-3' heavy-chain C-region-encoding genes.

Finally, Mongini et al. (31) addressed the question of effect of T cells on IgA and IgE responses. In these studies they reestablished at the clonal level an older finding that athymic animals had relatively poor IgA responses. In addition, they found that addition of T cells to inocula used to replete animals whose spleens were to be examined in the splenic-focus assay enhanced the frequency of IgA-expressing clones, but had only a slight enhancing effect on IgE-expressing clones. In addition, they observed that spleen fragments expressing either IgA and IgE antibodies did not usually co-express the various IgG subclass antibodies, even though these antibodies are encoded by genes located proximal to the IgE and IgA genes on the DNA strand. These studies, taken together, suggest that IgE and IgA C-region gene expression does not await IgG C-region expression and that T cells play an essential role in the switch process, at least as far as IgA is concerned.

The various observations on the role of T cells in general (IgG) B-cell development recounted earlier introduce (and support) a second theory of the origin of IgA B cells in the mucosal immune system, which is that IgA B-cell development is critically dependent on T-cell-derived class-specific signals that direct B cells into a pathway of IgA differentiation. This T-cell-centered theory of IgA B-cell development had its origin in the observation made a decade ago that thymectomized animals have decreased IgA antibody responses and that nude (congenitally athymic) mice have very low IgA levels, but more or less normal IgM and IgG levels (33,34). Much more recently, the importance of T cells to IgA B-cell development was reaffirmed as a result of an investigation of mitogen-induced regulatory T cells obtained from PP and other tissues. In the relevant studies, Elson and associates added T cells prestimulated with Con-A to indicator cultures consisting of B cells subjected to LPS stimulation (35). As expected, Con-A-exposed spleen T cells suppressed Ig synthesis of indicator cultures regardless of the Ig class under consideration; this undoubtedly was the result of Con-A activation of suppressor T cells in the spleen T-cell population. In contrast, whereas Con-A-exposed PP T cells also suppressed IgM and IgG synthesis, they greatly enhanced IgA synthesis. This effect was seen regardless of the B-cell source (i.e., spleen B cells also demonstrated enhanced IgA synthesis when co-cultured with PP T cells), indicating that the class-specific effects resided with the T cells, not with the B cells. These studies were therefore quite clear in showing that T cells do indeed have class-specific regulatory effects and that the PP is the locus of T cells that enhance IgA synthesis.

Further analysis of the role of T cells in IgA B-cell differentiation awaited the development of cloned T-cell populations whose regulatory effects could be precisely characterized. This was achieved by Kawanishi and associates, who adapted Con-A-stimulated T cells to long-term culture in IL-2-supplemented medium and then cloned the T cells by limiting dilution to obtain stable cloned T cells with defined growth requirements and stable phenotypic markers (36). In studies in which these cloned T cells were assessed for regulatory function, Kawanishi and associates observed that cells derived from PP (cloned PP T cells) influenced B-cell differentiation in a distinctive fashion. Thus, as shown in Table 1, when LPS-

TABLE 1. *Effects of cloned PP and spleen T cells on maturation of sIgM-bearing B cells in the presence of LPS stimulation* in vitro[a]

	Additions to cultures of sIgM PP B cells		
	LPS alone (%)	LPS + cloned PP T cells (%)	LPS + cloned spleen T cells (%)
sIgM	40[b]	36	40
sIgG	16	3	26
sIgA	<1	<43	<1

[a]From Kawanishi et al. (37).
[b]Percentage of cells bearing Ig indicated after 5 days of culture.

stimulated B cells were cultured in the presence of cloned PP T cells, cells bearing sIgG or producing IgG were greatly decreased, and, instead, very considerable numbers of cells bearing sIgA appeared, as compared with cultures in which B cells were cultured in the absence of T cells. In sharp contrast, when LPS-stimulated B cells were cultured in the presence of cloned spleen T cells, the numbers of sIgG-bearing and IgG-producing cells increased as compared with B cells cultured in the absence of T cells; in addition, under these circumstances, no sIgA-bearing B cells appeared. These data indicate that T cells present in PP (but not in the spleen) have the capacity to influence B cells (under a proliferative influence provided by LPS) to become IgA B cells, and they suggest that T-cell regulatory influences are indeed a requirement of IgA B-cell development.

The foregoing studies left open the important question whether cloned PP T cells act on sIgM-bearing B cells to actually effect an isotype switch to sIgA-bearing B cells or merely on sIgA-bearing B cells that have already formed to cause selective expansion of sIgA B-cell populations that have already switched. This question was addressed in studies in which B cells of a defined isotype were purified prior to culture with cloned PP T cells or cloned spleen T cells (37). It was found that co-culture of sIgM-bearing B cells and cloned PP T cells (in the presence of LPS) led to the appearance of sIgA-bearing B cells, whereas co-culture of sIgG-bearing B cells with cloned PP T cells (in the presence of LPS) did not lead to the appearance of sIgA-bearing B cells. Consistent with the studies of whole B-cell preparations mentioned earlier, cloned spleen T cells did not display an IgM-to-IgA switch in sIgM-bearing B-cell populations or an IgG-to-IgA switch in sIgG-bearing B-cell populations. In all, these data indicate that cloned PP T cells provide a true switch signal (which acts only on sIgM-bearing B cells), not a class-specific proliferation signal for B cells that have already switched to IgA; in other words, they appear to be IgA-class-specific switch T cells. These data are therefore distinct from the data gathered by Isakson and associates, which did not distinguish between a T-cell effect characterized by selective expansion of B cells that have spontaneously switched to an Ig class (or subclass) encoded by a more-3'-encoding gene and a T-cell effect on the switch process itself.

A final point concerning the action of switch T cells is that they do not bring about significant differentiation of B cells into Ig-producing plasma cells (37). That is, when B cells are cultured with cloned PP T cells along with LPS, there is decreased IgM and IgG secretion and little, if any, IgA secretion. Furthermore, co-cultures of sIgA-bearing B cells and cloned PP T cells did not cause proliferation of sIgA-bearing B cells above that brought about by LPS alone. These results are best explained by assuming that switch T cells cause B cells to shift away from IgM and IgG expression (and hence terminal differentiation) that is normally induced by LPS and into an IgA-expressing stage that stops short of IgA B-cell proliferation and terminal differentiation. As we shall see, it is likely that terminal differentiation requires additional T-cell influences not provided by switch T cells.

In summary, these studies on the regulatory function of cloned T cells obtained from PP strongly suggest that IgA B-cell development (at least that occurring in PP) is critically dependent on regulatory signals derived from T cells. Of the two theories of IgA B-cell development proposed earlier, the T-cell-centered theory appears to be better able to encompass the available data. This conclusion does not preclude the possibility that processes occurring within the B cell exclusive of T-cell activity are also necessary for the emergence of IgA B cells. In this latter regard, it is conceivable that B cells developing within the PP microenvironment become committed to IgA development, but such commitment becomes manifest only when the cells are exposed to appropriate T cells. We shall return to this possibility later.

Finally, whereas the foregoing data quite definitely establish a role for a special class of regulatory T cells in IgA B-cell development, they do not address the question why IgA-class-specific regulatory cells appear to be localized in mucosal follicles (and therefore confer on such follicles the status of IgA B-cell-generating areas). On the one hand, it is possible that T cells localizing in mucosal areas acquire switch-T-cell capability because of local influences, such as the secretion of T-cell differentiation factors by mucosa-specific epithelial cells; on the other hand, particular T cells with IgA switch capacity may preferentially home to mucosal tissues on the basis of their capacity to interact with vascular epithelial cells found only in PP lymphoid follicles. It is clear that additional work will be necessary before we can decide between these two possibilities.

Implications of Switch T Cells for B-Cell Differentiation and Activation

The studies of switch T cells described earlier raise a number of important questions concerning B-cell differentiation. The first question concerns the relation of switch events to antigen-specific B-cell activation: When during B-cell activation is a switch signal delivered? To put this question into perspective we must first recognize that B cells recognize antigen via antigen-specific Ig receptors, and it is the cross-linking of such receptors that is the first step in B-cell activation (5). One population of B cells recognizes antigen only when presented by antigen-specific T cells or factors derived from the latter (39). In this case, the T-cell–B-

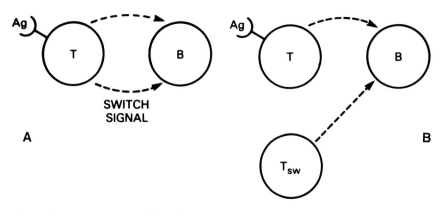

FIG. 4. Relation of the switch T cell to Ag-reactive cells. **A:** Antigen-reactive and switch T cells are identical. **B:** Antigen-reactive and switch T cells are distinct. The latter possibility assumes that the switch signal is not antigen-specific.

cell interaction is restricted by proteins (Ia antigens) encoded by genes located in the major histocompatibility complex (MHC), and there is joint recognition of antigen and MHC proteins. Following the antigen activation step, the B cell becomes susceptible to the action of T-cell-derived growth factors, the most important of which is B-cell growth factor (BCGF); it is likely that the latter interacts with specific receptors on the B cell to induce actual cell division (5). Another population of B cells is stimulated by certain antigens (type II antigens) either directly or by presenting T cells in an MHC-nonrestricted manner (39). Following such stimulation, these cells also require additional growth factors derived from T cells for proliferation. LPS (and other polyclonal activators) act mainly on the first population of B cells, and then only on those cells that have already received an initial activation signal via the Ig receptor (40). In general, therefore, the picture of B-cell activation that emerges is that antigen delivers an initial signal for B-cell activation, and T-cell factors and/or polyclonal stimulants are necessary for actual proliferation. In this situation it is reasonable to postulate that the switch signal is delivered to the cell after its initial activation by antigen at about the same time the signal provided by T-cell-derived growth factor is delivered. This is consistent with the fact that the switch signal appears to act only on LPS-stimulated cells, i.e., on cells having already interacted with antigen.

A second question concerns the nature of the switch T cell: Is the switch T cell an antigen-reactive cell that delivers the antigen signal to the B cell (in addition to the switch signal), or is the switch cell a separate cell, distinct from the antigen-reactive cell (Fig. 4), that is separately activated during the course of the mucosal immune response? In regard to the latter possibility, it is now well recognized that T cells can be activated in an antigen-nonspecific way by Ia antigens present on autologous B cells and/or macrophages that have themselves been stimulated by antigen. It has been suggested that such "autoreactive" cells have both positive and negative regulatory roles in the overall response (41). A variety of preliminary evidence suggests that the switch T cell is, in fact, a cell in the second category, i.e., a cell secondarily activated by interaction with autologous cells. First, attempts to find switch T cells among antigen-specific helper cells obtained from PP have been unsuccessful (42). Second, switch T cells do in fact proliferate when cultured with autologous B cells and macrophages (H. Kawanishi and W. Strober, *unpublished data*). Third, switch T cells have been demonstrated in a system that is propelled by polyclonal activators rather than antigens. Thus, the evidence is presently in favor of the view that the switch T cell and the antigen-specific T cell are separate cells arising from different elements of the mucosal immune response. However, additional study of this question will be necessary to resolve the issue.

A third question regarding switch T cells relates to the nature of the PP B cell undergoing switch to IgA expression. In particular, we must address the question mentioned earlier: whether or not the PP B cell is unique in the sense that it is precommitted to IgA differentiation and thus is better able to respond to IgA-class-specific switch T cells than B cells located elsewhere. The answer to this question depends ultimately on the nature of the switch-T-cell influence. On the one hand, it is possible that switch T cells actually influence intranuclear Ig heavy-chain C-region gene transcription, rearrangement, or deletion without reference to any preexisting B-cell differentiative events. On the other hand, it is possible that critical intracellular events necessary for switch to IgA expression have already occurred in PP B cells prior to T-cell signaling, with the function of the latter being merely to expand "pre-switched" cells that are appropriately prepared. In that switch T cells seem to act only on B cells bearing only IgM, the latter possibility appears unlikely, because we would have to postulate that "pre-switch" to IgA commitment can occur in cells that express only IgM on their surfaces and show no tangible evidence of α-gene activation. One way to resolve this issue is to study clonal IgM B-cell populations from a variety of tissue sources that are capable of being maintained in long-term culture and are inherently switchable. If such cells are induced to become IgA B cells only when influenced by IgA-specific switch T cells, we can conclude that the switch signal emanating from T cells is more than a signal to expand a particular B-cell subset; rather, it is a signal that directs B-cell differentiation.

A final question regarding switch T cells: What is the nature of the extracellular and intracellular molecular mechanisms that underlie the switch phenomenon? Concerning extracellular processes, we might presume that, in parallel with other T-cell–B-cell interactions, switch T cells act through a factor secreted by the T cells. Preliminary attempts to demonstrate such a factor have been unsuccessful, but the matter is by no means settled. If a switch factor is indeed found, progress toward identification and characterization of the recognition site on the sIgM B cell responsible for switch can be made.

Concerning intracellular processes, we must again return to the question of the level at which switch T cells operate. If such cells operate through effects on DNA rearrangements, it can be proposed that switch T cells somehow influence enzymes

TABLE 2. *Effects of BCDF on cytoplasmic Ig expression of post-switch PP B cells[a]*

	Additions to cultures of sIgM PP B cells		
1st culture	LPS (%)	LPS and cloned splenic T cells (%)	LPS and cloned PP T cells (%)
2nd culture	LPS + BCDF (%)	LPS + BCDF (%)	LPS + BCDF (%)
cIgM	48[b]	43	29
cIgG	24	12	8
cIgA	0	0	30

[a]Adapted from Kawanishi et al. (19).
[b]Percentage of cells with cytoplasmic Ig indicated after 5 days of culture.

that affect switch-site pairing conducive to IgA switches. Alternatively, if they operate on B cells precommitted to IgA expression, the switch influence may be a more superficial one that operates at the cell surface to cause expansion of cells that are somehow indicating (via a surface receptor?) that they are committed to IgA synthesis.

Post-Switch IgA B-Cell Differentiation

Isotype differentiation into sIgA-bearing B cells is by no means the only stage of B-cell development requiring T-cell influence. In this regard, it is now well known that the next stage of B-cell differentiation, that of terminal differentiation into plasma cells, is also under the direction of T cells. More specifically, it has been shown that terminal differentiation of all types of B cells requires the presence of T-cell-derived factors, termed T-cell replacing factors or B-cell differentiation factors (TRFs or BCDFs) (5,42). In recent studies, the relationships of such factors to switch events were explored in studies of terminal differentiation of B cells preexposed to various switching influences (38). In those studies it was shown that B cells exposed to LPS as well as to BCDF (a supernatant fluid derived from Con-A-stimulated mesenteric node or spleen T cells) did not go on to express or produce IgA; similarly, B cells exposed to LPS and cloned PP T cells made negligible amounts of IgA. In contrast, B cells exposed to all three components (LPS, cloned PP T cells, and BCDF) did produce substantial amounts of IgA (Table 2). This experiment was modified so that the switch step and the terminal differentiation step were separate: B cells could be first cultured with LPS and cloned PP T cells to effect switching of IgM cells to IgA B cells; the B cells could then be reisolated and cultured with LPS and BCDF. Under these conditions, IgA secretion was again obtained. In control studies in which cloned spleen T cells were used during the switch step, IgA production was not seen (Table 2). In general, then, these studies are compatible with the view that the emergence of IgA plasma cells requires two separate and distinct T-cell signals a switch signal and a terminal differentiation signal (Fig. 5).

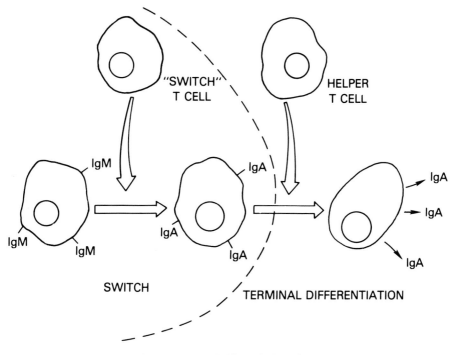

FIG. 5. IgA B-cell differentiation schema.

   The locus of development and action of the T cells capable of providing signals for terminal IgA B-cell differentiation is unclear. Because IgA plasma cells are not present in any significant numbers in PP, it can safely be assumed that terminal differentiation of IgA B cells does not occur at this lymphoid site. This does not mean, however, that T cells capable of influencing terminal B-cell differentiation do not develop in PP. On the contrary, the fact that IgA B-cell synthesis can be obtained *in vitro* by addition of PP T cells to B-cell populations [as shown in the experiments described earlier by Elson et al. (35)] indicates that whole PP T-cell populations contain all the cellular elements necessary for each of the steps of IgA B-cell differentiation. The nondevelopment of plasma cells in PP *in vivo* is best explained by assuming that sIgA-bearing B cells leave the patch prior to undergoing terminal differentiation. Finally, it should be noted that terminal differentiation of sIgA-bearing B cells can be brought about by cells or factors derived by mesenteric node and spleen T-cell populations. This implies that T cells necessary for terminal sIgA B-cell differentiation (as opposed to sIgA-specific switch T cells) are widely distributed.
   This brings us to the question of the class specificity of the terminal differentiation step. In the studies described earlier relative to the T cells or T-cell factors facilitating terminal differentiation of B cells, effects were seen on IgM and IgG B cells as well as IgA B cells. Because the T-cell influence studied did not involve

clonal T-cell populations, it could have derived from several different T-cell types, each with separate class-specific effects on B-cell differentiation; alternatively, the T-cell influence provided may have been class-nonspecific and capable of acting on any post-switch T cell. These studies were therefore indeterminate with respect to post-switch class specificity. Various other studies, however, have not supported the existence of T cells that facilitate class-specific terminal differentiation. Thus, Kiyono et al. (45) have developed antigen-specific T-cell clones that preferentially support IgA antibody synthesis, but have no effect on IgG antibody synthesis. It is clear that these T cells are not switch T cells, as described earlier, because their effect is only on B cells that already express IgA (45). In other studies, Mayer and associates have obtained human T-cell hybridomas that secrete factors that lead to terminal differentiation of sIgA-bearing B cells, but not other kinds of B cells (46). Here, as in the case of the studies by Kiyono and associates, clonal populations were also found that facilitated terminal differentiation of all B-cell types. Finally, Endoh et al. (47) have provided data that T cells bearing IgA Fc receptors help IgA B-cell differentiation in a class-specific manner. These various studies leave little doubt that terminal differentiation of IgA B cells can be a class-specific phenomenon and, as such, put IgA in line with other immunoglobulin classes in which similar effects have been seen (48–50). It need only be added that the mere existence of Ig-class-specific T-cell effects does not ensure the predominance of the latter, and it remains to be seen if class-specific or class-nonspecific helper effects are the major forms of post-switch T-cell influence.

The mechanism of IgA-specific T-cell regulation of terminal differentiation is poorly understood. One possibility relates to the fact that in the studies of Kiyono and those of Endoh, the cells that provided IgA-specific differentiation influences bore IgA Fc receptors. Inasmuch as studies by Ishizaka and associates have disclosed that IgE antibody production can be suppressed or enhanced by IgE-binding factors derived from cells bearing IgE Fc receptors (51,52), it is reasonable to suppose that IgA-binding factors perform a parallel function with regard to IgA B cells.

Class-Specific Suppression of sIgA B-Cell Terminal Differentiation

After isotype switch to IgA expression, sIgA-bearing B cells are subject to T-cell-mediated suppression as well as enhancement. As in the case of T-cell influences on IgA B-cell terminal differentiation, the regulation may be class-nonspecific or class-specific and may involve cells bearing IgA Fc receptors. In studies bearing on the possibility of class-specific suppression, Lynch and associates have shown that mice orally immunized with SRBCs and concomitantly injected with T cells bearing IgA Fc receptors show selective suppression of IgA anti-SRBC responses (53). The T cells that had this effect were obtained from animals bearing IgA plasmacytomas and appeared to arise in such animals as a feedback response to the raised IgA levels resulting from the plasmacytomas (54). The relation of cells bearing IgA Fc receptors to IgA responses is not unique to this Ig class, inasmuch as increased numbers of T cells bearing IgG and IgM Fc receptors are found in

IgG and IgM plasmacytoma-bearing aminals (54). In addition, there is evidence that T cells bearing IgG Fc receptors have negative class-specific effects on IgG antibody responses (55). Finally, we have already mentioned the fact that T cells bearing Fc receptors for IgE have suppressor and helper effects on IgE responses.

The mechanisms of action of cells bearing IgA Fc receptors and class-specific suppression are only now being elucidated. Yodoi et al. (56) have obtained a murine T-cell hybridoma (termed T_2D_4) that bears both IgG and IgA Fc receptors and that produces binding factors for IgG and IgA that are capable of causing class-specific suppression. Interestingly, the hybridoma cells do not release the binding factor unless incubated with IgA, and it is the factor that specifically binds to IgA that mediates suppression. This should not be taken to imply that it is necessarily the Fc receptor itself (or part of the Fc receptor) that is involved in suppression. In this regard, it has been shown in the IgE system that cells lacking IgE Fc receptors still produce binding factors capable of causing suppression.

T-cell-mediated class-specific suppression of IgA responses is not just a laboratory phenomenon. A subset of patients with IgA deficiency have circulating T cells that suppress production of IgA (but not IgG or IgM) induced by polyclonal stimulants (57). Although these T cells are not the cause of the IgA deficiencies (in that the patients also have profound IgA B-cell abnormalities), these T cells constitute evidence that class-specific suppressor T cells are a naturally occurring component of IgA regulation.

Relation of IgA B-Cell Regulation to Mucosal Responsiveness

As we have seen, IgA B-cell differentiation and IgA antibody formation are biological processes that are highly regulated by class-specific T cells, both at an early level of differentiation involving DNA rearrangements in the genome and at a later level of differentiation involving the help and suppression of B cells already bearing sIgA. In view of these facts it is reasonable to inquire if these IgA-related regulatory processes influence general responsiveness or lack of responsiveness of the mucosal immune system to orally administered antigens. In addressing this question, we must first point out that antigens impinging on the immune system via mucosal surfaces generally lead to unresponsiveness to subsequent parenteral challenge with the same antigen (58) (Fig. 6). As detailed by Tomasi and Plaut in another chapter, the mechanisms accounting for unresponsiveness are complex and involve the induction of suppressor T cells in mucosal lymphoid follicles, as well as direct inactivation or paralysis of antigen-responsive B cells. It is interesting to note, however, that in some instances the unresponsiveness induced by oral antigen has been class-specific. Thus, Challacombe and Tomasi have shown that systemic (IgG antibody) responses are diminished in orally stimulated animals, whereas secretory (IgA antibody) responses are intact (59). In a similar vein, Richman et al. (60) have shown that feeding of ovalbumin under certain conditions leads to simultaneous induction of suppressor cells for IgG antibody responses and helper cells for IgA antibody responses. These studies introduce the possibility that

1° ORAL ANTIGEN CHALLENGE

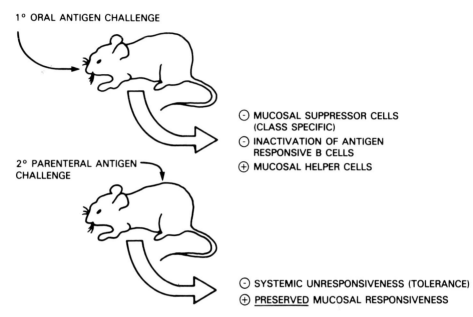

⊖ MUCOSAL SUPPRESSOR CELLS
(CLASS SPECIFIC)
⊖ INACTIVATION OF ANTIGEN
RESPONSIVE B CELLS
⊕ MUCOSAL HELPER CELLS

2° PARENTERAL ANTIGEN
CHALLENGE

⊖ SYSTEMIC UNRESPONSIVENESS (TOLERANCE)
⊕ PRESERVED MUCOSAL RESPONSIVENESS

FIG. 6. Responses of the mucosal and systemic immune systems to oral antigen.

independent (class-specific) regulation of IgA responses can result in novel immunoregulatory patterns wherein the mucosal response is stimulated at the same time that the systemic response is abrogated.

The potential advantage of such independent IgA regulation to the host is easily imagined. On the one hand, the individual is freed from the necessity to respond to many environmental materials that might otherwise engage the general immune system in reactions that are not protective and that could in fact lead to autoimmunity (in that many environmental antigens resemble self-antigens). On the other hand, the mucosal system could still form responses to common environmental materials in the mucosal environment that have host-protective roles at the mucosal surfaces and that aid in the exclusion of materials from the body via IgA-mediated mucosal exclusion and hepatic transport mechanisms. The demonstration that "split" regulation can occur should not, however, be taken to imply that all antigens impinging on the mucosal lymphoid tissue elicit such a form of regulation. On the contrary, it is possible that many or most antigens elicit across-the-board negative or positive responses. The fact is that we are just beginning to learn the "rules" governing regulation of the responses to particular antigens in the mucosal immune system. Knowledge of these rules will allow prediction of the precise response pattern we can expect following oral administration of a given antigen. In addition, such knowledge will govern approaches to the construction of oral vaccination programs and to the treatment of possible diseases that have their basis in abnormal regulation of the mucosal immune response.

CELLULAR MIGRATION IN THE MUCOSAL IMMUNE SYSTEM

The elaborate regulatory system controlling IgA responses discussed earlier would be to little avail if there did not also exist a mechanism for focusing IgA B cells at mucosal sites. It is clear that such a mechanism does exist, in that cells developing in organized mucosal lymphoid tissues (such as PP) and migrating out of these tissues have a strong tendency to return to the diffuse mucosal lymphoid tissues, the areas underlying mucosal epithelium. It is to this cell localization or homing pattern of mucosal cells that we shall now turn our attention.

The initial studies establishing cellular localization or homing in the mucosal immune system (other than the original study by Craig and Cebra mentioned earlier) were studies in which the fate of injected blast cells marked with DNA labels (^{3}H-thymidine or ^{125}I-iododeoxyuridine) was followed by autoradiography or direct tissue counting. These studies showed that blast cells obtained from thoracic duct lymph or from mesenteric lymph nodes localized in the gastrointestinal (GI) mucosa, whereas cells obtained from peripheral nodes did not (61,62). Cells taken from bronchial nodes also had a tendency to localize in mucosal areas, but here the localization pattern was weighted toward lung mucosa (63). Because the cells obtained from mucosa-associated nodes or the thoracic duct have their origin in mucosal follicles, it was at first confusing to find that cells obtained from PP had poor mucosa-localizing ability. However, this apparent discrepancy was resolved by the demonstration that PP cells do develop mucosa homing properties after residing for an appropriate time in mesenteric nodes. Thus, the mucosa homing capacity of mucosal follicular cells develops in draining nodes after the cells have left the follicle proper (64).

The nature of the blast cells migrating from mucosal follicles to diffuse mucosal areas was elucidated with double-marker studies in which blast cells with DNA labels were marked by an additional label consisting of either fluorescein-tagged anti-Ig or anti-T-cell antibodies to identify B cells and T cells, respectively. In such studies it was found that the majority (70–90%) of the migrating blast cells are B cells, most of which express IgA; however, if the cells have arisen in the bronchial lymphoid follicles, the migrating B-cell blast population may contain significant numbers of IgG B cells (63). T cells are also present among the migrating cells, composing a majority of the cells found in thoracic duct lymph, but less than 25% of the blast cells that finally localize in mucosal areas (65). This might indicate that T-cell blasts are less restricted to mucosal areas than are B-cell blasts. T cells, as opposed to B cells, settle in two distinct sites in the diffuse mucosal areas: in the lamina propria per se and between epithelial cells. The latter cells constitute a distinct cell population known as the intraepithelial lymphocytes (IEL).

Cell markers that identify resting B cells as well as blast B cells have also been used to trace mucosal cell migration. This was accomplished by Pierce and associates, who followed the migration and distribution of B cells with cholera toxin specificity by staining cell preparations and tissues with fluorescein-tagged cholera toxin (CT) (66,67). In those studies it was shown that oral immunization of animals with CT was followed within 60 to 120 hr by the appearance in the thoracic duct of a pulse of antitoxin-producing cells. This was followed, in turn, by appearance of CT-specific cells in the various mucosal tissues. The CT-specific cells included "memory" cells, because enhanced (secondary-type) responses could be elicited both at the site the antigen was initially applied and at mucosal sites that had never seen antigen. Finally, the cells marked by this technique appeared to consist of two populations in the sense that cells constantly circulating through the mucosal system could be identified, as well as cells fixed at a particular mucosal site; however, this distinction may be more apparent than real, because circulating cells become sessile on exposure to antigen. These studies with antibody-marked cells, at first sight, seem to conflict with studies with ^{51}Cr-labeled cells, because the latter fail to show mucosal homing of cells derived from mucosal follicles (62,68). However, this paradox is resolved when we realize that the ^{51}Cr labeling technique probably underestimates homing, because it tends to measure cell localization occurring over a very narrow time frame and because the ^{51}Cr labeling procedure may lead to labeling of many cells that do not have mucosal homing properties. In regard to this last point, when migrating cell populations in lymph rather than tissue-derived cell populations are labeled with ^{51}Cr, a mucosal homing pattern can in fact be discerned.

Several mechanisms have been proposed to explain the mucosal homing phenomenon, but none has yet been proved. Because surface proteins on the migratory cells are likely to be involved, IgA itself has been suggested as the homing signal. This is clearly not the case, however, because non-IgA-bearing cells (both B cells and T cells) exhibit homing. Similarly, histocompatibility antigens can hardly play a role, because we would not expect different organs in a given individual to differentially recognize these ubiquitous surface proteins. Certain tissue factors have been proposed as important homing mechanisms, such as blood flow patterns that favor a particular kind of lymphocyte migration pattern following oral antigen administration. Such a mechanism would not, however, explain the ongoing mucosal traffic exhibited by memory cells. Finally, on the assumption that homing is due to selective proliferation of cells in mucosal sites, it has been proposed that some aspects of homing could be due to T cells that preferentially expand migrating lymphocyte populations randomly moving through various tissues. This explanation of homing has a certain plausibility but lacks supporting evidence.

Another possible mechanism of homing that requires consideration is that homing is due to differential distribution of antigen. This follows from the realization that the presence of antigen to which a cell is sensitized would undoubtedly lead to stimulation of the cell and decreased migration. This mechanism, however, cannot account for the homing of blasts to mucosal sites, because such blasts also localize to antigen-free (fetal) intestinal tissue implanted in a site removed from antigen exposure (beneath the kidney capsule) (65). Evidence that resting cells also do not home because of contact with antigen is inherent in the observation that mice immunized initially in the colon with CT and then again exposed to the CT by infusion of the latter into a surgically isolated intestinal loop develop as many B cells with CT specificity in the lamina propria of a toxin-free intestinal loop as in the lamina propria of a toxin-exposed intestinal loop (66). Despite these data, it remains possible that antigen does play some role in the homing phenomenon. In this regard, it is possible that antigen acts on already homed cells to prevent their return to the migratory circuit. This would be consistent with the data of Husband, who has shown that although the numbers of intravenously injected cells with a particular antigen specificity appearing in the lamina propria of antigen-free and antigen-exposed surgically isolated intestinal loops are initially the same, the numbers of cells increase in the latter and decrease in the former (69). In all, the picture that emerges is that whereas initial entry of a cell into a mucosal site is probably not dependent on antigen, entrapment and expansion of cells having already entered are related to interaction with antigen.

A homing mechanism that more readily explains initial entry into a tissue, and one that now has considerable experimental support, is that mucosal homing is related to recognition sites on endothelial cells that lead first to binding of migrating cells to the endothelial cells and second to passage of lymphoid cells through the endothelial cells and into the tissues. This concept receives its main support from a series of studies conducted by Butcher and associates, who have shown that lymphoid cells bind to endothelial cells lining postcapillary venules (so-called high endothelial venules, HEV) (70). Furthermore, they have shown that organ specificity characterizes such binding, in that they have obtained a monoclonal antibody that inhibits the binding of lymphocytes to peripheral node HEV but has no effect on binding of lymphocytes to PP HEV (71). In addition, this antibody inhibits *in vivo* homing of lymphocytes to peripheral nodes, but not to PP. In related studies, this group has demonstrated that lymphoma cells (i.e., clonal lymphoid cell populations) bind either to peripheral node HEV or to PP HEV, but not to both kinds of HEV (70); this suggests that individual cells making up nonclonal cell populations also have a sharply defined capacity to bind to HEV of one tissue or another. In general, these data lead to the proposal that homing phenomena, in general, and mucosal homing, in particular, are related to specific interactions between migrating cells and HEV cells that do or do not result in passage of cells into the tissue proper (Fig. 7). If this is true, maturation of cells in mucosa-associated follicles is a process that includes the development of recognition sites specific for surface antigens present on endothelial cells in mucosal tissues. This theory suffers from the fact that HEV are not actually found in diffuse mucosal areas (as distinct from PP); however, it remains possible that the recognition is for vascular lining cells other than those present in HEV.

CELLULAR ORIGIN, MIGRATION, AND FUNCTION WITHIN THE MUCOSAL IMMUNE SYSTEM

On the basis of the information reviewed earlier, as well as information to be described, the following composite picture of cellular origin, migration, and function in the mucosal immune system can be constructed. Initially, cells present in

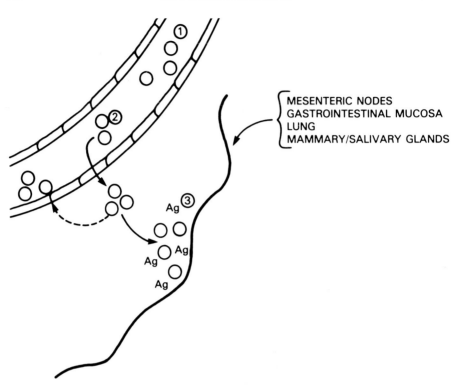

FIG. 7. Factors involved in homing of mucosal cells to mucosal sites: (1) circulation via blood and lymph; (2) efflux of migrating PP cells based on an interaction with the vascular endothelium; (3) interaction with antigen at local sites.

primordial lymphoid tissues such as bone marrow and thymus migrate to and populate PP and other mucosal follicles because of interactions with cells composing the HEV unique to the follicular tissue (72–74).

Antigen also enters the follicles, but it does so by a different route. It enters via specialized antigen-sampling and -transporting cells known as M cells, which are present on the dome of the follicles (75). Following entry into the follicle proper, antigen is taken up by functional PP macrophages and/or dendritic cells, and when presented to T cells and B cells it initiates the mucosal immune response (76). As discussed at length earlier, antigen-induced B-cell activation is accompanied by differentiation of sIgM-bearing B cells into sIgA-bearing B cells under the guidance of a special class of mucosa-associated regulatory T cells known as switch T cells. On this basis the germinal centers of mucosal follicles become populated with sIgA-bearing B cells that are the precursor cells of the IgA B cells and plasma cells ultimately found in diffuse mucosal tissues (77). Interestingly, cells actively producing IgA (or other immunoglobulins) are not found in PP, not because such cells have an intrinsic inability to become plasma cells (they can be induced to produce Ig *in vitro*), but because of rapid migration out of the patch (28,78). The reason for this outward movement, other than the fact that it is related in some way to an antigen-initiated event, is unknown. Finally, the migrating cells either are blast cells or are memory cells that mediate secondary-type responses on re-contact with antigen. As discussed earlier, these cells circulate through the mucosal immune system or reside (at least for a time) at mucosal sites; in either case, stimulation with antigen leads to tissue fixation.

Migration of cells out of mucosal follicles to all parts of the mucosal system has the effect of distributing cells sensitized in the GI or respiratory system to mucosal sites where they can participate in host defense function involving the very same antigens encountered in the GI and respiratory tracts. The most spectacular example of this is migration of sensitized cells from the GI tract to the lactating mammary gland (79,80). Because B cells in lactating mammary gland secrete products that find their way into the infant GI tract, mucosa-specific cell migration has the effect of transferring antibodies from the matured and developed maternal mucosal system to the immature and underdeveloped infant mucosal system.

The migratory pattern of cells within the mucosal system can consist of a pattern generalized to all mucosal areas or patterns that are organ-specific. Thus, we find that cells sensitized in bronchial lymphoid tissues have a predilection for respiratory mucosa, whereas cells sensitized in GI lymphoid follicles favor GI mucosa as their homing destination (63). In addition, there even appear to be suborgan circulatory patterns in that cells originating in colon have a greater tendency to return to the colon than to other parts of the GI tract (66). This suborgan circulation may be advantageous to the individual because it ensures that cells sensitized to a particular antigen will accumulate (or expand) at sites where that antigen is ultimately found.

T cells no less than B cells migrate out of mucosal follicles and home to diffuse mucosal sites. The parallel with B cells holds insofar as T cells appear to migrate out of follicles before they undergo terminal differentiation to effector cells (the equivalent of plasma cells). This is shown by the fact that when cells with cytotoxic effector function are induced in PP by feeding animals allogeneic cells, the cells do not demonstrate such function directly on removal from the patch, but only after *in vitro* restimulation (81). The migrating T cells include blast cells as well as small resting T cells that are analogous to resting cells in the B-cell population.

The functions of mucosal T cells are as varied as those of T cells found elsewhere in the immune system. We have already mentioned the fact that T cells have regulatory roles during the differentiation of B cells. In addition, mucosal T cells are involved in "exclusive" T-cell reactions such as delayed-type hypersensitivity reaction (DTH), reactions involving MHC-restricted cytotoxic T cells, and graft-versus-host reactions. The participation of mucosal T cells in DTH is inherent in the demonstration that ingestion of contactants capable of sensitizing the skin can prime the animal for systemic or GI DTH responses (82). Recently it has been shown that orally administered protein antigens can also elicit DTH, provided concomitant suppressor T-cell induction is prevented by administration of cyclophosphamide (83).

As far as reactions involving cytotoxic T cells are concerned, it has been found that oral or parenteral administration of allogeneic cells leads to the formation of alloantigen-specific cytotoxic T cells in the mucosal system. Thus, Sprent has shown that systemic (i.v.) injection of histoincompatible cells leads to the appearance in the thoracic duct of alloreactive blast cells that subsequently home to intestinal tissues (84). This result implies that alloantigen-bearing cells given parenterally gain access to the mucosal lymphoid follicles and induce cells with alloantigen-specific cytotoxic capability at these sites. Allogeneic cells are not, of course, the usual kind of antigen giving rise to MHC-restricted cytotoxic T cells in the mucosal immune system. The most common stimulants are probably virally altered autologous cells that induce the formation of cytotoxic T cells during infections with virus. This concept is supported by the observations of Ennis et al. (85), who have shown that immunization of mice with influenza virus via the respiratory tract leads to the formation of cytotoxic cells that have the capability of lysing autologous cells infected with the virus.

A final example of a mucosal immune response mediated exclusively by T cells, as mentioned earlier, is the graft-versus-host reaction (GVH reaction). In this regard, when parental lymphocytes are injected into F_1 recipient animals, a major component of the GVH reaction induced is infiltration of the intestinal mucosa with T cells. Guy-Grand et al. (86) have shown that the effector cells infiltrating the GI tract in such situations originate in PP. From these studies one might infer that the sequence of events occurring during intestinal GVH reactions includes the entry of parental cells into PP, induction at the latter site of cells reacting with F_1 histocompatibility antigens, and, finally, migration of sensitized cells from the patches to diffuse mucosal areas by the very same mechanisms governing other mucosal cell migrations.

One significant way in which the characteristics of dissemination of T cells in the mucosal system differ from the characteristics of B cells is that T cells also form a major part of a cell population mentioned earlier, the intraepithelial lymphocytes or IEL. The IEL population consists, in large part, of cells bearing characteristic T-cell surface markers (particularly Lyt-2); on this basis it comes as no surprise that IEL have been shown to be derived from (or be dependent on) T cells arising in PP (87). The T cells in the IEL population tend not to bear Thy-1 marker, a fact that may indicate that IEL T cells are significantly different from peripheral T cells.

Not all intraepithelial cells are T cells, and many may not even be lymphocytes. For instance, one population of intraepithelial cells are granulated cells that can be induced by appropriate stimuli to secrete mediators characteristic of mast cells (88). These cells, which are also found in the lamina propria, appear to be derived from non-T cells following exposure to T-cell factors (89). Undoubtedly, this is the population that is greatly expanded during mucosal helminth infections. In this instance we might postulate that the parasite initially causes T-cell stimulation and thus the release of most cell-related lymphokines; the latter then act on mast-cell precursors in the IEL population and in the lamina propria to induce maturation of large numbers of mucosal mast cells (90,91). A second intraepithelial cell population that may not be derived from T cells is the population having natural killer (NK) activity. In this regard, Tagliabue and associates have shown that there exists within the IEL large granular lymphocytes with clear-cut NK function (92). Whether or not such cells, as in the case of mast cells, also require T-cell factors for their development remains to be seen.

Cells in the IEL may play a critical role in both health and disease. For example, the NK cells in this population may constitute a first line of defense for elimination of virus-infected host epithelial cells. In addition, inasmuch as IEL numbers are increased in various mucosal diseases (93), IEL may be integral components of certain disease mechanisms.

CONCLUSION

In this chapter we have considered certain "cellular" aspects of the mucosal immune system. On the one hand, we have been concerned with the question why IgA B cells develop in relation to the mucosal system, whereas such cells are not at all prominent at systemic lymphoid areas. The general answer to this question put forward (and to some extent supported by evidence) is that an elaborate T-cell regulatory mechanism exists that is physically distributed in the mucosal lymphoid tissue and that directs B-cell development toward IgA expression and secretion. What is surprising about this regulatory T-cell system is that it acts at an unexpectedly early stage of B-cell differentiation, that is, by influencing the molecular events occurring in the B-cell nucleus during the differentiation process.

On the other hand, we have focused on the movement of cells within the mucosal immune system, particularly the tendency of cells arising in mucosal follicles to rapidly leave the follicle only to return to diffuse mucosal areas. The bipartite explanation of this phenomenon favored by the data presently available is that mucosal homing is due first to mucosa-specific interactions between migrating cells and vascular endothelium and second to selective proliferation of mucosally derived cells at mucosal sites because of antigen-induced proliferation. It appears likely that cells gain initial access to mucosal sites by the first mechanism and are retained at these sites by the second.

There can be little doubt that the ultimate explanation for the existence of mucosa-specific immune mechanisms is in the unique antigenic conditions prevalent in the mucosal environment. In this regard, the mucosal environment is replete with an extremely complex array of antigens and mitogens that mucosal lymphoid cells must either respond to or ignore, depending on whether or not the substance has pathologic significance. From the preceding discussion, some inkling of just how this is accomplished can be appreciated.

REFERENCES

1. Craig, S. W., and Cebra, J. J. (1981): Peyer's patches: An enriched source of precursors for IgA-producing immunocytes in the rabbit. *J. Exp. Med.* 134:188–200.
2. Kincade, P. W., Lee, G., Watanabe, T., Sun, L., and Scheid, M. P. (1981): Antigens displayed on murine B lymphocyte precursors. *J. Immunol.*, 127:2262–2268.
3. Cooper, M. D. (1981): Pre-B cells: Normal and abnormal development. *J. Clin. Immunol.*, 1:81–89.
4. Vittetta, E. S., and Uhr, J. W. (1975): Immunoglobulin receptors revisited. *Science*, 189:964–968.
5. Howard, M., and Paul, W. E. (1983): Regulation of B-cell growth and differentiation by soluble factors. *Annu. Rev. Immunol.*, 1:307–333.
6. Kuritani, T., and Cooper, M. D. (1982): Human B cell differentiation. III. Enhancing effect of monoclonal anti-immunoglobulin D antibody on pokeweed mitogen-induced plasma cell differentiation. *J. Immunol.*, 129:2490–2495.
7. Abney, E. R., Cooper, M. D., Kearney, J. F., Lawton, A. R., and Parkhouse, R. M. E. (1978): Sequential expression of immunoglobulins on developing mouse B lymphocytes: A systematic survey that suggests a model for the generation of immunoglobulin isotype diversity. *J. Immunol.*, 120:2041–2049.
8. Honjo, T. (1983): Immunoglobulin genes. *Annu. Rev. Immunol.*, 1:499–528.
9. Shimizu, A., Takahaoshi, N., Yaoita, Y., and Honjo, T. (1982): Organization of constant region gene family of the mouse heavy chain. *Cell*, 28:499–506.
10. Flanagan, J. G., and Rabbitts, T. H. (1982): Arrangement of human immunoglobulin heavy-chain constant region genes implies evolutionary duplication of a segment containing γ, ϵ, and α genes. *Nature*, 300:709–713.
11. Early, P., Huang, H., Davis, M., Calame, K., and Hood, L. (1980): An immunoglobulin heavy chain variable region gene is generated from three segments of DNA: V_H, D and J_H. *Cell*, 19:981–992.
12. Rabbitts, T. H. (1978): Evidence for splicing of interrupted immunoglobulin variable and constant region sequences in nuclear RNA. *Nature*, 275:291.
13. Moore, K. W., Rogers, J., Hunkapiller, T., Early, P., Nottenburg, C., Weissman, I., Bazin, H., Wall, R., and Hood, L. E. (1982): Expression of IgD may use both DNA rearrangement and RNA splicing mechanisms. *Proc. Natl. Acad. Sci. U.S.A.*, 78:1800–1804.
14. Maki, R., Traunecker, A., Sakano, H., Roeder, W., and Tonegawa, S. (1980): Exon shuffling generates an immunoglobulin heavy chain gene. *Proc. Natl. Acad. Sci. U.S.A.*, 77:2138–2142.
15. Honjo, T., Nishida, Y., Shimizu, A., Takahashi, N., Kataoka, T., Obata, M., Yamawaki-Kataoka, Y., Nikaido, T., Nakai, S., Yaoita, Y., and Ishida, N. (1982): Organization of immunoglobulin heavy chain genes and genetic mechanism for class switch. In: *Recent Advances in Mucosal Immunity*, edited by W. Strober, L. A. Hanson, and K. W. Sell, pp. 173–187. Raven Press, New York.
16. Davis, M. M., Kim, S. K., and Hood, L. E. (1980): DNA sequences mediating class switching in α-immunoglobulins. *Science*, 209:1360–1365.
17. Yaoita, Y., Kumagai, Y., Okumura, K., and Honjo, T. (1982): Expression of lymphocyte surface IgE does not require switch recombination. *Nature*, 297:697–699.
18. Cebra, J. J., Fuhrman, J. A., Gearhart, P. J., Horwitz, J. L., and Shahin, R. D. (1982): B lymphocyte differentiation leading to a commitment to IgA expression may depend on cell division and may occur during antigen-stimulated clonal expansion. In: *Recent Advances in Mucosal Immunity*, edited by W. Strober, L. A. Hanson, and K. W. Sell, pp. 155–171. Raven Press, New York.
19. Kawanishi, H., Saltzman, L., and Strober, W. (1983): Mechanisms regulating IgA class-specific immunoglobulin production in murine gut-associated lymphoid tissues. *J. Exp. Med.*, 158:649–669.
20. Klinman, N. R. (1972): The mechanism of antigenic stimulation of primary and secondary clonal precursor cells. *J. Exp. Med.*, 136:241–260.
21. Gearhart, P. J., and Cebra, J. J. (1979): Differentiated B lymphocytes. Potential to express particular antibody variable and constant regions depends on site of lymphoid tissue and antigen load. *J. Exp. Med.*, 149:216–227.
22. Fuhrman, J. A., and Cebra, J. J. (1981): Special features of the primary process for a secretory IgA response. B cell priming with cholera toxin. *J. Exp. Med.*, 153:534–544.
23. Cebra, J. J., Fuhrman, J. A., Gearhart, P. J., Horwitz, J. L., and Shahin, R. D. (1982): B lympho-

cyte differentiation leading to a commitment to IgA expression may depend on cell division and may occur during antigen-stimulated clonal expansion. In: *Recent Advances in Mucosal Immunity*, edited by W. Strober, L. A. Hanson, and K. W. Sell, pp. 155–171. Raven Press, New York.

24. Cebra, J. J., Cebra, E. R., Clough, E. R., Fuhrman, J. A., Komisar, J. L., Schweitzer P. A., and Shahin, R. D. (1983): IgA commitment: Models for B-cell differentiation and possible roles for T-cells in regulating B-cell development. *Ann. N.Y. Acad. Sci.*, 409:25–38.

25. Gearhart, P. J., Horwitz, J. L., and Cebra, J. J. (1980): Successive switching of antibody isotypes expressed within the lines of a B-cell clone. *Proc. Natl. Acad. Sci. U.S.A.*, 77:5424–5428.

26. Kuritani, T., and Cooper, M. D. (1982): Human B cell differentiation. I. Analysis of immuno-globulin heavy chain switching using monoclonal anti-immunoglobulin M, G, and A antibodies and pokeweed mitogen-induced plasma cell differentiation. *J. Exp. Med.*, 155:839–851.

27. Calvert, J. E., Kim, M. F., Gathings, W. E., and Cooper, M. D. (1983): Differentiation of B lineage cells from liver of neonatal mice: Generation of immunoglobulin diversity *in vitro. J. Immunol.*, 131:1693–1697.

28. Kagnoff, M. F. (1977): Functional characteristics of Peyer's patch lymphoid cells. IV. Effect of antigen feeding on the frequency of antigen-specific B cells. *J. Immunol.*, 118:992–997.

29. Mongini, P. K. A., Stein, K. E., and Paul, W. E. (1981): T cell regulation of IgG subclass antibody production in response to T-independent antigens. *J. Exp. Med.*, 153:1–12.

30. Mongini, P. K. A., Paul, W. E., and Metcalf, E. S. (1982): T cell regulation of immunoglobulin class expression in the antibody response to trinitrophenyl-Ficoll: Evidence for T cell enhancement of immunoglobulin class switch. *J. Exp. Med.*, 155:884–902.

31. Mongini, P. K. A., Paul, W. E., and Metcalf, E. S. (1983): IgG subclass IgE, and IgA anti-trinitrophenyl antibody production within trinitrophenyl-Ficoll-responsive B cell clones. Evidence in support of three distinct switching pathways. *J. Exp. Med.*, 157:69–85.

32. Isakson, P. C., Pure, E., Vitetta, E. S., and Kramer, P. H. (1982): T cell-derived B cell differen-tiation factor(s). Effect on the isotype switch of murine B cells. *J. Exp. Med.*, 155:734–748.

33. Clough, J. D., Mims, L. H., and Strober, W. (1971): Deficient IgA antibody responses to arsonilic acid bovine serum albumin (BSA) in neonatally thymectomized rabbits. *J. Immunol.*, 106:1624–1629.

34. Pritchard, H., Riddaway, J., and Micklem, H. S. (1973): Immune responses in congenitally thymus-less mice. II. Quantitative studies of serum immunoglobulin, the antibody response to sheep erythrocytes, and the effect of thymus allografting. *Clin. Exp. Immunol.*, 13:125–138.

35. Elson, C. C., Heck, J. A., and Strober, W. (1979): T-cell regulation of murine IgA synthesis. *J. Exp. Med.*, 149:632–643.

36. Kawanishi, H., Saltzman, L. E., and Strober, W. (1982): Characteristics and regulatory function of murine con A-induced, cloned T cells obtained from Peyer's patches and spleen. Mechanisms regulating isotype-specific immunoglobulin production by Peyer's patch B cells. *J. Immunol.*, 129:475–483.

37. Kawanishi, H., Saltzman, L., and Strober, W. (1983): Mechanisms regulating IgA class-specific immunoglobulin production in murine gut-associated lymphoid tissues. I. T cells derived from Peyer's patches that switch sIgM B cells to sIgA B cells *in vitro. J. Exp. Med.*, 157:437–450.

38. Kawanishi, H., Saltzman, L., and Strober, W. (1983): Mechanisms regulating IgA class-specific immunoglobulin production in murine gut-associated lymphoid tissues. II. Terminal differentiation of postswitch sIgA-bearing Peyer's patch B cells. *J. Exp. Med.*, 158:649–669.

39. Asano, Y., Singer, A., and Hodes, R. J. (1981): Role of major histocompatibility complex in T cell activation of B cell populations. MHC restricted and unrestricted B cell responses are mediated by distinct B cell subpopulations. *J. Exp. Med.*, 154:1100–1115.

40. Asano, Y., and Hodes, R. J. (1984): T cell regulation of B cell activation: MHC-restricted T augmenting cells enhance the B cell responses mediated by MHC-restricted cloned T helper cells. *J. Immunol.*, 132:1151–1157.

41. Kung, J. T., and Paul, W. E. (1983): B-lymphocyte subpopulations. *Immunology Today*, 4:37–41.

42. Quagliata, J. M., Roux, M. E., Arny, M., Kelly-Hatfield, P., McWilliams, M., and Lamm, M. E. (1983): Migration and regulation of B-cells in the mucosal immune system. *Ann. N.Y. Acad. Sci.*, 409:194–203.

43. Schimpl, A., and Wecker, E. (1975): A third signal in B cell activation given by TRF. *Transplant. Rev.*, 23:176–188.

44. Kiyono, H., McGhee, J. R., Mosteller, L., Eldridge, J., Koopman, W. J., Kearney, J. F., and

Michalek, S. M. (1982): Murine Peyer's patch T cell clones. Characterization of antigen-specific helper T cells for immunoglobulin A responses. *J. Exp. Med.*, 156:1115–1130.

45. Kiyono, H., Cooper, M. D., Kearney, J. F., Mosteller, L. M., Michalek, S. M., Koopman, W. J., and McGhee, J. R. (1984): Isotype specificity of helper T cell clones. *J. Exp. Med.*, 159:798–811.

46. Maver, L., Shu Man Fu, and Kunkel, H. G. (1982): Human T cell hybridomas secreting factors for IgA-specific help, polyclonal B cell activation, and B cell proliferation. *J. Exp. Med.*, 156:1860–1865.

47. Endoh, M., Sakai, H., Nomoto, Y., Tomino, Y., and Kaneshigi, H. (1981): IgA-specific helper activity of T cells in human peripheral blood. *J. Immunol.*, 127:2612–2613.

48. Kishimoto, T., and Ishizaka, K. (1973): Regulation of antibody response *in vitro*. VI. Carrier-specific helper cells for IgG and IgE antibody response. *J. Immunol.*, 111:720–732.

49. Martinez-Alonso, C., Coutinho, A., and Augustin, A. A. (1980): Immunoglobulin C-gene expression. I. The commitment to IgG subclass of secretory cells is determined by the quality of the non-specific stimuli. *Eur. J. Immunol.*, 10:698–702.

50. Rosenberg, Y. J., and Chiller, J. M. (1979): Ability of antigen-specific helper cells to effect a class-restricted increase in total Ig-secreting cells in spleen after immunization with the antigen. *J. Exp. Med.*, 150:517–530.

51. Suemura, M., and Ishizaka, K. (1979): Potentiation of IgE response in vitro by T cells from rats infected with *Nippostrongylus brasiliensis*. *J. Immunol.*, 123:918–924.

52. Hirashima, M., Yodoi, J., and Ishizaka, K. (1980): Regulatory role of IgE-binding factors from rat T lymphocytes. III. IgE-specific suppressive factors with IgE-binding activity. *J. Immunol.*, 125:1442–1448.

53. Hoover, R. G., and Lynch, R. G. (1983): Isotype-specific suppression of IgA: Suppression of IgA responses in BALB/c Mice by T α cells. *J. Immunol.*, 130:521–523.

54. Hoover, R. G., Gebel, H. M., and Dieckgraefe, B. K. (1981): Occurrence and potential significance of increased numbers of T cells with Fc receptors in myeloma. *Immunol. Rev.*, 56:115–139.

55. Bich Thuy, L. T., and Revillard, J. P. (1982): Selective suppression of human B lymphocyte differentiation into IgG-producing cells by soluble Fc receptors. *J. Immunol.*, 129:150–152.

56. Yodoi, J., Adachi, M., Teshigawara, K., Miyama-Inaba, M., Masuda, T., and Fridman, W. H. (1983): T cell hybridomas coexpressing Fc receptors (FcR) for different isotypes. II. IgA-induced formation of suppressive IgA binding factor(s) by a murine T hybridoma bearing FcγR and FcαR. *J. Immunol.*, 131:303–310.

57. Waldmann, T. A., Broder, S., Krakauer, R., Derm, M., Meade, B., and Goldman, C. (1976): Defect in IgA secretion and in IgA specific suppressor cells in patients with selective IgA deficiency. *Trans. Assoc. Am. Physicians*, 89:219–224.

58. Strober, W., Richman, L. K., and Elson, C. O. (1981): The regulation of gastrointestinal immune responses. *Immunology Today*, 2:156–161.

59. Challacombe, S. J., and Tomasi, T. B., Jr., (1980): Systemic tolerance and secretory immunity after oral immunization. *J. Exp. Med.*, 152:1459–1472.

60. Richamn, L. K., Graeff, A. S., Yarchoan, R., and Strober, W. (1981): Simultaneous induction of antigen-specific IgA helper T cells and IgG suppressor T cells in the murine Peyer's patches after protein feeding. *J. Immunol.*, 126:2079–2083.

61. Halstead, T. E., and Hall, J. G. (1972): The homing of lymph-borne immunoblasts to the small gut of neonatal rats. *Transplantation*, 14:339–346.

62. McWilliams, M., Phillips-Quagliata, J. M., and Lamm, M. E. (1975): Characteristics of mesenteric lymph node cells homing to gut associated lymphoid tissue in syngeneic mice. *J. Immunol.*, 115:54–58.

63. McDermott, M., and Bienenstock, J. (1979): Evidence for a common mucosal immunologic system. I. Migration of B immunoblasts into intestinal, respiratory and genital tissues. *J. Immunol.*, 122:1892–1898.

64. Roux, M. E., McWilliams, M., Phillips-Quagliata, J. M., and Lamm, M. E. (1981): Differentiation pathways of Peyer's patch precursors of IgA plasma cells in the secretory immune system. *Cell. Immunol.*, 61:141–153.

65. Guy-Grand, D., Griscelli, C., and Vassalli, P. (1974): The gut-associated lymphoid system: Nature and properties of the large dividing cells. *Eur. J. Immunol.*, 4:435–443.

66. Pierce, N. F., and Cray, W. C., Jr. (1972): Determinants in the localization, magnitude, and duration of a specific mucosal IgA plasma cell response in enterically immunized rats. *J. Immunol.*, 128:1311–1315.

67. Pierce, N. F., Cray, W. C., Jr., Sacci, J. B., Jr., Craig, J. P., Germanier, R., and Furer, E. (1983): Oral immunization against experimental cholera: The role of antigen form and antigen combination in evoking protection. *Ann. N.Y. Acad. Sci.*, 409:724–733.

68. de Frietas, A. A., Rose, M. L., and Parrott, D. M. V. (1977): Mesenteric and peripheral lymph nodes: A common pool of small T cells. *Nature*, 270:731–733.

69. Husband, A. J. (1982): Kinetics of extravasation and redistribution of IgA-specific antibody-containing cells in the intestine. *J. Immunol.*, 128:1355–1359.

70. Butcher, E. C., Scollary, R. G., and Weissman, I. L. (1980): Organ specificity of lymphocyte migration: Mediation by highly selective lymphocyte interaction with organ-specific determinants on high endothelial venules. *Eur. J. Immunol.*, 10:556–561.

71. Gallatin, W. M., Weissman, I. L., and Butcher, E. C. (1983): A cell-surface molecule involved in organ-specific homing of lymphocytes. *Nature*, 304:30–34.

72. Waksman, B. H. (1973): The homing pattern of thymus-derived lymphocytes in calf and neonatal mouse Peyer's patches. *J. Immunol.*, 111:878–884.

73. Barg, M., and Draper, L. R. (1975): Migration of thymus cells to the developing gut-associated lymphoid tissues of the young rabbit. *Cell. Immunol.*, 20:177–186.

74. Howard, J. C., Hunt, S. V., and Gowans, J. L. (1972): Identification of marrow-derived and thymus-derived small lymphocytes in the lymphoid tissue and thoracic duct lymph of normal rats. *J. Exp. Med.*, 136:200–219.

75. Wolf, J. L., Rubin, D. H., Finberg, R., Kauffman, R. S., Sharpe, A. H., Trier, J. S., and Fields, B. N. (1981): Intestinal M cells: A pathway for entry of reovirus into the host. *Science*, 212:471–472.

76. Richman, L. K., Graeff, A. S., and Strober, W. (1981): Antigen presentation by macrophage-enriched cells from the mouse Peyer's patch. *Cell. Immunol.*, 62:110–118.

77. Butcher, E. C., Rouse, R.V., Coffman, R. L., Nottenbury, C. N., Hardy, R. R., and Weissman, I. L. (1982): Surface phenotype of Peyer's patch germinal center cells: Implications for the role of germinal centers in B cell differentiation. *J. Immunol.*, 129:2698–2707.

78. Bienenstock, J., and Dolezel, J. (1971): Peyer's patches. Lack of specific antibody-containing cells after oral and parenteral immunization. *J. Immunol.*, 106:938–945.

79. Weisz-Carrington, P., Roux, M. E., McWilliams, M., Phillips-Quagliata, J. M., and Lamm, M. E. (1979): Organ and isotype distribution of plasma cells producing specific antibody after oral immunization. Evidence for a generalized secretory immune system. *J. Immunol.*, 123:1705–1708.

80. Roux, M. E., McWilliams, M., Phillips-Quagliata, J. M., Weisz-Carrington, P., and Lamm, M. E. (1977): Origin of IgA-secreting plasma cells in the mammary gland. *J. Exp. Med.*, 146:1311–1321.

81. Kagnoff, M. F. (1978): Effects of antigen-feeding in intestinal and systemic immune responses. I. Priming of precursor cytotoxic T cells by antigen feeding. *J. Immunol.*, 120:395–399.

82. Asherson, G. L., Perera, M. A. C. C., Thomas, W. R., and Zembala, M. (1979): Contact-sensitizing agents and the intestinal tract: The production of immunity and unresponsiveness by feeding contact-sensitizing agents and the role of suppressor cells. In: *Immunology of Breast Milk*, edited by P. O. Ogra and D. Dayton, pp. 19–36. Raven Press, New York.

83. Mowat, M. I. A., Strobel, S., Drummond, H. E., and Ferguson, A. (1982): Immunological responses to fed protein antigens in mice. I. Reversal of oral tolerance to ovalbumin by cyclophosphamide. *Immunology*, 45:105–113.

84. Sprent, J. (1976): Fate of H2-activated T lymphocytes in syngeneic hosts I. Fate in lymphoid tissues and intestines traced with ^{3}H-thymidine, ^{125}I-deoxyuridine and ^{51}chromium. *Cell. Immunol.*, 21:278–302.

85. Ennis, F. A., Wells, M. A., Butchko, G. M., and Albrecht, P. (1978): Evidence that cytotoxic T cells are part of the host's response to influenza pneumonia. *J. Exp. Med.*, 148:1241–1250.

86. Guy-Grand, D., Griscelli, C., and Vassalli, P. (1978): The mouse gut T lymphocyte, a novel type of T cell. Nature, origin and traffic in mice in normal and graft-versus-host conditions. *J. Exp. Med.*, 148:1661–1676.

87. Parrott, D. M. V., Tait, C., MacKenzie, S., Mowat, A. M., Davies, M. D. J., and Micklem, H. S. (1983): Analysis of the effector functions of different populations of mucosal lymphocytes. *Ann. N.Y. Acad. Sci.*, 409:307–320.

88. Bienenstock, J., Befus, A. D., Pearce, F., Denburg, J., and Goodacre, R. (1982): Mast cell

heterogeneity: Derivation and function with emphasis on the intestine. *J. Allergy Clin. Immunol.*, 70:407–412.

89. Haig, D. M., McMenamin, C., Gunneberg, C., Woodbury, R., and Jarrett, E. E. E. (1983): Stimulation of mucosal mast cell growth in normal and nude rat bone marrow cultures. *Proc. Natl. Acad. Sci. U.S.A.*, 80:4499–4503.

90. Befus, A. D., and Bienenstock, J. (1982): Host resistance to parasites at mucosal surfaces. *Prog. Allergy*, 31:76–77.

91. Mayrhofer, G., and Fisher, R. (1979): Mast cells in severely T-cell depleted rats and the response to infestation with *Nippostrongylus brasiliensis. Immunology*, 37:145–155.

92. Tagliabue, A., Befus, A. D., Clark, D. A., and Bienenstock, J. (1982): Characteristics of natural killer cells in the murine intestinal epithelium and lamina propria. *J. Exp. Med.*, 155:1785.

93. Ferguson, A., McClure, J. P., and Townley, R. R. W. (1976): Intraepithelial lymphocyte counts in small intestinal biopsies from children with diarrhea. *Acta Paedr. Scand.*, 65:541–546.

Advances in Host Defense Mechanisms, Vol. 4,
edited by J. I. Gallin and A. S. Fauci.
Raven Press, New York © 1985.

Humoral Aspects of Mucosal Immunity

*Thomas B. Tomasi and **Andrew G. Plaut

*Department of Cell Biology, University of New Mexico School of Medicine,
Albuquerque, New Mexico 81713; and **Department of Medicine, Tufts–New England
Medical Center, Boston, Massachusetts 02111

In this chapter we shall focus on recent advances in the study of mechanisms of immune regulation at mucosal surfaces. The chapter will begin with a brief overview of mucosal immunity, but because of space limitations it will not be all-inclusive, and we recommend to the reader who seeks more detail a number of books and articles (5,13,85,96,114,164,167).

The mucosal tissues of the body provide an extensive surface on which potentially pathogenic microorganisms make their initial contact with the host. A variety of mechanisms, including both immune and nonimmune factors, have evolved to prevent colonization, invasion, and local disease. Predominant among the immune mechanisms (the primary focus of this chapter) is the occurrence of secretory antibodies in the fluids that bathe mucosal membranes. These antibodies have critical biological and medical implications, because they interact with a large variety of viable and nonviable substances that are deposited on mucous surfaces. In addition, the elicitation of mucosal antibodies by active immunization could lead to effective methods of immunoprophylaxis against a variety of bacterial, viral, and parasitic infections for which vaccines are not currently available.

It has been known for nearly 20 years (170) that IgA is the predominant class of immunoglobulins in various mucosal secretions. Following the original description of the predominance of IgA plasma cells at mucosal sites, a variety of studies have quantitated the classes of the Ig-containing cells in various secretory as well as peripheral lymphoid tissues, as reviewed elsewhere (85,164). More recently, Kutteh et al. (81) have found that intestinal lamina propria cells secrete the largest amounts of polymeric IgA (although these cells also produce monomeric IgA), whereas cultured spleen and bone marrow cells produce predominantly monomeric (7S) IgA. There is also a positive correlation between the amount of polymeric IgA produced and the presence of cytoplasmic J chain (*vide infra*). These authors suggested that the bone marrow may be a major source of serum 7S IgA. Crago et al. (28) have shown that human spleen, tonsils, bone marrow, and peripheral lymphoid tissues contain predominantly IgA_1-staining cells (75–90%), whereas the small and large intestines and salivary and lacrimal glands exhibit approximately equal numbers of IgA_1 and IgA_2 plasma cells. Larger numbers of cells staining for

31

J chain have been found in mucosal tissues, and a higher percentage of the IgA_2 cells contained J chain than did IgA_1-positive cells. Thus, it appears that the proportions of IgA_1 and IgA_2 molecules in serum and secretions are similar to the tissue distributions of the cells containing the two subclasses. These studies on the cellular contents of tissues strengthen the evidence for local production of the majority of secretory IgA. Recent studies (37) suggest that less than 2% of the total salivary polymeric IgA originates from plasma, which is consistent with older studies (170) as well as recent work (4) indicating that only a small portion of salivary IgA in patients with myeloma of the IgA class is derived from the circulating monoclonal protein.

Transport of dimeric IgA is facilitated by complexing with membrane-bound secretory component (SC), which functions as a receptor. IgM is transported by a similar route, but how IgG, IgE, and IgD are secreted is not definitely known. The binding of IgA to SC serves not only to facilitate transport but also to stabilize the IgA molecule to proteolytic degradation. Increased resistance to proteolysis may be of considerable importance to antibodies functioning in fluids in which degradative enzymes are abundant. Recently it has been found that dimeric IgA may be transported across the hepatic cell from serum into bile, and again SC appears to be involved in the transport process *(vide infra)*. In this regard, Halsey et al. (59) reported significant transport of IgA into the mammary secretions of mice. Similarly, Sheldrake et al. (151) found that the bulk of IgA in sheep milk was derived from serum during early and middle lactation, whereas during mammary involution, IgA was locally produced. Concomitant studies on sheep intestinal IgA production suggested that the vast majority was locally produced. Brandtzaeg (14) has carefully studied human mammary glands and concluded that milk IgA is synthesized in cells intrinsic to the lactating gland; the densities of IgA-producing cells and the daily outputs of IgA per kilogram wet weight of tissue are similar for salivary tissues and lactating mammary tissues. These apparently conflicting data can be rationalized on the following basis: Transport of IgA from serum depends on (a) the concentration of dimeric IgA in serum, (b) the ability of dimeric IgA to permeate the capillaries of a particular tissue, and (c) the availability of SC locally to mediate transport across the epithelial cells of a particular tissue. In ruminants, such as the sheep, serum IgA is primarily dimeric (derived largely from the gut), whereas in humans, 90% of the serum IgA is monomeric. Therefore, the interstitial regions of the sheep mammary glands should contain large amounts of potentially transportable dimeric IgA derived from serum. Thus, an inverse correlation might be expected between the extent of local production and serum transport; i.e., in tissues such as the gastrointestinal (GI) tract, where IgA-producing cells (and therefore dimeric IgA) are abundant, the SC is unavailable for transporting any molecules derived from serum, because it is "preempted" or occupied by locally produced IgA. If this concept is valid, then biliary transport should not be a unique mechanism for removal of IgA from serum. Because the liver does not produce IgA, the hepatic cell plasma membrane receptor (SC on the sinusoidal surface) should be freely available to transport serum IgA without competition from any locally produced dimer. However, in the rat, very few cells are found in the lactating breast, and yet dimeric IgA is reportedly not transferred to milk (34). Here we could invoke a particularly active "competitive" biliary transport (known to occur in this species) that would rapidly remove serum dimeric IgA and/or the relative impermeability of the mammary capillaries of this species to dimeric IgA. Obviously, additional studies are needed to evaluate how much of a given antibody is produced in cells indigenous to the tissues versus the amount derived from serum.

The origin of the cells in mucous membranes is reviewed in more detail in another chapter and will be briefly mentioned here in order to set the stage for a discussion of antibody production, secretion, and function. It should be emphasized that the mucosal system, and particularly the gut, contains more lymphoid tissue than the spleen and peripheral lymph nodes. Of the mucosal tissues, the gut has been most extensively studied, and the lamina propria has been shown to contain B cells, plasma cells, macrophages, and T cells; the latter mediate help, alloreactivity, and cytotoxicity. In intraepithelial locations, large granular lymphocytes predominate, and they have been shown to be involved in antibody-dependent cell-mediated cytotoxicity (ADCC) and natural killer (NK) activity. Key components of the lymphoid tissues of the gut are focal collections of lymphoid cells scattered throughout the small intestine, of which Peyer's patches (PP) are the most prominent. Similar lymphoid follicles are present in the lung (bronchial-associated lymphoid tissues) and perhaps the eye and tonsils. Most, but not all, of the large variety of antigens that are ingested are absorbed through the specialized epithelium covering the PP called microfold or M cells (120). Although lymphoid cells are first sensitized in PP, production of antibody does not begin until the B cells leave the patches and migrate to other sites. Sensitized cells undergo a remarkable journey that involves migration to the mesenteric lymph nodes, and then via the thoracic duct to the circulation. These cells subsequently seed not only the whole length of the gut lamina propria but also other mucosal tissues (6,29,187). Such migratory phenomena have important implications, because deposition of antigens in the GI tract (and possibly the respiratory tract) can elicit antibodies at distant mucosal sites. A similar migration pattern has been described for T cells, but localization in this case occurs predominantly in the intraepithelial regions of the mucosal membranes (57). Several laboratories are currently attempting to devise means of immunization via the gut and respiratory tract that will take advantage of these migratory patterns. It should be mentioned that although oral immunization may lead to secretory immunity, in some circumstances there is concomitant suppression of the systemic immune response to the same antigen (oral tolerance) *(vide infra)*.

It is clear that defects in the secretory system (seen in patients with a selective deficiency of IgA), if not compensated for by the secretion of other immunoglobulin classes, can lead to both recurrent infections and "leaky" mucous membranes that will allow the absorption of a multitude of ingested and inhaled antigens. These antigens may elicit the formation of antibodies (in classes other than IgA), which could result in the formation of immune complexes and autoimmune syndromes.

More subtle defects may occur in the secretory immune system in a variety of diseases, including other immune deficiencies, autoimmune syndromes, and inflammatory bowel disease. Studies of the role of the secretory system in these diseases are just beginning.

SECRETORY IMMUNOGLOBULINS

Secretory IgA (sIgA) is an 11S molecule (MW 390,000) consisting of two IgA monomers covalently bonded by a joining chain (J chain) and complexed to one molecule of SC.

J chain has a molecular weight of 15,600 and is covalently associated with polymeric immunoglobulins (IgA and IgM) (61,186,189). A single J chain is present per mole of polymeric Ig, regardless of the polymer size (dimer, trimer, tetramer, or pentamer). The carbohydrate portion of J chain consists of a single asparagine-linked oligosaccharide composing approximately 7.5% of its molecular weight. The primary structure of the polypeptide portion of the J chain has been elucidated (103), and the complete structure of the carbohydrate moiety has recently been established (3). Analysis of the interaction of monomer Ig to form polymers *in vitro* suggests that J chain is probably involved in the initiation of polymerization. In IgM and higher polymers of IgA, J chain binds via a disulfide linkage to the penultimate cysteine residue of the two monomer heavy chains. Apparently this association with J chain results in a dimer conformation that tends to promote interaction with additional monomeric subunits, giving rise to higher-order IgA polymers and the pentameric IgM molecule (61,76). Little J chain is present in unstimulated B cells, but following exposure to mitogen or antigen there is a marked increase (100–200-fold) in intracellular J chain (77). However, the presence of J chain has been described (by immunoelectron microscopy and radioimmunoassay) in pre-B cells and in HLA-DR$^+$ null cell leukemias (58,95), suggesting that J-chain expression precedes antigen-induced events. Thus, J-chain expression may be one of the earliest markers for differentiation along the B-cell pathway, because it is not detectable in malignant cells of the T or myeloid lineages. All Ig-secreting plasmacytomas, regardless of their Ig class, contain detectable amounts of J chain, but it is incorporated into Ig and secreted only in IgM- and polymeric-IgA-producing cells. The presence of J chain in cells other than IgM and IgA suggests that once the J-chain gene is activated, it continues to be expressed during the subsequent heavy-chain class switches. There is some evidence that J chain is rapidly degraded in cells producing monomeric Ig (104). Genetic analysis (191) indicates that there is a single J-chain gene in the mouse haploid genome located on chromosome 5 that is unlinked to any of the Ig genes. The same gene product must therefore be used for polymerization in both IgM and IgA. The locations of the genes for J chain and heavy (H) and light (L) chains on different chromosomes suggest that activation of polymeric Ig production in B cells is mediated by mechanisms that can generate either three separate signals or one signal that subsequently affects loci on the other chromosomes. It should be emphasized that although polymers lacking J chain (168) are capable of binding secretory component, they do so in smaller amounts and with lesser affinity than those containing J chain. Thus, the conformation induced by J chain may be optimal for the subsequent binding of SC. In addition to J chain, there is recent evidence (145) that an enzyme present in stimulated, but not unstimulated, B lymphocytes catalyzes polymer assembly. Analysis of the polymerization reactions suggests that the enzyme is a sulfhydryl oxidase directly catalyzing the oxidation of disulfide bonds rather than an interchange reaction, as previously postulated.

SC is a glycoprotein of approximately 80,000 MW that is synthesized in epithelial cells of mucous membranes (167,170). Human milk SC contains 23.4% carbohydrate (133), and the precise structure of the carbohydrate moiety has recently been reported (102,127). In addition to bound SC (in IgA and IgM), SC is also present in a free or unbound form in secretions from the digestive, respiratory, and other exocrine glands (169). By immunohistochemical localization, SC is found predominantly, but not exclusively, in serous cells of epithelial and exocrine glands. It is also present in certain ductal epithelial cells, including those of the salivary, bile, and pancreatic ducts. In human IgA and IgM the majority of SC is complexed by disulfide bonds (not directly involving J chain) to a single-monomer subunit (174), but in the rabbit a significant portion of the SC is noncovalently bound (22). Free SC has been shown to complex *in vitro* with polymeric IgA and IgM, and this does not require the formation of a covalent bond (12,167,185). The reaction is not species-restricted: Human SC complexes with IgA from a variety of species, including chicken (91). The affinity constant for the binding of free SC to the intact IgA dimer in solution is approximately 10^8 M^{-1} (78), but the apparent affinity constant for both mammary gland and liver membranes is significantly higher ($K_a = 10^9$ M^{-1}). The binding of ^{125}I-labeled IgA dimer to membranes is saturable and reversible and is a time- and temperature-dependent process. The number of measurable IgA dimer binding sites per epithelial cell varies (260–7,000 sites per mammary cell) and is directly related to the number of unoccupied receptor (SC) molecules in the membrane (79).

TRANSPORT AND DISTRIBUTION OF IgA ANTIBODIES

IgA moves from one body compartment to another by highly specific transport mechanisms that allow for an orderly distribution of antibodies into those secretions where they are required. As already mentioned, transcellular passage involves the direct participation of SC, a protein synthesized by many mucosal epithelial cells that binds specifically to the Fc region of polymeric IgA and IgM. SC is asymmetrically distributed in the membranes of epithelial cells in such a way that binding of IgA is followed by an orderly, vectorial transport of the antibody to the opposite side of the cell, a process ensuring efficient delivery of antibody into secretions and apparently preventing its encounter with degradative organelles, e.g., lysosomes. A comprehensive view of mucosal immunity and the physiology of IgA requires not only consideration of lymphocytes, macrophages, plasma cells, and mediators of inflammation but also consideration of the biology of epithelial cells. Variations in IgA transport among mammalian species and among different tissues of a given species are recognized, and generalizations regarding mechanisms may therefore be misleading.

Secretion of dimeric IgA requires a transcellular transport pathway, because junctional complexes exclude all but small ions from direct passage via the intercellular space. SC is not limited in distribution to mucosal epithelial cells but is also present on hepatocyte membranes of certain species, where it allows for the transport of IgA and immune complexes involving IgA through the liver cells into the biliary system. This route will be examined in greater detail later, but the general properties and function of SC appear to be the same in all mucosal and glandular tissues thus far examined. SC production is characteristic of fully differentiated cells, and human colonic polyps and adenomas show reduction in SC expression when the cells become dedifferentiated (dysplastic) (144).

Much remains to be learned about SC expression and function, and other mechanisms for Ig transport into secretions may be important (60). Although the milk of most mammals contains large amounts of IgA, there is some debate about the relative importance of serum and locally synthesized IgA, or even macrophages, in contributing to this output (14,59,128). It has also been suggested by Wira and associates that movement of IgA across cells may be modified by hormones (160). Their studies in rats have shown that estrogen administration increases the accumulation of polymeric IgA in uterine secretions, possibly mediated by increases in membrane SC.

Comparisons of SC isolated from deoxycholate-solubilized plasma membranes from rabbit liver and mammary gland have revealed a heterogeneous population of molecules in two size ranges: one group with a molecular weight of approximately 100,000, and the other 80,000. This raises the possibility that a portion of SC occurs as a large transmembrane form anchored in the lipid bilayer of the membrane. Charge-shift electrophoresis has shown that free SC is not affected by cationic and anionic detergents, whereas the mobility of the protein isolated from membranes is shifted in the presence of detergents. This indicates the presence of a hydrophobic domain on the membrane-associated molecule (80). Mostov and Blobel (105,108) have identified transmembrane and secreted forms of SC using a cell-free translation system supplemented with dog pancreatic microsomal membranes. High-molecular-weight SC precursors have also been noted in rat hepatocyte Golgi membranes (162). Studies of the structure of SC have been extended by analysis of a human adenocarcinoma cell line (HT-29) that synthesizes SC (64). Brown and associates demonstrated that HT-29 cells have polarity and are capable of binding dimer IgA at the basal and lateral plasma membranes and translocating IgA across the cell to the luminal membrane (110). Using a subclone (HT-29E10) that produces significantly larger amounts of SC than the parent line, Mostov et al. (105,106) showed by cell-free translation and pulse-labeling experiments that SC is made as a larger precursor (MW 95,000, but converted to MW 100,000 by the addition of peripheral sugars) that is a transmembrane protein containing cytoplasmic, membrane-spanning, and ectoplasmic domains. Messenger RNA extracted from HT-29E10 cells and translated in a cell-free system (wheat germ) produced proteins that when precipitated with anti-SC and analyzed by SDS-PAGE gave a primary product of MW 80,000. However, when microsomal vesicles from the dog pancreas were added to the translation reaction, the primary product was MW 95,000. Addition of trypsin posttranslationally resulted in a reduction in the size of the 95,000 MW molecule, suggesting that the precursor molecule contained a trypsin-sensitive domain as well as membrane-protected portions. The undigested precursor (MW 95,000), free SC (MW 80,000), and the intracellular cleavage product (MW 80,000) of the precursor form all have the same *N*-terminal amino acid sequence. This result suggests that the 80,000 MW form of SC (free SC and that complexed with IgA and IgM) is proteolytically cleaved from the *N*-terminal (ectoplasmic) domain of the precursor molecule. Figure 1 represents a hypothetical model for the transport pathway of Ig across the epithelial cell. SC is synthesized on polysomes as a transmembrane protein that is integrated into the rough endoplasmic reticulum (RER), with its ectoplasmic domain projecting into the lumen of the RER. After transport to the Golgi (where terminal saccharide units are added), SC is inserted into the basal lateral region of the epithelial cell membrane. The ectoplasmic domain of the transmembrane protein projects from the cell surface and acts as a receptor for polymeric Igs. After complexing with J-chain-containing polymers (IgA and IgM), endocytosis is initiated, and Ig is transported across the cell within vesicles that ultimately fuse with the apical plasma membrane. Because colchicine has little effect on binding and internalization of IgA (53), but does effect translocation, it has been suggested that microtubules are involved in vesicular movement across the cell. There are no data suggesting fusion of these vesicles with lysosomes, but this has not been excluded. Somewhere along this transcytotic process the transmembrane Ig complex is proteolytically cleaved, releasing soluble sIgA and leaving behind the residual membrane-protected and cytoplasmic domains. The location and characteristics of the proteolytic enzyme that is responsible for this cleavage are unknown, but the cleavage may be highly specific, similar to that of IgA protease *(vide infra)*. The SC attached to IgA (and IgM) as well as free SC is of MW 80,000, and therefore the portion remaining in the cell is approximately 20,000 MW. Most of the residual SC represents an unusually large intracytoplasmic domain (compared with other transmembrane proteins). This scheme is consistent with previous fluorescence studies localizing SC and IgA to identical regions of the basal lateral plasma membrane of intestinal cells and is consistent with the finding of IgA and SC in membrane-bound intracytoplasmic vesicles (15,18,27,110). Similar transport mechanisms may be operative in the transfer of dimeric IgA from serum to bile *(vide infra)*, in which the sinusoidal plasma membrane is equivalent to the basal lateral membrane of the intestinal epithelial cell, and the bile canaliculus corresponds to the apical (luminal) membrane. The various historical models suggested for the transport of IgA and IgM have been reviewed by Brandtzaeg (13). These models basically represent a continual refinement of the original proposal (170): SC is synthesized by epithelial cells and mediates

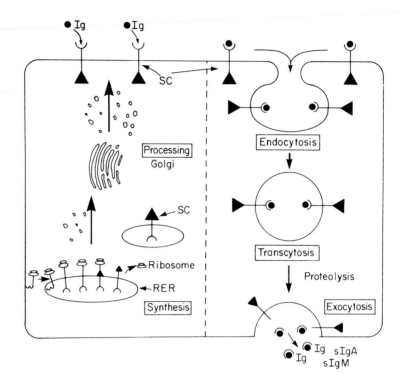

BASAL - LATERAL or SINUSOIDAL

LUMINAL or BILE CANALICULAR

FIG. 1. Model for transport of IgA and IgM across the mucosal epithelial cell or hepatocyte. The synthesis of SC *(left side)* and the steps in the transport of Ig across the cell *(right side)* are graphically represented. SC is synthesized on membrane-bound polysomes (RER) as a trans-membrane protein (~95,000 MW) and is co-translationally inserted into the RER. Further processing may occur in the Golgi (including the addition of terminal sugars). SC then becomes integrated into the basal (and lateral) plasma membranes of the mucosal epithelial cell or the sinusoidal membrane of the hepatocyte. The transmembrane SC ( )——▶) consists of three domains: (a) cytoplasmic (▶), (b) membrane-spanning (———), and (c) ectoplasmic ( )). The ectoplasmic domain acts as the external receptor for J-chain-containing polymeric Igs, such as IgA and IgM (●Ig). Endocytosis of the receptor is probably continuously occurring (escalator model) and carries Ig into the cell. Transcytosis of Ig occurs in vesicles (endosomes) that probably do not fuse with lysosomes but do fuse with the plasma membrane, thus carrying the Ig-receptor complex to the luminal surface. Proteolysis occurs at an unknown stage, leaving behind the cytoplasmic and membrane-spanning portions (MW~20,000). The Ig is secreted with the ectoplasmic domain (MW~80,000) covalently attached to $_R$IgA or $_R$IgM. Further details are available elsewhere (7,17,106).

the transport of IgA across the epithelial level after forming a complex at or near the lateral (intraepithelial) surface. A very recent study (107) reported the complete amino acid sequence of the polymeric Ig receptor deduced from its gene sequence and derived from rabbit liver and lactating mammary glands. The entire SC receptor consists of 773 amino acids (aa) and includes: an 18-aa signal peptide, a 629-aa ectoplasmic domain, a 23-aa (largely hydrophobic) membrane-spanning segment, and a 103-aa cytoplasmic tail. The extracellular portion consists of five highly conserved domains of 100 to 115 aa. A sixth domain is somewhat more distantly related and includes the membrane-spanning portion. When the domains were compared with each other and with other proteins using the Dayhoff Protein Data Bank, homologies were found with immunoglobulins as well as related proteins such as Thy-1. The most significant homologies were found between IgK–V regions (an average 28% identical aa, and when compared on the basis of similar side chains, the homology increased to 56%). A striking feature was a highly conserved 18-residue consensus sequence that was found in each of the five domains and closely resembled a segment that had been reported (116) to represent the primordial building block of immunoglobulin heavy-chain variable regions. The similarity of the receptor and its ligand is not unique to immunoglobulins and could indicate that domains on the receptor and ligand (Ig) interact via a mechanism similar to the interaction between immunoglobulin domains in polymeric Ig molecules (61). Alternatively, the receptor may have V-region-like specificity for a site on polymeric IgA and IgM. In any case, these homologies, if biologically relevant, could have implications for other receptors, particularly those involved in transport of Ig (e.g., across the neonatal intestine and placenta). Whether or not the Fc receptor on various cells or even the T-cell receptor for antigen will show properties similar to those mentioned earlier (i.e., homologies with Ig) is an interesting topic for future work.

The SC-mediated transport of immunoglobulins differs from that in other types of receptor-mediated systems in several respects (7,17,50,68,106,122–125,147,182). Some receptors, such as those for low-density lipoproteins and insulin, are recycled to the cell surface, where they are reused, whereas others (e.g., epidermal growth factor) are largely degraded in lysosomes. The transport of IgA described earlier is similar to the transport of Ig from the intestinal lumen to the circulation in the neonate and from the placenta to the fetus, in that the transported Ig molecule passes through the cell and is not utilized within the cell. Whether a receptor accompanies the transport of Ig in these systems or is recycled, as has been suggested (143), has not been established. However, as indicated earlier, SC cannot be recycled, because it undergoes limited proteolysis, and a part of it is released with the Ig. The fates of the cell-associated residual intramembranous and cytoplasmic domains after cleavage are unknown, but they are probably rapidly degraded. The evolution of a transport system in which a portion of the receptor remains attached to the ligand may be beneficial in the immunoglobulin system, because SC appears to protect the Ig molecule (a) from degradation in its passage through the cell and (b) from the mucosal contents once SC reaches the lumen. In addition, sIgA may interact with epithelial ductal cells and/or the mucous blanket on the surface of the epithelium, and it has been suggested (180,181) that IgA antibodies coating the luminal surfaces of epithelia act as a barrier to the entrance of antigens *(vide supra)*.

HEPATOBILIARY TRANSPORT OF IgA

While studies were being performed to elucidate the mechanism of mucosal transepithelial passage of IgA, Vaerman and associates made the important observation that the polymeric IgA in rat serum is rapidly cleared by the liver and delivered into bile (65). Similar observations were made by Orlans et al. (119). This hepatobiliary transport pathway shows pronounced species variation, but in the rat, intravascularly infused dimeric IgA from a variety of species (rat, mouse, rabbit, human) is passed into bile (peaking 30–120 min after injection), and membrane-bound SC on the sinusoidal surface of the hepatocyte is required for transport (45,117,155). In contrast, sheep are incapable of transporting human or IgA dimers, but they readily transport the homologous protein. However, as Orlans et al. (118) have pointed out, there is no obvious phylogenetic relationship involved in transport of one species' IgA by another. IgA undergoes endocytosis, is transported through the hepatocyte in vesicles that fuse with the canalicular membrane, and is passed into the bile and hence to the proximal intestine. The details are probably very similar to those described earlier for the epithelial cell and depicted schematically in Fig. 1. This transport mechanism occurs against a blood/bile concentration gradient but is not specifically dependent on IgA, because IgG anti-SC antibodies are transported (45). This shows the critical role of SC cross-linking in the transport phenomenon that may be accomplished by dimeric but not monomeric IgA or by divalent antibody (but not univalent Fab antibodies). As expected, bile duct ligation causes rapid and sustained elevation of polymeric IgA in rat serum.

Hepatobiliary transport of IgA in humans is much less certain; human hepatocytes apparently do not synthesize or express SC, at least in amounts detectable by the methods applied to date. However, studies of biliary transport of IgA in patients with indwelling bile duct T tubes indicate that 160 to 400 mg of IgA enter the bile in a 24-hr period (82). Moreover, transport from serum to bile of polymeric IgA is approximately 10 times greater than that of monomeric IgA. Also, the transport of IgA into bile is on the order of 50 times less in humans than in rats (38). In addition, serum polymeric IgA levels are high in parenchymal liver disease (82,99,112). The significance of this with respect to IgA transport is unclear, because common bile duct obstruction does not result in elevated serum IgA in humans (35), although levels of SC are markedly elevated in obstructive diseases, especially biliary cirrhosis (31,38). The source of biliary IgA in humans is unclear; some may be locally synthesized by plasma cells in the bile ducts or gallbladder, but indirect evidence, such as the high fractional catabolic rate of polymeric versus monomeric IgA (38), suggests that plasma clearance through some as yet undefined transport mechanism probably occurs. Although the existence of SC in bile ducts suggests that epithelial cells may play a key role in transport, several workers (24,30) have suggested a dual role of the liver and bile duct in transporting serum IgA. The possibility that hepatic receptors other than SC may be involved in transport in the human has also been suggested (82).

In attempting to identify an animal model that mimics the human biliary transport system, Delacroix et al. (36) have found that the dog secretes biliary polymeric IgA against a concentration gradient. This IgA is bound to SC, and the coefficient of biliary excretion of ^{125}I-polymeric-IgA relative to that of infused albumin (as control) was found to be 9.2; the corresponding figure in humans is 4.9 (37). Both these values are far below the 1,060 and 320 figures for rat and rabbit, respectively, and they correlate well with the fractional catabolic rate for human and dog for polymeric IgA (26–36% per day, as compared with 100% per hour in the rat) (35,36). Because neither dogs nor humans express hepatocyte SC, both species may transport IgA through a transbiliary ductule route, as originally proposed by Nagura et al. (111). Thus, the dog deserves further evaluation as a model for biliary IgA secretion in the human.

To more clearly define the difference between SC-mediated uptake by rat liver cells and the lysosomal degradative pathway for glycoproteins on the same cells, Underdown et al. (175) used an isolated perfused rat liver preparation. They found that chloroquine, which interrupts the lysosomal pathway, had no influence on IgA uptake and transport but markedly inhibited uptake and processing of ^{131}I-asialo-orosomucoid. However, as mentioned earlier, SC protects IgA from degradation, so that lysosomal enzymes may, if involved, be unable to completely degrade IgA complexed to SC. The converse was true when taurocholic acid was added to the perfusion medium, but how this bile acid impairs IgA transport is unknown. A contrasting view was put forth by Stockert et al. (159), who showed that the polymeric IgA of human serum competed for binding sites on the rat hepatic binding protein involved in clearance of asialoglycoproteins from the circulation. Binding of IgA_1 exceeded that of IgA_2, presumably because only IgA_1 proteins express the terminal galactose residue required for hepatocyte binding. These experiments do not exclude rat hepatocyte SC in IgA binding, but they raise questions as to its exclusive role in mediating IgA interaction with liver cell plasma membranes.

Although several unresolved issues related to the hepatobiliary transport of IgA remain, this pathway in rodents is apparently an efficient route for antigen disposal into the gut. Russell et al. (148) demonstrated that TNP-human serum albumin complexed with TNP-specific mouse IgA myeloma protein MOPC-315 was efficiently transported into mouse bile from the blood, but similar complexes involving IgG and IgM antibodies were not. In these studies, more than half the recovered biliary radioactivity was in high-molecular-weight IgA fractions representing antigen-antibody complexes. Pneumococcal type III capsular antigens were similarly transported when complexed with polymeric IgA myeloma proteins or hybridoma antibody (149). These transport processes were not blocked by asialofetuin, suggesting that asialoglycoprotein receptors were not involved. Also, there was little radioactivity in other secretions or tissues that would indicate alternative secretory pathways. The size of circulating complexes is important in the biliary transport mechanism, because exceptionally large complexes exceeding 10^6 daltons are inefficiently cleared and may be degraded by the reticuloendothelial system of the liver (142,154). In some species the liver-bile pathway may be a major route of elimination of foreign proteins that gain access to the body. Diseases of the hepatobiliary system may significantly disrupt this pathway, leading to an accumulation of antigens and immune complexes in the circulation (150).

ANTIGEN UPTAKE AND PROCESSING

It has been known for some time that newborns of certain species are able to absorb large amounts of ingested proteins and that each species has a characteristic time at which gross absorption ceases (2–3 days in ruminants, 18–20 days in mice and rats), as reviewed by Brambell (11). It is less well known that even in the adult, small but significant absorption of proteins and even particulate matter (2-μm latex particles) occurs across the intestine. For example, up to 2% of the dose of an ingested soluble protein appears in an antigenically recognizable form in the circulation (146). It seems likely that antigen absorption occurs to some extent directly across the intestinal epithelial cell, and particularly rapid absorption has been found following inhalation of antigens in the lower reaches of the lung (137). Bockman and Winborn (10) first demonstrated the pinocytosis of macromolecules from the intestinal lumen through the absorbtive cell into the capillaries of the lamina propria. It has been suggested that the route of mucosal absorption of antigens may be the anatomic antithesis of that for secretion of IgA, i.e., plasma membrane endocytosis into vesicles and then across the cytoplasm to be discharged via the basal lateral membranes into the interstitial space (183). However, most macromolecular absorption (including soluble proteins and particulate matter) probably occurs via the M cells of the PP, as shown by the work of Bockman and Cooper (9) involving ferritin tracers in animals and the electron microscopic studies of Owen and Jones (121) in humans. Also, after oral infection with *Salmonella* (21), the bacteria are first found in the PP before their dissemination to systemic tissues. Thus, the PP may be critical tissues in determining the access of infectious agents and the success of oral immunization with killed or attenuated vaccines. As will be discussed later, it has been shown that uptake of antigenic material in the adult is modulated by antibody (180).

Macrophages are present in both the PP and the lamina propria (6). We have found that in the mouse, approximately 5% of the cells in PP are phagocytic, and 3.8% are glass-adherent. Within the adherent cell population, only approximately 15% of the cells are phagocytic in PP, whereas some 30% of the adherent cells from spleen and lymph nodes are phagocytic. However, there is considerable variation in these figures, depending on the manner in which PP are obtained. A significant problem in interpreting these data is whether or not there is contamination by surrounding lamina propria. Whether or not macrophages transport antigens to other sites and have traffic patterns similar to those discussed for T and B cells remains to be determined.

It was originally proposed by Kagnoff and Campbell (67) that the relative absence of antibody-containing cells in PP was secondary to a lack or defect in accessory cells. A key finding in this study was the ability of the PP to synthesize antibodies *in vitro* only after addition of peritoneal-exudate-adherent cells. More recently it was reported (166) that adherent cells isolated from murine PP were unable to present antigen effectively, but that antigen-presenting cells were present in whole PP and were enriched in the nonadherent population. These studies also showed that PP lacked classic dendritic cells, using techniques that were effective in demonstrating numbers of dendritic cells in the spleen similar to the numbers reported by Steinman and Cohn (158). However, other workers found that nonadherent cell populations contained cells with dendritic morphology (40). Treatment of PP by enzymatic dissociation (Dispase) produced Ia-positive cells having accessory function in an oxidative mitogenic assay. The accessory cell activity was attributable to radioresistant cells that resided primarily in the nonadherent fraction and lacked Fc receptors (FcR), whereas spleen accessory activity was predominantly in the adherent FcR population. Mitogenesis was inhibited by anti-Ia, and it was reported that adherent FcR-bearing cells (macrophages) were inactive as stimulators in the mitogenic assay (156). Richman et al. (140) used collagenase and obtained adherent cells (macrophages) from PP that presented antigen, although in our laboratory we have been unable to reproduce this finding. In summary, it is probably most accurate to state that the nature of the antigen-presenting cell in PP remains to be defined. It has not been excluded that several cell types that have been implicated in other tissues may be involved in presentation, including Ia-positive macrophages (173), dendritic cells (179), and B cells (25). In fact, in recent work (T. Tomasi, *unpublished data*), a population derived from PP having the greatest antigen-presenting activity has been enriched for B blasts. In this regard, lipopolysaccharides (LPS) that are present in the gut of conventionally fed mice have a dramatic effect on the activation of B cells for presentation of antigen (25). Moreover, the role of LPS in regulating both local and systemic immune receptors has recently been emphasized (100).

ORAL TOLERANCE

It has been known since the work of H. G. Wells in 1911 (188) that animals fed soluble proteins lose their ability to respond to the specific antigen on subsequent systemic challenge. Systemic suppression after oral feeding has been demonstrated with a variety of thymic-dependent antigens, including heterologous erythrocytes, haptenes, and various soluble proteins (165). For example, mice fed sheep red blood cells show decreased numbers of splenic PFC and a diminished delayed hypersensitivity reaction. Hyporesponsiveness is antigen-specific and is suppressed in its generation. Some workers ascribe suppression to soluble serum factors, particularly antigen-IgA-antibody complexes (2,66). Some have reported antigen-specific suppressor cells (Ts) (94), and other investigators have implicated at least two distinct T-cell-derived soluble suppressive factors (93).

Oral tolerance to soluble proteins [human gammaglobulin (HGG), ovalbumin (OVA), bovine serum albumin (BSA), keyhole limpet hemocyanin (KLH)] involves both humoral and T-cell-mediated reactions, such as antigen-induced proliferative responses. Tolerance in this system has also been attributed to elicitation of antigen-specific Ts, as demonstrated by adoptive transfer (23,113,139). Suppressor cells first appear in the gut associated lymphoid tissues (PP and mesenteric lymph nodes) and subsequently migrate to systemic sites such as the spleen, where they are presumably responsible for systemic tolerance. Although T cells can definitely transfer suppression, it is not certain that Ts are required for either development or maintenance of oral tolerance. In one study (138), Ts were shown to disappear from the spleen and thymus by 30 days after tolerance induction, even though the animals remained tolerant for several months. In our work (166), treatment with cytoxan or colchicine prior to ingestion of antigen had no effect on the subsequent development of systemic tolerance. In recent studies by Silverman et al. (152,153), evidence was presented that although *in vitro* antigen-induced proliferation could not be detected in whole lymphocyte populations from peripheral lymph nodes or spleen from orally tolerized animals, treatment with anti-Lyt-1^+ plus complement resulted in a significant proliferative response. These authors hypothesized that the Ts elicited by oral immunization was of the Lyt-1^+ phenotype. Previous studies (88) had suggested that the Ts capable of inhibiting the cellular response to influenza virus was Lyt-1^+2^- and that suppression of the immediate response to *Leishmania tropica* (87) and to sheep erythrocytes (89,134) was also mediated by Lyt-1^+ cells. An alternative, although less likely, possibility is that treatment with anti-Lyt-1^+ enriches for proliferating Lyt-1^-2^+ Ts known to be induced by oral immunization (141). Functional neutralization of Lyt-1^+ and Lyt-2^+ cells in whole-cell populations has been postulated (71), and the contrasuppressor system originally described by Gershon et al. (49) has been reported (54) to operate locally in PP. Thus, after removal of contrasuppressors with anti-I-J + C suppression (by Lyt-2^+ I-J$^-$) becomes manifest in PP in co-culture experiments with normal spleen cells. Thus, failure to observe Ts activity in adoptive transfer and co-culture experiments may be due to the use of a whole population of cells in which suppressor activity is contraregulated. Therefore, in studies attempting to elucidate the mechanisms of suppression in oral tolerance, the activity and migration patterns of isotype-specific T helper and suppressor cells, as well as suppressor inducers and components of the contrasuppressor circuit, must all be considered. Many (or all) of these cells may have different migratory patterns to various lymphoid tissues at different times following immunization, and thus a detailed analysis is necessary to dissect out the relative roles of each cell type. One commonly suggested scenario (165) is that oral immunization leads to isotype-specific Ts for IgG and IgM that first appear in the gut and subsequently migrate to systemic lymphoid tissues, while T_H for IgA remain locally in the intestine. Some workers doubt the existence of antigen-specific Ts for IgA (92).

It should also be noted that oral tolerance applies primarily (or solely) to T-dependent antigens, that the B cell is not tolerized, and that tolerance is maintained at the T-cell level. It is possible that active suppression may be present for longer periods of time than the adoptive-transfer studies indicate. In this regard, suppressive factors have been found in extracts of spleen taken from HGG-tolerant animals as long as 4 months after induction, whereas Ts disappears (by adoptive transfer) in 90 to 120 days. It may be that only low levels of suppressor activity are necessary to maintain T-cell unresponsiveness late in tolerance. Although it is difficult to reconcile the results discussed earlier into a unified mechanism for the development of oral tolerance, it is nevertheless important to recognize that oral immunization may concomitantly lead to production of secretory immunity and systemic unresponsiveness (23). Thus, whatever the mechanisms involved, ingested antigens may elicit a complete dissociation between the secretory and systemic immune systems.

A critical point concerning oral tolerance is that its induction is dependent on the prior immunologic status of the animal. Thus, if antigen is first administered parenterally, subsequent feeding either has no tolerizing effect or may actually boost serum IgG and IgE antibody titers. This is probably attributable to the fact that early in feeding some antigen is absorbed, and this leads to a secondary systemic response. Because absorption of antigen progressively decreases with oral immunization (immune exclusion), it may be that tolerance would eventually develop if antigen were continuously administered over a long period of time. A recent study (84) suggests that subsequent feeding can abrogate the antibody response (including IgE) induced by parenteral immunization. This point is important in terms of the potential of treating previously sensitized patients by the oral route.

There also appear to be differences between antigens regarding their abilities to induce oral tolerance that may depend on their chemical structures. For example, soluble proteins lead to long-lasting systemic tolerance and an active mucosal immune response. Moreover, *in vitro* antigen-induced proliferative reactions in PP cells are absent following ingestion of soluble proteins. Tolerance to more complex antigens such as whole *Streptococcus mutans* or their cell walls requires large amounts of antigen (10^9–10^{10} cells) for induction and is of relatively short duration, disappearing in 2 to 4 weeks. A significant proliferative response is seen in the PP by 10 days after feeding, and it is difficult to demonstrate splenic Ts cells in adoptive-transfer assays at any time after feeding. Thus, as is the case with the antigens derived from cholera (126), the role of antigen structure may be critical in the elicitation of an immune response versus tolerance. This is also illustrated by the effect of adjuvants on orally administered antigens. For example, Genco et al. (48) have been able to induce a salivary IgA response with a protein antigen (BSA) in the absence of an appreciable serum IgG or IgM response only after incorporating the antigen into liposomes that are given orally. The mechanism of action of these adjuvants is unclear but may involve the binding of the antigen by a hydrophobic region of the liposome, with subsequent attachment of the liposome-antigen complex to the dome epithelial cells, where it may be taken up and "processed" in a more immunogenic (and less tolerogenic) fashion. Another complicating feature is the role of bacterial LPS in modulating immune tolerance. It is known that LPS can promote unresponsiveness (172), and, as discussed earlier, some evidence has been presented that LPS produced by intestinal bacteria modulate immunity and tolerance in the gut (100). Still another factor that may affect immune regulation and tolerance *(vide supra)* is the nature of the antigen-presenting cell. It has not been excluded that the IgA system utilizes a different presenting cell than that for IgG or IgM and/or that structural forms of various antigens might be handled differently. The relative uniqueness of the gut-associated lymphoid tissues (GALT) is evidenced by the fact that despite the presence of T and B cells in proportions similar to those in the spleen, it has not been possible to directly stimulate the production of antibodies in PP by any route of immunization.

A major unresolved question concerning oral tolerance is whether it is a unique form of tolerance or simply another route of administration of antigen. Perhaps small amounts of monomer or fragments of antigen that are highly tolerogenic are absorbed from the gut, and systemic tolerance results from the same mechanisms as does parenteral tolerance. If, as mentioned earlier, Ts are formed early in the immune response in the gut and later migrate to the spleen, or if the reports of serum factors (IgA antibody-antigen complexes) are verified, then these mechanisms suggest a unique form of tolerance. Also, initial studies (166) have shown that oral tolerance may be different from systemic tolerance in its genetic control. Ranges and Azar (135) have shown that both H-2 and non-H-2 genes influence systemic tolerance to parenterally administered deaggregated human gammaglobulin (DHGG). Our results indicate that within the H-2^k haplotype there are significant differences in the ease of induction of oral tolerance to DHGG, suggesting that non-H-2-linked genes are also important in oral tolerance. Interestingly, however, differences are seen in the ease of induction of oral tolerance and systemic tolerance when BALB/c and DBA/2 strains are compared. These results, if confirmed and extended to other strains, would suggest differences in the mechanisms of induction of tolerance via the oral versus parenteral route. Such differences could possibly be related to variation in the types of macrophages (particularly in their FcR) in the gut versus peripheral lymphoid tissues. It is known that among various mice strains, susceptibility to tolerance induction is related to the efficiency of macrophages in processing and presenting antigen, and these in turn are related to the presence of FcR for the Ig subclasses (26).

The occurrence of an active secretory immune response concomitant with systemic tolerance following ingestion (or inhalation?) of antigen could function to inhibit absorption of antigens that are potentially allergenic or autoantigenic. Speculatively, oral tolerance could be visualized as a defense against the development of certain hypersensitivity and autoimmune diseases by preventing reactions to antigens that have escaped immune exclusion. This thesis is indirectly supported by clinical evidence suggesting that sensitization in atopic persons may occur in early life when the secretory immune system is immature, allowing access of potential allergens to systemic lymphoid tissues. This thesis is consistent with the clinical observation that patients who have defective secretory systems have circulating immune complexes containing ingested antigens and develop a high incidence of allergies and autoimmune diseases. Whereas it has generally been assumed that the high titers of antibodies to food antigens in patients with mucosal deficiencies result from failure of immune exclusion, it is also possible that they lack the capacity to develop oral tolerance because of a defective secretory system. There have been a few studies addressing the important question whether or not normal adults are "naturally tolerant" to environmental antigens such as ingested food and milk proteins. Korenblat et al. (75) have presented evidence that the low incidence of detectable antibodies against BSA among adults is in part due to an acquired immunologic tolerance. From studies in mice, we have evidence (166) that there is at least a partial tolerance to bovine milk proteins in adult mice, and these proteins are constituents of mouse chow. Thus, BSA is a much poorer antigen (the mice are partially tolerant) than human serum albumin (HSA); if BSA is removed from their food, then HSA and BSA are equivalent antigens. Thus, there may be a degree of tolerance in adult animals to certain environmental antigens. Defects in this acquired tolerance could lead to continuing immune responses resulting from the repeated challenges with ubiquitous environmental antigens, and these responses could have potentially harmful results.

EFFECTOR FUNCTIONS OF MUCOSAL ANTIBODIES

The effector functions of mucosal antibodies, particularly IgA, have been a topic of debate for some years (20,72,190). Although generally regarded as those properties of antibodies that are recruited for antigen disposal once binding has occurred, a broader view of the effector functions is useful to account for the unique ability of antibodies to distribute themselves in specific tissue compartments. Both IgA and IgM have properties that ensure efficient translocation across epithelial membranes, and these are central to their actions.

IgA antibodies are largely silent as mediators of inflammatory reactions. This is particularly notable when IgA is compared with IgG and IgM antibodies of similar specificity that participate in an array of inflammatory functions, such as complement activation, neutrophil chemotaxis, and phagocytosis (72,190). Although the failure of IgA to participate in inflammatory events was originally regarded as puzzling (some reports questioned the biological value of IgA), it is now recognized that IgA mediates an "escort" function involving efficient disposal of antigens through a mechanism of inhibition of adherence or transport from one body compartment to another. As will be reviewed later, the mucosal immune system is part of a comprehensive local systemic defense mechanism in which IgA plays a major role by disposing of microbial and dietary antigens locally and/or preventing them from entering the blood. The fact that continuous encounters with antigen do not trigger vigorous inflammatory responses can be regarded as advantageous.

Neither secretory nor serum IgA monomers or dimers activate complement *in vivo*. Several laboratories have described complement activation by IgA *in vitro* (8,19,39,55), but these experiments typically involved aggregation or proteolytic disassembly of the protein. Activation of complement by IgA seems to have a marginal biological role, if any, and there is even experimental and theoretical evidence showing that circulating IgA antibodies will block immune (complement-mediated) lysis of *Neisseria meningitidis* by otherwise effective IgG and IgM antibodies (55). Serum IgA blocks complement-mediated immune effector mechanisms (56), and it has been suggested that it functions as an antiinflammatory Ig (176). In diseases such as IgA nephropathy and dermatitis herpetiformis involving tissue deposition of IgA autoantibodies or immune complexes, either complement components are absent or associated deposits of complement-activating IgG or IgM can be demonstrated. The significance of the components of the alternative pathway (properdin, etc.) that are seen in association with IgA deposits in certain diseases is unclear (132). However, at present there is no definitive evidence that IgA antibodies can mediate immunologic tissue damage through a complement-dependent mechanism.

The absence of opsonic activity of IgA antibodies has frequently been cited, but here again the issue is not clear. The binding of human IgA myeloma proteins (of both subclasses) and secretory IgA to peripheral blood polymorphonuclear leukocytes has been demonstrated by several investigators (44,86), but there is debate over the importance of these IgA receptors in promoting phagocytosis of infectious agents. For example, Van Epps and associates reported that polymeric IgA paraproteins inhibited chemotaxis of neutrophils (178) and eosinophils (136), using a modified Boyden chamber technique, and these proteins also suppressed the bactericidal activity of neutrophils without interfering with cell metabolism, membrane fluidity, or the ability of the neutrophils to participate in the lysis of IgG-coated avian erythrocytes in an antibody-dependent cytotoxicity system (177). Fanger et al. (42) reported that although circulating human neutrophils were unable to phagocytose erythrocytes sensitized by specific rabbit IgA antibodies, neutrophils recovered from mucosal sites, such as the gingival crevices of teeth, were able to phagocytose such cells. They also demonstrated that more gingival neutrophils (62%) than peripheral blood neutrophils (35%) had IgA receptors, that the presence of IgA evoked both an increase in the number of IgA receptors per neutrophil and an increase in the overall number of receptor-positive cells, and that simultaneous sensitization of erythrocytes with IgA and IgG lowered the requirement of IgG needed to promote phagocytosis. Further examination of these issues is clearly needed because of the obvious importance of the neutrophil in the host response to diverse bacterial infections of mucosal tissues.

Several investigators have studied the binding of IgA to lymphocytes, monocytes, and macrophages and have defined the biologic consequences of such interactions. Earlier studies had failed to show cytophilic attachment of IgA to spleen macrophages, and this was consistent with the lack of opsonization of specific IgA antibodies (169). However, using as a model mice infected with the parasite *Nippostrongylus brasiliensis*, Gauldie et al. (47) found that on the second day of infection, when parasites were passing through the lung, resident macrophages having IgA receptors increased their numbers from 14% to 29%. Such cells were activated, as measured by secretion of plasminogen activator, and they had an enhanced ability to ingest TNP-coated erythrocytes sensitized by the mouse IgA myeloma protein MOPC-315. Studies with MOPC-315 may underestimate phagocyte activation, because Stafford et al. (157) have shown that dimeric IgA bearing secretory component binds to monocytes more efficiently than does monomeric IgA. Weaver et al. (184) reported that macrophages, which represent approximately 90% of cells in human milk, were able to phagocytose *Escherichia coli* (serotype 07KL) preopsonized by human serum, and in so doing the macrophages released 50% of their intracellular IgA. These workers proposed that phagocytosis and IgA release may continue to occur by ingested macrophages that become resident in the intestine of the nursing infant. The potential value of cells of the monocyte/ macrophage system in defending mucosal surfaces was also suggested by the studies of Lowell et al. (90), who demonstrated that circulating, nonadherent mononuclear cells in patients recovering from type C meningococcal infections were cidal for the infecting organism in the presence of serum IgA antibodies. This activity was complement-independent and was not found after immunization of normal individuals with type C polysaccharide vaccine. Fanger et al. (43) were also able to demonstrate IgA binding to human circulating monocytes using ox erythrocytes sensitized by rabbit IgA as the test system, and employing a sensitive assay involving cytofluorographic analysis of the binding of FITC-labeled human myeloma IgA. These investigators also showed that proteins of IgA_2 isotype bound to peripheral mononuclear cells, but IgA_1 proteins did not. The explanation for this differential binding of the two human IgA isotypes, both of which are present in serum and secretions, is not clear.

The availability of receptors for IgA binding on peripheral mononuclear cells is apparently a variable function that depends on circulating levels of IgA. Twice-daily injection of BALB/c mice with the murine myeloma protein MOPC-315 was shown by Hoover et al. (62) to induce an expansion of a pool of T lymphocytes ($Lyt-1^-2^+$) that have IgA receptors ($T\alpha$). This cell has a suppressor phenotype in the mouse. They also showed that $T\alpha$ cells could be expanded in a pool of BALB/ c spleen cells incubated with MOPC-315 *in vitro*, a phenomenon that was dependent on both DNA and protein synthesis. This group has also shown that $T\alpha$ cells are increased in patients with IgA myeloma, and cells with IgE receptors are elevated in rats having high circulating levels of IgE, indicating that increased expression of Ig receptors is neither species- nor isotype-specific (63). Adachi et al. (1), using a rosetting assay involving MOPC-315, showed that IgA-deficient individuals had only 5.1% (but normal individuals had 12.5%) receptor-positive lymphocytes for IgA after incubation with the indicator erythrocytes for 18 hr. The defect in the patients' lymphocytes could be corrected by incubation in a preconditioned medium derived from normal cells, indicating that the deficient cells were not intrinsically unable to generate IgA receptors. The low level of receptor-positive cells in normal persons was attributed to the dominance of monomeric IgA in normal human blood. In patients with IgA nephropathy, characterized by higher levels of serum polymeric IgA (171), IgA receptors were found to be already activated *in vivo* and required only 1 hr of incubation with indicator erythrocytes for expression. The expression of IgA receptors apparently represents an unusual example of "up-regulation" by ligand. Although the significance of these findings for the functions of IgA antibodies and effector cells of both the lymphocytic and monocytic macrophage systems is not completely clear, it has been suggested that Tα cells are involved in isotype-specific helper activity (41), as well as suppressor functions (62). Thus, the observed changes in Tα may represent regulatory factors for IgA production. A recent study (162) demonstrated *in vitro* cell-mediated antibacterial activity of GALT lymphocytes against *Shigella X16* (a hybrid strain between the enteric pathogen *S. flexneri* and *E. coli*). Importantly, murine lymphocytes from GALT, but not other tissues (thymus or popliteal lymph nodes), exerted natural antibacterial activity, and sIgA specifically increased cytotoxic activity. The type of cell involved was not defined, but some evidence was presented that a null or K lymphocyte (not a macrophage) was mediating the ADCC by sIgA. If this work should be verified, it would represent an important new role for sIgA in protecting the host against infectious agents at the mucosal level.

IgA antibodies have been shown to have several effector functions that are not dependent on phagocytic cells, lymphocytes, and complement; also, these biological properties may be of crucial importance in defense against mucosal pathogens and undesirable gastrointestinal absorption of ingested antigenic materials. Most of these are well known and have been extensively reviewed (97). They will be mentioned here only for completeness. Mucosal IgA neutralizes viruses, as exemplified by the extensive studies of Ogra and associates on poliovirus immunization by the oral route (115). In the case of bacterial infections, IgA blocks the attachment of pathogens to relevant mucosal tissues and cells, and such an adherence inhibition function has been demonstrated in several experimental models and in humans, particularly with reference to the oral microflora (51), major intestinal pathogens, e.g., *E. coli* and *Vibrio cholerae* (46), and urinary tract pathogens (161).

New work of note has been reported by Porter and Linggood (131), who have shown that mucosal antibodies may eliminate ("cure") plasmids coding for K88 adhesive determinants in *E. coli* strains that are common intestinal pathogens of pigs. These antibodies are not directed at K88 or serotype antigens themselves, and bacteria exposed to immune sow's milk do not recover the ability to synthesize K88 antigens even when recultured in the absence of antibody. Confirmation that plasmids are lost is apparent by the concomitant loss of the ability of *E. coli* strain 0149:K91 to ferment raffinose, the raf$^+$ gene and K88ac genes being present on the same plasmid. The phenomenon of sustained plasmid elimination represents a potentially important function of mucosal antibody, because it may reduce the virulence of bacterial strains in the environment. However, the mechanisms involved in plasmid exclusion are presently unknown.

Another biologically relevant function of mucosal antibodies is the binding and subsequent inhibition of absorption of soluble macromolecular antigens (immune exclusion), as shown in extensive studies by Walker and Bloch (180). Everted gut sacs of rats orally immunized with BSA or horseradish peroxidase showed an antigen-specific reduction in passage of the immunizing antigen to the serosal surface. The mechanism was thought to involve immune-complex formation, followed by subsequent rapid degradation of these complexes by proteolytic enzymes of pancreatic origin. These investigators also showed that intestinal inflammation in the rat (by *N. brasiliensis* infection) or intestinal anaphylaxis caused enhanced uptake into the systemic circulation of intestinal "bystander" macromolecules. It has been postulated that immune exclusion is mediated by antibodies bound to the surface of the mucosal epithelium, although other ultrastructural studies have suggested that IgA does not bind to the apical plasma membrane of normal or neoplastic colon cells (18,110). A clinical counterpart of immune exclusion may exist in IgA-deficient individuals who have high levels of serum antibody to food antigens, particularly bovine milk proteins. Cunningham-Rundles (32) has identified dietary proteins in circulating immune complexes in such individuals, presumably because they experience chronic hyperabsorption of macromolecules that remain antigenically intact. An interesting recent observation (33) is that a small but significant fraction of the immune complexes in IgA-deficient serum involves idiotype–antiidiotype interactions. Because antiidiotype antibodies have been shown to have both suppressive and stimulatory activity on idiotype production, and both idiotype and antiidiotype Ts have been defined, the foregoing findings have potential implications for regulation of immune reactivity to environmental antigens.

IgA$_1$ PROTEASES

A medically important group of bacterial pathogens produce IgA$_1$ proteases, extracellular enzymes that are highly substrate-specific in that they cleave only human IgA$_1$ proteins (98,109,130). The enzymes are metal-dependent (Mg^{2+}), and some evidence has been presented (83) that specificity may depend on the combination of a protease and a dextran sucrase. Bacteria releasing these proteases include the two pathogenic *Neisseria* (*N. meningitidis* and *N. gonorrhoeae*), *Haemophilus influenzae*, *Streptococcus pneumoniae*, and pathogens involved in dental caries and periodontal infections: *Streptococcus sanguis* and *Bacteroides melaninogenicus* (129). In addition, IgA$_1$ protease activity has recently been found among fresh clinical isolates of *E. coli* and certain other urinary tract pathogens (101), but enzyme output by these strains apparently falls after repeated subculture. Among *Neisseria* and *Haemophilus* species, IgA$_1$ protease activity is confined to the human pathogens; nonpathogens within these two genera are not only enzyme-negative but also do not have the gene specifying the enzyme in their chromosomal DNA (16). Because IgA$_1$ proteases are found only among bacteria capable of causing human infections, are present in infected secretions, and exhibit substrate specificity for human IgA$_1$, it is likely that they take part in the infectious process, although the precise mechanisms have not been defined.

The IgA$_1$ proteases are variably antigenic in humans and experimental animals; for example, high titers of antibodies that inhibit the catalytic function of the neisserial IgA$_1$ proteases are found in the secretory IgA purified from normal human colostrum (52), and serum antibody titers (of the IgG class) rise markedly in patients convalescent from meningococcal meningitis. Inhibiting antibodies are present at low titers in all normal sera, but the role these play in normal resistance is unknown. In marked contrast, the IgA$_1$ proteases of *S. sanguis* are not antigenic for humans. These variations in antigenicity reflect the pronounced differences among the enzymes (70) that is also apparent at the genetic level *(vide infra)*. At present, the IgA$_1$ proteases, considered as a group, all have the same substrate specificity but differ structurally when the enzymes from different organisms are compared. The extent and nature of the differences will require purified proteases in greater amounts than are presently available.

Each IgA$_1$ protease identified to date cleaves a single peptide bond in the hinge region in the IgA$_1$ heavy polypeptide chain, and proline residues invariably contribute the carboxyl group to the bond cleaved. There are multiple such Pro-R bonds in the hinge region of IgA$_1$ because of the unique proline-rich stretch of 16 amino acids that represents the duplication of an octapeptide having the composition Thr-Pro-Pro-Thr-Pro-Ser-Pro-Ser. IgA$_2$ proteins have a deletion of 13 hinge residues and are therefore resistant to protease hydrolysis. Although each bacterial isolate cleaves one bond, several types of specificities are found among certain species, e.g., *N. meningitidis* and *H. influenzae* (69), and the specificity is strongly correlated with the capsular serotype. Of considerable interest is the fact that synthetic peptide analogues of the IgA$_1$ hinge region are not susceptible to hydrolysis, indicating that the IgA$_1$ proteases undoubtedly interact with segments of the substrate distant from the hinge region and/or that the carbohydrate moieties are critical. These relationships have been discussed in a recent review of these enzymes (129).

Production of active IgA$_1$ protease is encoded by a single gene on the chromosomal DNA of both *N. gonorrhoeae* (74) and *H. influenzae* (16). But in both cases, when these were subcloned into a vector and introduced into *E. coli*, the bacteria produced lower enzyme activity than did the donor strain in transformation experiments, and the *Haemophilus* enzyme accumulated in the periplasm and was not secreted. It is possible that secretion is a function requiring additional genes that were excised when preparing the donor DNA. DNA probes prepared from the cloned genes of both strains showed strong homology with DNA restriction fragments of bacterial species from within the respective genera, but homology was marginal with DNA of other protease-positive bacteria. This suggests that the IgA$_1$ proteases from various bacteria will have structural differences, a result consistent with the biochemical diversity discussed earlier. Genetic studies of these enzymes have not yet revealed their functions. A *N. gonorrhoeae* mutant produced by reintroduction of a physically modified (deleted) gene failed to produce the active enzyme but was found phenotypically indistinguishable from its protease-positive but otherwise isogenic counterpart (73). The participation of IgA$_1$ protease function in virulence could be tested with a protease-negative strain transfected with the protease gene, but the paucity of animal models of infection by these strictly human pathogens is a continuing impediment to such studies.

ACKNOWLEDGMENTS

The authors wish to acknowledge the excellent secretarial assistance of Mrs. Mary Overmier. This work was supported in part by USPHS NIH grants AM-31448, HD-17013, and DE-06048.

REFERENCES

1. Adachi, M., Yodoi, J., Masuda, T., Takatsuki, K., and Uchino, H. (1983): Altered expression of lymphocyte Fcα receptor in selective IgA deficiency and IgA nephropathy. *J. Immunol.*, 131:1246.
2. André, C., Heremans, J. F., Vaerman, J. P., and Cambiaso, C. L. (1975): A mechanism for the induction of immunological tolerance by antigen feeding: Antigen-antibody complexes. *J. Exp. Med.*, 142:1509.
3. Baenziger, J. U. (1979): Structure of the oligosaccharide of human J chain. *J. Biol. Chem.*, 254:4063.
4. Bertoli, L. F., Kubagawa, H., Koopman, W. F., Mestecky, J., and Cooper, D. (1983): Presence of monoclonal immunoglobulins in saliva of myeloma patients. *Fed. Proc.*, 42:840.
5. Bienenstock, J., and Befus, A. D. (1980): Musocal immunology. *Immunology*, 41:249.
6. Bienenstock, J., and Dolezel, J. (1971): Peyer's patches: Lack of specific antibody-containing cells after oral and parenteral immunization. *J. Immunol.*, 106:938.
7. Blobel, G. (1980): Intracellular protein topogenesis. *Proc. Natl. Acad. Sci. U.S.A.*, 77:1496.
8. Boackle, R. J., Caughman, G. B., and Carsgo, E. A. (1978): The partial isolation and function of salivary factors which interact with the complement system: A possible role in mucosal immunity. In: *Secretory Immunity and Infections*, edited by J. R. McGhee, J. Mestecky, and J. L. Babb, pp. 411–421. Plenum Press, New York.
9. Bockman, D. E., and Cooper, M. D. (1973): Pinocytosis by epithelium associated with lymphoid follicles in the bursa of Fabricius, appendix, and Peyer's patches. An electron microscopic study. *Am. J. Anat.*, 136:455.
10. Bockman, D. E., and Winborn, W. B. (1966): Light and electron microscopy of intestinal ferritin absorption. Observations in sensitized and non-sensitized hamsters *(Mesocricetus auratus)*. *Anat. Rec.*, 155:603.
11. Brambell, F. W. R. (1970): *The Transmission of Passive Immunity from Mother to Young.* North-Holland, Amsterdam.
12. Brandtzaeg, P. (1974): Characteristics of SC-Ig complexes formed *in vitro*. In: *The Immunoglobulin A System*, edited by J. Mestecky and A. R. Lawton, pp. 87–97. Plenum Press, New York.
13. Brandtzaeg, P. (1981): Transport models for secretory IgA and secretory IgM. *Clin. Exp. Immunol.*, 44:221.
14. Brandtzaeg, P. (1983): The secretory immune system of lactating human mammary glands compared with exocrine organs. In: *The Secretory Immune System, Vol. 409*, edited by J. R. McGhee and J. Mestecky, pp. 353–382, New York Academy of Science, New York.
15. Brandtzaeg, P., and Baklien, K. (1977): Intestinal secretion of IgA and IgM: A hypothetical model. In: *Immunology of the Gut,(CIBA Foundation Symp.)*, pp. 77. Elsevier, Amsterdam.
16. Bricker, J., Mulks, M. H., Plaut, A. G., Moxon, E. R., and Wright, A. (1983): IgA$_1$ proteases of *Hemophilus influenzae*: Cloning and characterization in *E. coli* K-12. *Proc. Natl. Acad. Sci. U.S.A.*, 80:2681.
17. Brown, M. S., Anderson, R. G., and Goldstein, J. L. (1983): Recycling receptors: The round-trip itinerary of migrant membrane proteins. *Cell*, 32:663.
18. Brown, W. R., Isobe, Y., and Nakane, P. K. (1976): Studies on translocation of immunoglobulins across intestinal epithelium. II. Immunoelectronmicroscopic localization of immunoglobulins and secretory component in human intestinal mucosa. *Gastroenterology*, 71:985.
19. Burritt, M. F., Calvanico, N. J., Mehta, S., and Tomasi, T. B. (1977): Activation of the classical complement pathway by Fc fragment of human IgA. *J. Immunol.*, 118:723.
20. Calvanico, N. J., and Tomasi, T. B. (1979): Effector sites on antibodies. In: *Immunochemistry of Proteins, Vol. 3*, edited by M. Z. Atassi, pp. 1–85. Plenum Press, New York.
21. Carter, P. B., and Collins, F. M. (1974): The route of enteric infection in normal mice. *J. Exp. Med.*, 139:1189.
22. Cebra, J. J., and Small, P. A. (1967): Polypeptide chain structure of rabbit immunoglobulins. III. Secretory γA-immunoglobulin from colostrum. *Biochemistry*, 6:503.
23. Challacombe, S. J., and Tomasi, T. B. (1980): Systemic tolerance and secretory immunity after oral immunization. *J. Exp. Med.*, 152:1459.
24. Chandy, K. G., Hübscher, S. G., Elias, E., Berg, J., Khan, M., and Burnett, D. (1983): Dual role of the liver in regulating circulating polymeric IgA in man: Studies on patients with liver disease. *Clin. Exp. Immunol.*, 52:207.
25. Chesnut, R. W., Colon, S. M., and Grey, H. M. (1982): Antigen presentation by normal B cells, B cell tumors and macrophages: Functional and biochemical comparison. *J. Immunol.*, 128:1764.

26. Cowing, C., Garabedian, C., and Leskowitz, S. (1979): Strain differences in tolerance induction to human γ-globulin subclasses: Dependence on macrophages. *Cell. Immunol.*, 47:407.

27. Crago, S. S., Kulhavy, R., Prince, S. J., and Mestecky, J. (1978): Secretory component on epithelial cells is a surface receptor for polymeric immunoglobulins. *J. Exp. Med.*, 147:1832.

28. Crago, S. S., Kutteh, W. H., Moro, I., Allansmith, M. R., Radl, J., Haaijman, J. J., and Mestecky, J. (1984): Distribution of IgA_1^-, IgA_2^- and J chain containing cells in human tissues. *J. Immunol.*, 132:16.

29. Craig, S. W., and Cebra, J. J. (1975): Rabbit Peyer's patches, appendix, and popliteal lymph node B lymphocytes: A comparative analysis of their membrane immunoglobulin components and plasma cell precursor potential. *J. Immunol.*, 114:492.

30. Cuadrado, E., Arenas, J. I., Echaniz, P., Garcia-Gonzales, M., and Damiano, A. (1983): Rapid decrease of secretory IgA serum levels in extrahepatic obstructive jaundice after surgical relief of the bile duct obstruction. *Gastroenterology*, 84:203.

31. Culp, K. S., Anderson, W. L., Dickson, E. R., and Tomasi, T. B. (1981): Secretory component (SC) elevations in primary biliary cirrhosis. *Gastroenterology*, 80:1130.

32. Cunningham-Rundles, C. (1981): The identification of specific antigens in circulating immune complexes by an enzyme linked immunoabsorbent assay: Detection of bovine k-casein in IgG complexes in human sera. *Eur. J. Immunol.*, 11:504.

33. Cunningham-Rundles, C. (1983): Isolation and analysis of anti-idiotypic antibodies from IgA-deficient sera. In: *The Secretory Immune System, Vol. 409*, edited by J. R. McGhee and J. Mestecky, pp. 469–477. New York Academy of Sciences, New York.

34. Dahlgren, U. Ahlstedt, S., Hedman, L., Wadsworth, C., and Hanson, L. (1981): Dimeric IgA in the rat is transferred from serum into bile but not into milk. *Scand. J. Immunol.*, 14:95.

35. Delacroix, D. L., Elkon, K. B., Geubel, A. P., Hodgson, H. F., Dive, C., and Vaerman, J. P. (1983): Changes in size, subclass, and metabolic properties of serum immunoglobulin A in liver diseases and in other diseases with high serum immunoglobulin A. *J. Clin. Invest.*, 71:358.

36. Delacroix, D. L., Furtado-Barreira, G., de Hemptinne, B., Goudswaard, J., Dive, C., and Vaerman, J. P. (1983): The liver in the IgA secretory immune system. Dogs, but not rats and rabbits, are suitable models for human studies. *Hepatology*, 3:980.

37. Delacroix, D. L., Hodgson, H. J. F., McPherson, A., Dive, C., and Vaerman, J. P. (1982): Selective transport of polymeric IgA in bile: Quantitative relationships of monomeric and polymeric IgA, IgM and other proteins in serum, bile and saliva. *J. Clin. Invest.*, 70:230.

38. Delacroix, D. L., and Vaerman, J. P. (1983): Function of the human liver in IgA homeostasis in plasma. In: *The Secretory Immune System, Vol. 409*, edited by J. R. McGhee and J. Mestecky, pp. 383–401. New York Academy of Sciences, New York.

39. Eddie, D. S., Shulkind, M. L., and Robbins, J. B. (1971): The isolation and biological activities of purified secretory IgA and IgG anti-*Salmonella typhimurium* "O" antibodies from rabbit intestinal fluid and colostrum. *J. Immunol.*, 106:181.

40. Eldridge, J. H., Lee, Y., Kiyono, H., Spalding, D. M., Gollahon, K. A., Wood, G. W., Koopman, W. J., and McGhee, J. R. (1983): Peyer's patch accessory cells bear I-A. In: *The Secretory Immune System, Vol. 409*, edited by J. R. McGhee and J. Mestecky, pp. 819–821. New York Academy of Sciences, New York.

41. Endoh, M., Sakai, H., Nomoto, Y., Tomino, Y., and Kaneshige, H. (1981): IgA-specific helper activity of Tα cells in human peripheral blood. *J. Immunol.*, 127:2612.

42. Fanger, M. W., Goldstine, S. N., and Shen, L. (1983): The properties and role of receptors for IgA on human leukocytes. In: *The Secretory Immune System, Vol. 409*, edited by J. R. McGhee and J. Mestecky, pp. 552–563. New York Academy of Sciences, New York.

43. Fanger, M. W., Goldstine, S. N., and Shen, L. (1983): Cytofluorographic analysis of receptors for IgA on human polymorphonuclear cells and monocytes and the correlation of receptor expression with phagocytes. *Mol. Immunol.*, 20:1019.

44. Fanger, M. W., Shen, L., Pugh, L., and Bernier, G. M. (1980): Subpopulations of human peripheral granulocytes and monocytes express receptors for IgA. *Proc. Natl. Acad. Sci. U.S.A.*, 77:3640.

45. Fisher, M. M., Nagy, B., Bazin, H., and Underdown, B. J. (1979): Biliary transport of IgA: Role of secretory component. *Proc. Natl. Acad. Sci. U.S.A.*, 76:2008.

46. Freter, R., and Jones, G. W. (1983): Models for studying the role of bacterial attachment in virulence and pathogenesis. *Rev. Infect. Dis.*, 5:S647.

47. Gauldie, J., Richards, C., and Lamontagne, L. (1983): Fc receptors for IgA and other immuno-globulins on resident and activated alveolar macrophages. *Mol. Immunol.*, 20:1029.
48. Genco, R. J., Linzer, R., and Evans, R. T. (1983): Effect of adjuvants on orally administered antigens. In: *The Secretory Immune System, Vol. 409*, edited by J. R. McGhee and J. Mestecky, pp. 650–668. New York Academy of Sciences, New York.
49. Gershon, R. K., Eardley, D. D., Durum, D., Green, D. R., Shen, F. W., Yamauchi, K., Cantor, H., and Murphy, D. B. (1981): Contrasuppression—a novel immunoregulatory activity. *J. Exp. Med.*, 153:1533.
50. Geuze, H. J., Slot, J. W., and Strous, G. J. (1983): Intracellular site of asialoglycoprotein receptor-ligand uncoupling: Double-label immunoelectron microscopy during receptor-mediated endocytosis. *Cell*, 32:277.
51. Gibbons, R. J., and Van Houte, J. (1975): Bacterial adherence in oral microbial ecology. *Annu. Rev. Microbiol.*, 29:19.
52. Gilbert, J. V., Plaut, A. G., Longmaid, B., and Lamm, M. E. (1983): Inhibition of microbial IgA proteases by human secretory IgA and serum. *Mol. Immunol.*, 20:1039.
53. Goldman, I. S., Jones, A. L., Hradek, G. T., and Huling, S. (1983): Hepatocyte handling of immunoglobulin A in the rat: The role of microtubules. *Gastroenterology*, 85:130.
54. Green, D. R., Gold, J., St. Martin, S., Gershon, R., and Gershon, R. K. (1982): Microenvironmental immunoregulation: Possible role of contrasuppressor cells in maintaining immune receptor in gut-associated lymphoid tissues. *Proc. Natl. Acad. Sci. U.S.A.*, 79:889.
55. Griffiss, J. M. (1982): Epidemic meningococcal disease: Synthesis of a hypothetical immunoepidemiologic model. *Rev. Infect. Dis.*, 4:159.
56. Griffiss, J. M. (1983): Biologic function of serum IgA system: Modulation of complement-mediated effector mechanisms and conservation of antigenic mass. In: *The Secretory Immune System, Vol. 409*, edited by J. R. McGhee and J. Mestecky, pp. 697–707. New York Academy of Sciences, New York.
57. Guy-Grand, D., Griscelli, C., and Vassali, P. (1978): The mouse gut T lymphocyte, a novel type of T cell. *J. Exp. Med.*, 148:1661.
58. Hajdu, I., Moldoveanu, Z., Cooper, M. D., and Mestecky, J. (1983): Ultrastructural studies of human lymphoid cells. *J. Exp. Med.*, 158:1993.
59. Halsey, J. F., Johnson, B. F., and Cebra, J. J. (1980): Transport of immunoglobulins from serum into colostrum. *J. Exp. Med.*, 151:767.
60. Halsey, J. F., Mitchell, C., Meyer, R., and Cebra, J. J. (1982): Metabolism of Immunoglobulin A in lactating mice: Origins of immunoglobulin A in milk. *Eur. J. Immunol.*, 12:107.
61. Hauptman, S. P., and Tomasi, T. B. (1975): Mechanisms of immunoglobulin A polymerization. *J. Biol. Chem.*, 250:3891.
62. Hoover, R. G., Dieckgraefe, B. K., and Lynch, R. G. (1981): T cells with Fc receptors for IgA: Induction of Tα cells *in vivo* and *in vitro* by purified IgA. *J. Immunol.*, 127:1560.
63. Hoover, R. G., Hickman, S., Gebel, H. M., Rebbe, N., and Lynch, R. G. (1981): Expansion of Fc receptor-bearing T lymphocytes in patients with immunoglobulin G and immunoglobulin A myeloma. *J. Clin. Invest.*, 67:308.
64. Huang, S. W., Fogh, J., and Hong, R. (1976): Synthesis of secretory component by colon cancer cells. *Scand. J. Immunol.*, 5:263.
65. Jackson, G. D. F., Lamaitre-Coelho, I., Vaerman, J. P., Bazin, H., and Beckers, A. (1978): Rapid disappearance from serum of intravenously injected rat myeloma IgA and its secretion into bile. *Eur. J. Immunol.*, 8:123.
66. Kagnoff, M. F. (1978): Effects of antigen-feeding on intestinal and systemic immune responses. III. Antigen-specific serum-mediated suppression of humoral and antibody responses after antigen feeding. *Cell. Immunol.*, 40:186.
67. Kagnoff, M. F., and Campbell, S. (1974): Functional characteristics of Peyer's patch lymphoid cells. I. Induction of humoral antibody and cell-mediated allograft reactions. *J. Exp. Med.*, 139:398.
68. Kaplan, J. (1981): Polypeptide-binding membrane receptors: Analysis and classification. *Science*, 212:14.
69. Kilian, M. (1981): Degradation of immunoglobulin A_1, A_2, and G by suspected principal periodontal pathogens. *Infect. Immun.*, 34:757.
70. Kilian, M., Thomsen, B., Petersen, T. E., and Bleeg, H. (1983): Molecular biology of *Haemophilus influenzae* IgA_1 proteases. *Mol. Immunol.*, 20:1051.

71. Kim, B. S., and Greenberg, J. A. (1981): Mechanisms of idiotype suppression. IV. Functional neutralization in mixtures of idiotypespecific suppressor and hapten-specific suppressor T cells. *J. Exp. Med.*, 154:809.

72. Klein, M., Haeffner-Cavaillon, N., Isenman, D. E., Rivat, C., Navia, M. A., Davies, D. R., and Dorrington, K. J. (1981): Expression of biological effector functions by immunoglobulin G molecules lacking the hinge region. *Proc. Natl. Acad. Sci. U.S.A.*, 78:524.

73. Kommey, J. M., Gill, R. E., and Falkow, S. (1982): Genetic and biochemical analysis of gonococcal IgA₁ protease: Cloning in *Escherichia coli* and construction of mutants of gonococci which fail to produce the activity. *Proc. Natl. Acad. Sci. U.S.A.*, 79:7881.

74. Koomey, J. M., and Falkow, S. (1984): Nucleotide sequence homology between the immunoglobulin A₁ protease genes of *Neisseria gonorrhoeae, Neisseria meningitidis*, and *Hemophilus influenzae. Infect. Immun.*, 43:101.

75. Korenblat, P. E., Rothberg, R. M., Minden, P., and Farr, R. S. (1968): Immune responses of human adults after oral and parenteral exposure to bovine serum albumin. *J. Allergy*, 41:226.

76. Koshland, M. E. (1975): Structure and function of the J chain. In: *Advances in Immunology, Vol. 20*, edited by F. J. Dixon and H. G. Kunkel, pp. 41–69. Academic Press, New York.

77. Koshland, M. E. (1983): Presidential address. Molecular aspects of B cell differentiation. *J. Immunol.*, 131:i.

78. Kühn, L. C., and Kraehenbuhl, J. P. (1979): Interaction of rabbit secretory component with rabbit IgA dimer. *J. Biol. Chem.*, 254:11066.

79. Kühn, L. C., and Kraehenbuhl, J. P. (1979): Role of secretory component, a secreted glycoprotein, in the specific uptake of IgA dimer by epithelial cells. *J. Biol. Chem.*, 254:11072.

80. Kühn, L. C., and Kraehenbuhl, J. P. (1981): The membrane receptor for polymeric immunoglobulin is structurally related to secretory component. Isolation and characterization of membrane secretory component from rabbit liver and mammary gland. *J. Biol. Chem.*, 256:12490.

81. Kutteh, W. H., Prince, S. J., and Mestecky, J. (1982): Tissue origins of human polymeric and monomeric IgA. *J. Immunol.*, 128:990.

82. Kutteh, W. H., Prince, S. J., Phillips, J. D., Spenney, J. G., and Mestecky, J. (1982): Properties of immunoglobulin A in serum of individuals with liver diseases and in hepatic bile. *Gastroenterology*, 82:184.

83. Labib, R. S., Calvanico, C., and Tomasi, T. B. (1978): Studies on extracellular proteases of *Streptococcus sanguis*: Purification and characterization of a human IgA₁ specific protease. *Biochim. Biophys. Acta*, 526:547.

84. Lafont, S., André, C., André, F., Gillon, J., and Fargier, M. C. (1982): Abrogation by subsequent feeding of antibody response, including IgE, in parenterally immunized mice. *J. Exp. Med.*, 155:1573.

85. Lamm, M. E. (1976): Cellular aspects of immunoglobulins. In: *Advances in Immunology, Vol. 22*, edited by F. J. Dixon and H. G. Kunkel, pp. 223–290. Academic Press, New York.

86. Lawrence, D. A., Weigle, W. O., and Spiegelberg, H. L. (1975): Immunoglobulins cytophilic for human lymphocytes, monocytes and neutrophils. *J. Clin. Invest.*, 55:368.

87. Liew, F. Y., Hale, C., and Howard, J. G. (1982): Immunologic regulation of experimental cutaneous leishmaniasis. V. Characterization of effector and specific suppressor T cells. *J. Immunol.*, 128:1917.

88. Liew, F. Y., and Russell, S. M. (1980): Delayed-type hypersensitivity to influenza virus. Induction of antigen specific suppressor T cells for delayed-type hypersensitivity to hemagglutinin during influenza virus infection in mice. *J. Exp. Med.*, 151:799.

89. Liew, F. Y., Sia, D. Y., Parish, C. R., and McKenzie, I. F. (1980): Major histocompatibility gene complex (M.H.C.)-coded determinants of antigen-specific suppressor factor for delayed type hypersensitivity and surface phenotypes of cells producing the factor. *Eur. J. Immunol.*, 10:305.

90. Lowell, G. H., MacDermott, R. P., Summers, P. L., Reeder, A. A., Bertovich, M. J., and Formal, S. B. (1980): Antibody-dependent cell-mediated antibacterial activity: K lymphocytes, monocytes, and granulocytes are effective against shigella. *J. Immunol.*, 125:2778.

91. Mach, J. P. (1970): *In vitro* combination of human and bovine free secretory component with IgA of various species. *Nature*, 228:1278.

92. Mattingly, J. A. (1983): Cellular circuitry involved in orally induced systemic tolerance and local antibody production. In: *The Secretory Immune System, Vol. 409*, edited by J. R. McGhee and J. Mestecky, pp. 204–213. New York Academy of Sciences, New York.

93. Mattingly, J. A., Kaplan, J. M., and Janeway, C. A., Jr. (1980): Two distinct antigen-specific suppressor factors induced by the oral administration of antigen. *J. Exp. Med.*, 152:545.

94. Mattingly, J. A., and Waksman, B. H. (1978): Immunologic suppression after oral administration of antigen. I. Specific suppressor cells formed in rat Peyer's patches after oral administration of sheep erythrocytes and their systemic migration. *J. Immunol.*, 121:1878.

95. McCune, J. M., Fu, S. M., and Kunkel, H. G. (1981): J chain biosynthesis in pre-B cells and other possible precursor B cells. *J. Exp. Med.*, 154:138.

96. McGhee, J. R., and Mestecky, J. (editors) (1983): *Annals of the New York Academy of Sciences, Vol. 409.* New York Academy of Sciences, New York.

97. McNabb, P., and Tomasi, T. B. (1981): Host defense mechanisms at mucosal surfaces. *Annu. Rev. Microbiol.*, 35:477.

98. Mehta, S. K., Plaut, A. G., Calvanico, N. J., and Tomasi, T. B. (1973): Human immunoglobulin A: Production of an Fc fragment by an enteric microbial proteolytic enzyme. *J. Immunol.*, 111:1274.

99. Mestecky, J., Kutteh, W. H., Brown, T. A., Russell, M. W., Phillips, J. O., Moldoveanu, Z., Moro, I., and Crago, S. S. (1983): Function and biosynthesis of polymeric IgA. In: *The Secretory Immune System, Vol. 409*, edited by J. R. McGhee and J. Mestecky, pp. 292–305. New York Academy of Sciences, New York.

100. Michalek, S. M., McGhee, J. R., Kiyono, H., Colwell, D. E., Eldridge, J. H., Wannemuehler, M. J., and Koopman, W. J. (1983): The IgA response: Inductive aspects, regulatory cells, and effector functions. In: *The Secretory Immune System, Vol. 409*, edited by J. R. McGhee and J. Mestecky, pp. 48–71. New York Academy of Sciences, New York.

101. Miluzzo, F. H., and Delisle, G. J. (1984): Immunoglobulin A proteases in Gram-negative bacteria isolated from human urinary tract infections. *Infect. Immun.*, 43:11.

102. Mizoguchi, A., Mizuochi, T., and Kobata, A. (1982): Structures of the carbohydrate moieties of secretory component purified from human milk. *J. Biol. Chem.*, 257:9612.

103. Mole, J. E., Bhown, A. S., and Bennett, J. C. (1977): Primary structure of human J chain: Alignment of peptides from chemical and enzymatic hydrolyses. *Biochemistry*, 16:3507.

104. Mosmann, T. R., Gravel, Y., and Williamson, A. R. (1978): Modification and fate of J chain in myeloma cells in the presence and absence of polymeric immunoglobulin secretion. *Eur. J. Immunol.*, 8:94.

105. Mostov, K. E., and Blobel, G. (1982): A transmembrane percursor of secretory component. The receptor for transcellular transport of polymeric immunoglobulins. *J. Biol. Chem.*, 257:11816.

106. Mostov, K. E., and Blobel, G. (1983): Transcellular transport of polymeric immunoglobulin by secretory component: A model system for studying intracellular protein sorting. In: *The Secretory Immune System, Vol. 409*, edited by J. R. McGhee and J. Mestecky, pp. 441–451. New York Academy of Sciences, New York.

107. Mostov, K. E., Friedlander, M., and Blobel, G. (1984): The receptor for transepithelial transport of IgA and IgM contains multiple immunoglobulin-like domains. *Nature*, 308:37.

108. Mostov, K. E., Kraehenbuhl, J. P., and Blobel, G. (1980): Receptor-mediated transcellular transport of immunoglobulin: Synthesis of secretory component as multiple and larger transmembrane forms. *Proc. Natl. Acad. Sci. U.S.A.*, 77:7257.

109. Mulks, M. H., and Plaut, A. G. (1978): IgA protease production as a characteristic distinguishing pathogenic from harmless *Neisseriaceae. N. Engl. J. Med.*, 299:973.

110. Nagura, H., Nakane, P., and Brown, W. R. (1979): Translocation of dimeric IgA through neoplastic colon cells *in vitro. J. Immunol.*, 123:2359.

111. Nagura, J., Smith, P. D., Nakane, P. K., and Brown, W. R. (1981): IgA in human bile and liver. *J. Immunol.*, 126:587.

112. Newkirk, M. M., Klein, M. H., Katz, A., Fisher, M. M., and Underdown, B. J. (1983): Estimation of polymeric IgA in human serum: An assay based on binding of radiolabeled human secretory component with applications in the study of IgA nephropathy, IgA monoclonal gammopathy and liver disease. *J. Immunol.*, 130:1176.

113. Ngan, J., and Kind, L. S. (1978): Suppressor T cells for IgE and IgG in Peyer's patches of mice made tolerant by the oral administration of ovalbumin. *J. Immunol.*, 120:861.

114. Ogra, P. L., and Dayton, D. H. (1979): *Immunology of the Breast Milk.* Raven Press, New York.

115. Ogra, P. L., Karzon, D. T., Righthand, F., and McGillivray, M. (1968): Immunoglobulin response in serum and secretions after immunization with live and inactivated poliovaccine and natural infection. *N. Engl. J. Med.*, 279:894.

116. Ohno, S., Matsunaga, T., and Wallace, R. B. (1982): Identification of the 48-base-long primordial

building block sequence of mouse immunoglobulin variable region genes. *Proc. Natl. Acad. Sci. U.S.A.*, 79:1999.

117. Orlans, E., Peppard, J., Fry, J. R., Hinton, R. H., and Mullock, B. M. (1979): Secretory component as the receptor for polymeric IgA on rat hepatocytes. *J. Exp. Med.*, 150:1577.

118. Orlans, E., Peppard, J. V., Payne, A. W. R., Fitzharris, B. M., Mullock, B. M., Hinton, R. H., and Hall, J. G. (1983): Comparative aspects of the hepatobiliary transport of IgA. In: *The Secretory Immune System, Vol. 409,* edited by J. R. McGhee and J. Mestecky, pp. 411–426. New York Academy of Sciences, New York.

119. Orlans, E., Peppard, J., and Reynolds, J. (1978): Rapid active transport of immunoglobulin A from blood to bile. *J. Exp. Med.*, 147:588.

120. Owen, R. L. (1977): Sequential uptake of horseradish peroxidase by lymphoid follicle epithelium of Peyer's patches in the normal unobstructed mouse intestine: An ultrastructural study. *Gastroenterology*, 72:440.

121. Owen, R. L., and Jones, A. L. (1974): Epithelial cell specialization within human Peyer's patches: An ultrastructural study of intestinal lymphoid follicles. *Gastroenterology*, 63:1160.

122. Palade, G. (1975): Intracellular aspects of the process of protein synthesis. *Science*, 189:347.

123. Pastan, I. H., and Willingham, M. C. (1981): Journey to the center of the cell: Role of the receptosomes. *Science*, 214:504.

124. Pearse, B. M. (1976): Clathrin: A unique protein associated with intracellular transfer of membrane by coated vesicles. *Proc. Natl. Acad. Sci. U.S.A.*, 73:1255.

125. Pearse, B. M. (1978): On the structural and functional components of coated vesicles. *J. Mol. Biol.*, 126:803.

126. Pierce, N. F., Cray, W. C., and Sacci, J. B. (1983): Oral immunization against experimental cholera: The role of antigen form and antigen combinations in evoking protection. In: *The Secretory Immune System, Vol. 409,* edited by J. R. McGhee and J. Mestecky, pp. 724–733. New York Academy of Sciences, New York.

127. Pierce-Cretel, A., Pamblanco, M., Strecker, G., Montreuil, J., Spik, G., Dorland, L., Van Halbeek, H., and Vliegenthart, J. F. G. (1982): Primary structure of the *N*-glycosidically linked sialoglycans of secretory immunoglobulins A from human milk. *Eur. J. Biochem.*, 125:383.

128. Pittard, W. B., Polmer, S. H., and Fanaroff, A. A. (1977): The breast milk macrophages: A potential vehicle for immunoglobulin transport. *J. Reticuloendothel. Soc.*, 22:597.

129. Plaut, A. G. (1983): The IgA$_1$ proteases of pathogenic bacteria. *Annu. Rev. Microbiol.*, 37:603.

130. Plaut, A. G., Gilbert, J. V., Artenstein, M. S.,and Capra, J. D. (1975): *Neisseria gonorrhoeae* and *Neisseria meningitidis*: Extracellular enzyme cleaves human immunoglobulin A. *Science*, 190:1103.

131. Porter, P., and Linggood, M. A. (1983): Novel mucosal anti-microbial functions interfering with the plasmid-mediated virulence determinants of adherence and drug resistance. In: *The Secretory Immune System, Vol. 409,* edited by J. R. McGhee and J. Mestecky, pp. 564–579. New York Academy of Sciences, New York.

132. Provost, T. T., and Tomasi, T. B. (1974): Evidence for the activation of complement via the alternate pathway in skin diseases. II. Dermatitis herpetiformis. *Clin. Immunol. Immunopathol.*, 3:178.

133. Purkayastha, S., Rao, C. V. N., and Lamm, M. E. (1979): Structure of the carbohydrate chain of free secretory component from human milk. *J. Biol. Chem.*, 254:6583.

134. Ramshaw, I. A., McKenzie, I. F., Bretscher, P. A., and Parish, C. R. (1977): Discrimination of suppressor T cells of humoral and cell-mediated immunity by anti-Ly and anti-Ia sera. *Cell. Immunol.*, 31:364.

135. Ranges, G. E., and Azar, M. M. (1979): Inheritance of tolerance susceptibility to human γ-globulin in congenic mice. *J. Immunol.*, 123:1151.

136. Reed, K. J., Van Epps, D. E., and Williams, R. C., Jr. (1979): Inhibition of human eosinophil chemotaxis by IgA paraproteins. *Inflammation*, 3:405.

137. Richardson, J., Bouchard, T., and Ferguson, C. C. (1976): Uptake and transport of exogenous proteins by respiratory epithelium. *Lab. Invest.*, 35:307.

138. Richman, L. K. (1979): Immunological unresponsiveness after enteric administration of protein antigens. In: *Immunology of Breast Milk*, edited by P. L. Ogra and D. H. Dayton, pp. 49–62. Raven Press, New York.

139. Richman, L. K., Chiller, J. M., and Brown, W. R. (1978): Enterically induced immunologic tolerance. I. Induction of suppressor T lymphocytes by intragastric administration of soluble proteins. *J. Immunol.*, 121:2429.

140. Richman, L. K., Graeff, A. S., and Strober, W. (1981): Antigen presentation by macrophage enriched cells from the mouse Peyer's patch. *Cell. Immunol.*, 62:110.
141. Richman, L. K., Graeff, A. S., Yarchoan, R., and Strober, W. (1981): Simultaneous induction of antigen-specific IgA helper T cells and IgG suppressor T cells in the murine Peyer's patch after protein feeding. *J. Immunol.*, 126:2079.
142. Rifai, A., and Mannik, M. (1983): Clearance kinetics and fate of mouse IgA immune complexes prepared with monomeric or dimeric IgA. *J. Immunol.*, 130:1826.
143. Rodewald, R. (1980): Distribution of immunoglobulin G receptors in the small intestine of the young rat. *J. Cell Biol.*, 85:18.
144. Rognum, T. O., Fausa, O., and Brandtzaeg, P. (1982): Immunohistochemical evaluation of carcinoembryonic antigen, secretory component, and epithelial IgA in tubular and villous large-bowel adenomas with different grades of dysplasia. *Scand. J. Gastroenterol.*, 17:561.
145. Roth, R. A., and Koshland, M. E. (1983): Identification of a lymphocyte enzyme that catalyzes pentamer immunoglobulin M assembly. *J. Biol. Chem.*, 256:4633.
146. Rothberg, R. M., Kraft, S. C., Farr, R. S., Kriebel, G. W., and Goldberg, S. S. (1971): Local immunologic responses to ingested protein. In: *The Secretory Immunologic System*, edited by P. A. Small, D. H. Dayton, R. M. Chanock, H. E. Kaufman, and T. B. Tomasi, pp. 293–307. U.S. Government Printing Office, Washington, D.C.
147. Rothman, J. E. (1981): The Golgi apparatus: Two organelles in tandem. *Science*, 213:1212.
148. Russell, M. W., Brown, T. A., Claflin, J. L., Schroer, K., and Mestecky, J. (1983): Immunoglobulin A-mediated hepatobiliary transport constitutes a natural pathway for disposing of bacterial antigens. *Infect. Immun.*, 42:1041.
149. Russell, M. W., Brown, T. A., Kulhavy, R., and Mestecky, J. (1983): IgA-mediated hepatobiliary clearance of bacterial antigens. In: *The Secretory Immune System, Vol. 409*, edited by J. R. McGhee and J. Mestecky, pp. 871–872. New York Academy of Sciences, New York.
150. Sancho, J., Egido, J., Sanchez-Crespo, M., and Blasco, R. (1981): Detection of monomeric and polymeric IgA containing immune complexes in serum and kidney from patients with alcoholic liver disease. *Clin. Exp. Immunol.*, 47:327.
151. Sheldrake, R. F., Husband, A. J., Watson, D. L., and Cripps, A. W. (1984): Selective transport of serum-derived IgA into mucosal secretions. *J. Immunol.*, 132:363.
152. Silverman, G. A., Peri, B. A., Fitch, F. W., and Rothberg, R. M. (1983): Enterically induced regulation of systemic immune responses. I. Lymphoproliferative responses in mice suppressed by ingested antigen. *J. Immunol.*, 131:2651.
153. Silverman, G. A., Peri, B. A., Fitch, F. W., and, Rothberg, R. M. (1983): Enterically induced regulation of systemic immune responses. II. Suppression of proliferating T cells by an Lyt-1$^+$,2$^-$ T effector cell. *J. Immunol.*, 131:2656.
154. Skogh, T. (1982): Tissue distribution of intravenously injected dinitrophenylated human serum albumin (DNP-HSA) preparations. Effects of specific IgG and IgA antibodies. *Scand. J. Immunol.*, 16:465.
155. Socken, D. J., Jeejeebhoy, K. N., Bazin, H., and Underdown, B. J. (1979): Identification of secretory component as an IgA receptor on rat hepatocytes. *J. Exp. Med.*, 150:1538.
156. Spalding, D. M., Koopman, W. J., and McGhee, J. R. (1983): Identification of a nonadherent accessory cell in murine Peyer's patches. In: *The Secretory Immune System, Vol. 409*, edited by J. R. McGhee and J. Mestecky, pp. 880–881. New York Academy of Sciences, New York.
157. Stafford, H. A., Knight, K. L., and Fanger, M. W. (1982): Receptors for IgA on rabbit lymphocytes. II. Characterization of their binding parameters for IgA. *J. Immunol.*, 128:2201.
158. Steinman, R. M., and Cohn, Z. A. (1973): Identity of novel cell type in peripheral lymphoid organs of mice. I. Morphology, quantitation and tissue distribution. *J. Exp. Med.*, 137:1142.
159. Stockert, R. J., Kressner, M. S., Collins, J. C., Sternlieb, I., and Morell, A. G. (1982): IgA interaction with asialoglycoprotein receptor. *Proc. Natl. Acad. Sci. U.S.A.*, 79:6229.
160. Sullivan, D. A., and Wira, C. R. (1983): Variations in free secretory component levels in mucosal secretions of the rat. *J. Immunol.*, 130:1330.
161. Svanborg, E., Freter, C. R., Hagbert, R., Hull, R., Hull, S., Leffler, H., and Schoolnik, G. (1982): Inhibition of experimental ascending urinary tract infection by receptor analogue. *Nature*, 298:560.
162. Sztul, E. S., Howell, K. E., and Palade, G. E. (1983): Intracellular and transcellular transport of secretory component and albumin in rat hepatocytes. *J. Cell Biol.*, 97:1582.
163. Tagliabue, A., Nencioni, L., Villa, L., Keren, D. F., Lowell, G. H., and Boraschi, D. (1983):

Antibody-dependent cell-mediated antibacterial activity of intestinal lymphocytes with secretory IgA. *Nature*, 306:184.

164. Tomasi, T. B. (1976): *The Immune System of Secretions*. Prentice-Hall, Englewood Cliffs, N.J.
165. Tomasi, T. B. (1980): Oral tolerance. *Transplantation*, 29:353.
166. Tomasi, T. B., Barr, W. G., Challacombe, S. J., and Curran, G. (1983): Oral tolerance and accessory-cell function of Peyer's patches. In: *The Secretory Immune System, Vol. 409*, edited by J. R. McGhee and J. Mestecky, pp. 145–163. New York Academy of Sciences, New York.
167. Tomasi, T. B., and Bienenstock, J. (1968): Secretory immunoglobulins. In: *Advances in Immunology, Vol. 9*, edited by F. J. Dixon, Jr., and H. G. Kunkel, pp. 2–96. Academic Press, New York.
168. Tomasi, T. B., and Czerwinski, D. S. (1976): Naturally occurring polymers of IgA lacking J chain. *Scand. J. Immunol.*, 5:647.
169. Tomasi, T. B., and Grey, H. M. (1972): Structure and function of immunoglobulin A. In: *Progress in Allergy, Vol. 16*, edited by P. Kallos, B. H. Waksman, and A. de Weck, pp. 81–213. S. Karger, New York.
170. Tomasi, T. B., Tan, E. M., Solomon, A., and Prendergast, R. A. (1965): Characteristics of an immune system common to certain external secretions. *J. Exp. Med.*, 121:101.
171. Trascasa, M. L., Egido, J., Sancho, J., and Hernando, L. (1980): IgA glomerulonephritis (Berger's disease): Evidence of high serum levels of polymeric IgA. *Clin. Exp. Immunol.*, 42:247.
172. Uchimaya, T., and Jacobs, D. M. (1978): Modulation of immune responses by bacterial lipopolysaccharide (LPS): Cellular basis of stimulatory and inhibitory effects of LPS on the *in vitro* IgM antibody response to a T-dependent antigen. *J. Immunol.*, 121:2347.
173. Unanue, E. R., Beller, D. I., Lu, C. Y., and Allen, P. M. (1984): Antigen presentation: Comments on its regulation and mechanism. *J. Immunol.*, 132:1.
174. Underdown, B. J., Derose, J., and Plaut, A. G. (1977): Disulfide bonding of secretory component to a single monomer subunit in human secretory IgA. *J. Immunol.*, 118:1816.
175. Underdown, B. J., Schiff, J. M., Nagy, B., and Fisher, M. M. (1983): Differences in processing of polymeric IgA and asialoglycoproteins by the rat liver. In: *The Secretory Immune System, Vol. 409*, edited by J. R. McGhee and J. Mestecky, pp. 402–410. New York Academy of Sciences, New York.
176. Van Epps, D. E., and Brown, S. L. (1981): Inhibition of formylmethionylleucyl-phenylalanine-stimulated neutrophil chemiluminescence by human immunoglobulin A paraproteins. *Infect. Immun.*, 34:864.
177. Van Epps, D. E., Reed, K., and Williams, R. C., Jr. (1978): Suppression of human PMN bacterial activity by human IgA paraproteins. *Cell. Immunol.*, 36:363.
178. Van Epps, D. E., and Williams, R. C. (1976): Suppression of leukocyte chemotaxis by human IgA myeloma components. *J. Exp. Med.*, 144:1227.
179. Van Voorhis, W. C., Witmer, M. D., and Steinman, R. M. (1983): The phenotype of dendritic cells and macrophages. *Fed. Proc.*, 42:3114.
180. Walker, W. A., and Bloch, K. J. (1983): Intestinal uptake of macromolecules: *In vitro* and *in vivo* studies. In: *The Secretory Immune System, Vol. 409*, edited by J. R. McGhee and J. Mestecky, pp. 593–601. New York Academy of Sciences, New York.
181. Walker, W. A., Wu, M., Isselbacher, K. J., and Bloch, K. J. (1975): Intestinal uptake of macromolecules. III. Studies on the mechanism by which immunization interferes with antigen uptake. *J. Immunol.*, 115:854.
182. Walter, P., and Blobel, G. (1983): Disassembly and reconstitution of signal recognition particle. *Cell*, 34:525.
183. Warshaw, A. L., Walker, W. A., Cornell, R., and Isselbacher, K. J. (1971): Small intestinal permeability to macromolecules: Transmission of horseradish peroxidase into mesentric lymph and portal blood. *Lab. Invest.*, 25:675.
184. Weaver, E. A., Tsuda, H., Goldblum, R. M., Goldman, A. S., and Davis, C. P. (1982): Relationship between phagocytosis and immunoglobulin A release from human colostral macrophages. *Infect. Immun.*, 38:1073.
185. Weicker, J., and Underdown, B. J. (1975): A study on the association of human secretory component with IgA and IgM proteins. *J. Immunol.*, 114:1337.
186. Weinheimer, P. F., Mestecky, J., and Acton, R. T. (1971): Species distribution of J chain. *J. Immunol.*, 107:1211.
187. Weisz-Carrington, P., Roux, M. E., McWilliams, M., Phillips-Quagliata, J. M., and Lamm, M. E.

(1978): Hormonal induction of the secretory immune system in the mammary gland. *Proc. Natl. Acad. Sci. U.S.A.*, 75:2928.

188. Wells, H. G. (1911): Studies on the chemistry of anaphylaxis. III. Experiments with isolated proteins, especially those of the hens egg. *J. Infect. Dis.*, 9:147.

189. Wilde, C. E., and Koshland, M. E. (1973): Molecular size and shape of the J chain from polymeric immunoglobulins. *Biochemistry*, 12:3218.

190. Winkelhake, J. L. (1978): Immunoglobulin structure and effector functions. *Immunochemistry*, 15:695.

191. Yagi, M., D'Eustachio, P., Ruddle, F. H., and Koshland, M. E. (1982): J chain is encoded by a single gene unlinked to other immunoglobulin structural genes. *J. Exp. Med.*, 155:647.

Advances in Host Defense Mechanisms, Vol. 4,
edited by J. I. Gallin and A. S. Fauci.
Raven Press, New York © 1985.

Host Defenses Against Adhesion of Bacteria to Mucosal Surfaces

Soman N. Abraham and Edwin H. Beachey

*Veterans Administration Medical Center, and Department of Medicine, University of
Tennessee Center for the Health Sciences, Memphis, Tennessee 38104*

The mucosal surfaces of the host provide an extensive substratum for adhesion of a wide variety of microorganisms. Soon after birth, the mucosal surfaces of the upper respiratory tract, the intestinal tract, and the lower genital tract become colonized by a variety of bacteria and other microorganisms contained in inspired air, ingested food, and fecal excretions, respectively. Most of these organisms become established as the indigenous microflora, the so-called normal flora. Other mucosal surfaces, such as the lower respiratory, biliary, and urinary tracts, are normally sterile in the healthy host. During states of good health, all of the mucosal surfaces contain remarkable barriers against attachment of invading bacterial pathogens. When these barriers break down, however, pathogenic bacteria can quickly gain a foothold and colonize large areas of the mucosal surfaces that are normally sterile or are occupied by the indigenous microflora. From these colonized sites, pathogenic bacteria produce infectious diseases either by invading into deeper tissues or excreting toxins that damage local and distant tissues.

The pathogenesis of bacterial infectious diseases arising from mucosal surfaces involves a number of distinct interactions between the host and the bacterial pathogen. Virulence factors of the bacteria enable the organisms to attach to and multiply on mucosal surfaces and to evade the defense mechanisms of the host, both at these surfaces and in deeper tissues into which the organisms may invade. To counter the virulence factors of the invading bacteria, the host has developed remarkable barriers, including chemical and mechanical modalities, as well as specific and nonspecific humoral and cellular elements.

In this chapter we shall review some of the mucosal defense mechanisms directed against bacterial adhesion, colonization, and invasion. Possible approaches to the prevention of bacterial infections at the earliest adherence and colonization steps of the infectious process will be discussed.

ADHERENCE OF BACTERIA TO MUCOSAL SURFACES

The infectious process is initiated when a successful bacterial pathogen first encounters the mucosal surfaces of the host. The result of the initial encounter

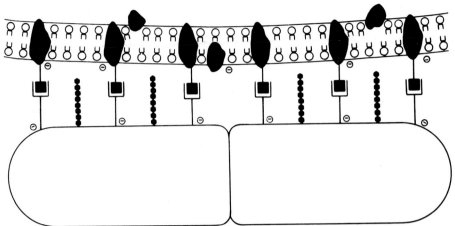

FIG. 1. Attachment of a bacterial cell *(bottom)* via specific adhesins *(branching vertical lines)* to complementary receptors *(black squares)* on the host-cell membrane *(top)*. To overcome the net negative charges *(circled minus signs)* on both the bacterial and host-cell surfaces, hydrophobic molecules *(hexagons)* on the surfaces of the bacteria are attracted toward the hydrophobic phospholipid molecules *(rows of circles)* in the lipid-bilayer membrane. The irregular black structures represent proteins or glycoproteins incorporated into the host-cell membrane. (From Beachey, ref. 7, with permission.)

depends on the ability of the organism to adhere to the mucosal surface; nonadherent bacteria are simply swept away in the fluids that constantly flow across the mucous membranes. Not only must the bacteria adhere, they also must be able to multiply at a rate sufficient to overcome the cleansing effect brought about by the desquamation of colonized epithelial cells. Once the pathogen has established stable colonies, invasive organisms penetrate into deeper tissues and set up local or systemic infectious disease. Certain bacteria (i.e., *Vibrio cholerae* or *Corynebacterium diphtheriae*) do not themselves invade, but rather elaborate toxins that penetrate the mucosal barrier and produce local and systemic tissue injury. In order to deliver these toxins in the most efficient manner, the organisms must be attached to the epithelial cells of the mucosae. In this way the excreted toxins evade destructive enzymes in the mucosal secretions and are delivered in concentrated form directly to toxin receptors on the epithelial cells.

The ability of bacteria to adhere to the mucosal epithelium is dependent on the expression of special adhesive structures called adhesins that bind the organisms in a lock-and-key fashion to complementary molecular structures (called receptors) on mucosal cells (7,8,53). Bacterial adhesion consists of a two-step process. In the first step the bacteria are nonspecifically and transiently adsorbed in a loose association with the mucosal cells. The loose association permits organisms that possess adhesins on their surfaces to bind to complementary receptors on the mucosal cells in a highly specific lock-and-key or induced-fit interaction (Fig. 1) (7,52). A number of specific molecules of recognition of bacterial (adhesins) and host-cell (receptors) origin have now been identified (Table 1).

TABLE 1. *Examples of adhesins and receptors mediating attachment of pathogenic bacteria to mucosal surfaces*

Microorganism	Adhesin	Receptor	Ref.
Escherichia coli	Type 1 fimbriae	D-Mannose	28,33
	p-fimbriae	α-D-Gal$p$-(1-4)-β-Gal$p$	55,61
	K88 fimbriae	β-D-Gal or Glc, Gal, and Fuc (GM$_1$ ganglioside)	36
	K99 fimbriae	GalNacβ(1-4)Galβ(1-4)GlcCer 2NeuAc (GM$_2$ ganglioside)	32,36
	CFA 1 fimbriae	GalNacβ(1-4)Galβ(1-4)GlcCer 2NeuAc (GM$_2$ ganglioside)	32,36
Pseudomonas aeruginosa	Fimbriae	Sialic acid residues	82
Vibrio cholerae	Fimbriae	Fucose	52,53
Neisseria meningitidis	Fimbriae	?	21,53
Neisseria gonorrhoeae	Fimbriae	Galβ(1-3)GalNacβ(1-4)Gal	21,53
Bordetella pertussis	Fimbriae	?	105
Staphylococcus aureus	Lipoteichoic acid	?Fibronectin	19
Streptococcus pyogenes	Lipoteichoic acid-M Protein complex (fibrillae)	Fibronectin	70,95
Streptococcus pneumoniae	?	Galβ(1-4)GlcNacβ(1-3)Lac	98,99
Streptococcus salivarius	Cell surface lectin	Galactose (on *A. viscosus*)	41
Streptococcus sanguis	Lipoteichoic acid	Sialic acid residues	65
Streptococcus mutans	Glucan-binding protein	Glucan	41
Actinomyces viscosus	Fimbriae	Galactose (on *S. sanguis*)	22,30,41
Actinomyces naeslundii	Fimbriae	Galactose (on *S. sanguis*)	23,30,41

Bacterial Adhesins

A variety of molecular structures serve to bind bacteria to host cells (7,8,53). Among the best described are the fimbriae of Gram-negative bacteria. These organelles consist of proteinaceous filaments radiating from the bacterial cell surfaces (28,79) (Fig. 2). Based on differing morphologies and binding specificities, several types of fimbriae have been distinguished among various species of *Enterobacteriaceae* and other pathogenic bacteria (Table 1) (79).

Type 1 fimbriae mediate the attachment of bacteria to D-mannose-containing receptors on eukaryotic cells (28). They consist of a single-subunit species arranged in a low-pitched, right-handed helix to form a hollow filament approximately 200 nm in length and 7 nm in diameter. Type 1 fimbriae are thought to bind to D-mannose residues on host cells, because of all the sugars tested, only D-mannose and its derivatives inhibit adhesion of these organelles to eukaryotic cells (33,70). Evidence that type 1 fimbriae are involved in adhesion is based on the observation that type 1 fimbriated organisms are adhesive, whereas their nonfimbriated counterparts usually are not (28,70). Moreover, isolated type 1 fimbriae inhibit the

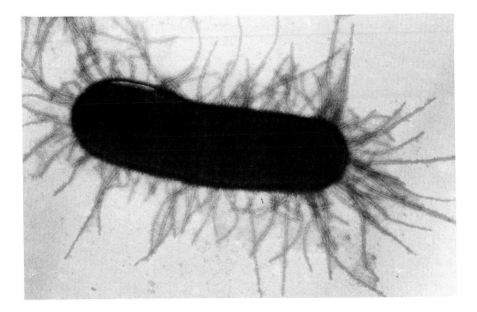

FIG. 2. Electron micrograph of type 1 fimbriated *E. coli*. Note the fairly rigid fimbriae radiating uniformly from the surface of the bacterium.

adhesion of type 1 fimbriated bacteria, and they exhibit the same adhesive characteristics as type 1 fimbriated organisms (28,70).

Although most bacteria appear to contain only one adhesin, some bacteria may simultaneously express two or more adhesins with distinct binding specificities. The ability to produce more than one distinct adhesin increases the range of specific receptors and host cells to which the organisms can attach. Examples of bacteria expressing more than one adhesin can be found among the uropathogenic *Escherichia coli*; over 70% of such bacterial isolates express both type 1 fimbriae and p-fimbriae (75,97,101). As opposed to the type 1 fimbriae that are recognized by D-mannose residues of glycoproteins, the p-fimbriae are recognized by α-D-Gal$p$-(1-4)-β-Gal$p$ residues on glycolipid molecules of host cells (54,55,61). The phenotypic expression of both types of fimbriae appears to be regulated by an on–off switch at the DNA transcriptional level resulting in shifts from nonfimbriate to fimbriate phases (or vice versa) (29,84). In *E. coli*, the switch frequency for the production of type 1 fimbriae is very high (1 per 1,000 bacteria per generation). Thus, at any given time during growth, bacterial populations contain both fimbriated and nonfimbriated organisms (29). The ability to undergo such rapid phenotypic variation may be one of the most important determinants of the virulence of bacteria that attack the host through mucosal surfaces. Whereas the adhesive organisms serve to maintain infections on mucosal surfaces where attachment is vital, nonadhesive organisms serve to disperse the pathogen to distant sites. Moreover, the presence of certain adhesins may be detrimental to bacteria that

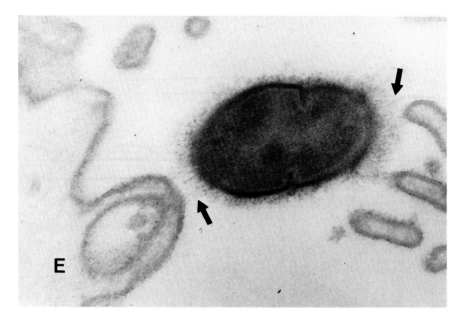

FIG. 3. Electron micrograph of ultrathin section of group A streptococcal cell *(center)* adherent to villi of pharyngeal epithelial cell (E). The surface fibrillar network composed of protein–lipoteichoic acid complexes appears to mediate the attachment of organisms to the epithelial cell membrane. (From Beachey and Ofek: *J. Exp. Med.*, 143:759–771, 1976, with permission.)

invade into deeper tissues. On encountering professional phagocytes containing receptors for their adhesins, the bacteria can be recognized, ingested, and destroyed (97).

Unlike Gram-negative bacteria, many Gram-positive organisms employ a complex of surface structures as adhesins (21). Perhaps the best-described complex adhesins are the fibrillae on the surfaces of *Streptococcus pyogenes* cells (70,72) (Fig. 3). These fibrillae are thought to consist of an ionic complex of lipoteichoic acid (LTA) and M protein or other LTA-binding protein (70). Streptococcal LTA is composed of a highly charged polymer of polyglycerol phosphate substituted to varying degrees with alanine residues, and capped at one end with a lipid moiety (glycerophosphoryl-diglucosyl/diglyceride). The lipid moiety imparts the adhesive properties to LTA (24,72). The LTA molecule is stabilized on the surface of the streptococcus by forming ionic complexes with clusters of positive charges on surface proteins such as the M protein (70). Recently, several investigators have described LTA as an adhesin also for *Staphylococcus aureus* and *Streptococcus sanguis* (19,47).

These are but a few examples of the bacterial adhesins that have been described to date. More detailed reviews are available (8,21).

Host-Cell Receptors

The presence on host mucosal surfaces of receptors that interact in a complementary manner with specific bacterial adhesins is an important determinant of stable bacterial adherence. If the receptors on the mucosal cells are present at low density, are inaccessible, or are not expressed at all, binding of bacteria and subsequent colonization cannot take place.

The receptivity of epithelial cells for various bacterial adhesins has been associated, for the most part, with carbohydrate residues (Table 1). Most of the receptors described thus far have been identified by employing techniques of inhibition of bacterial adhesion (28,33,52). In this way, many simple sugars have been demonstrated to block bacterial attachment in a highly specific manner. The conclusion from such studies has been that the inhibitory sugars are represented in the cell surface receptor structures presumed to be composed of glycoproteins or glycolipids (21,52). The precise orientation of the sugar moieties in the receptor structure and the presence of neighboring submolecular structures determine the binding affinities and specificity of the receptor for its complementary adhesins (33).

Differences in the specificity and in the distribution of receptors account for tissue tropisms wherein different bacterial species attach selectively to one tissue niche in preference to another. For example, *E. coli* bacteria are the most common cause of urinary tract infections and are seldom found in the upper respiratory tract. Conversely, *S. pyogenes* organisms are the most common cause of bacterial pharyngitis and are seldom found in the urinary tract. The binding of *E. coli* to the uroepithelium has been related to the presence of mannose residues and glycolipid receptors, respectively, for the binding of type 1 and p-fimbriated *E. coli* to uroepithelial cells (26,55,61,70). Similarly, the binding of *S. pyogenes* to the upper respiratory tract has been associated with the presence of fibronectin on the surfaces of upper respiratory epithelial cells (2,95,109,110). Interestingly, fibronectin appears to serve as a receptor on oral epithelial cells for *S. pyogenes*, but appears to hinder the adhesion of *Pseudomonas aeruginosa* and *E. coli* (2,109,110). The mechanism by which fibronectin hinders adherence of the latter organisms remains unclear. It can be speculated, however, that while providing receptors for the attachment of streptococci, fibronectin masks the receptors for these Gram-negative bacteria (2,109).

The presence of specific receptors on the cells of a host appears to be genetically determined. For example, Sellwood et al. (93) have shown that the intestinal epithelial cells of pigs that are highly resistant to diarrheagenic K88 fimbriated *E. coli* lack complementary receptors, whereas those from susceptible pigs are rich in K88 receptors. Cross-breeding of resistant and susceptible pigs has demonstrated that susceptibility is coded by autosomal-dominant genes (93).

Equally intriguing observations have been made in humans. The presence of specific glycolipid receptors on the membranes of human uroepithelium that recognize the p-fimbriae of uropathogenic *E. coli* appears to be genetically determined (54,55). Recent studies have shown that the quantity of these glycolipid receptors varies from person to person, and the relative susceptibility to pyelonephritogenic *E. coli* is related to the relative density of these structures on the host-tissue cells (54,55,98).

Developmental changes also may have an important bearing on the bacterial receptivity of a particular host cell. For example, Ofek et al. (71) demonstrated that oral epithelial cells of newborn infants were poor binders of streptococci (71). Within 3 days, however, the epithelial cells rapidly gained the capacity to bind adult levels of streptococci.

In addition to naturally occurring receptors for bacteria, new receptors that recognize different species have been observed as cells infected with certain viruses (89,90). Thus, a previously resistant host may be rendered susceptible to the adherence of pathogenic bacteria during certain viral infections. These intriguing findings have important implications with regard to the association of secondary bacterial infections following viral infections, the classic example being influenza infections followed by bacterial pneumonias.

In summary, bacteria possess specific adhesive structures that are recognized to varying degrees by mucosal surfaces, depending on the relative receptivity displayed by that surface for the adhesins of a particular bacterial species. The expression, density, accessibility, and specificity of the respective host and bacterial adhesive structures are important determinants of host and bacterial survival during a bacterial infection. It must be remembered, however, that in states of good health of the immune host, the final adhesin–receptor interaction is subject to obstruction or interruption by a number of nonspecific and specific forces prevailing in the mucosal milieu. These forces constitute the host's defenses against bacterial adherence.

NONSPECIFIC DEFENSES AGAINST BACTERIAL ADHERENCE

An almost impenetrable array of specific and nonspecific defenses is erected against the initial encounter between the bacterial pathogen and the mucosal surfaces. Among the nonspecific defenses are the cleansing mechanisms of the fluid flow of the secretions and luminal contents, the desquamation of heavily colonized mucosal cells, the barrier functions of luminal mucus, and the antagonistic actions of the commensal microbial flora of the mucosa (40,66,73,98). The specific defenses include the presence of inhibitory elements in the mucosal milieu that prevent the interaction of bacterial adhesins with complementary host-cell receptors. Some of these inhibitory compounds are of nonimmune origin and include food lectins that compete with bacterial adhesins for binding to specific sugar receptors on host cells (34,38,39). In addition, mucus secretions contain soluble compounds that bind, in a competitive way, to bacterial adhesins (37). Bacteria that bind to such soluble receptor analogues are unable to bind to the epithelial cells and thus are easily cleared (37,74). Predominant among the specific immune defenses is secretory IgA (sIgA) in mucosal secretions. Adhesin-specific sIgA prevents bacterial adherence by blocking the recognition of the adhesin by host-cell receptors (44,66).

Hydrokinetic Defense Factors

The flushing action of mucosal secretions and luminal contents mechanically dislodges and eliminates loosely adherent microorganisms from mucosal surfaces.

The potency of this mechanism of bacterial elimination is perhaps most evident in the urinary tract, where the forceful flow of urine creates an environment unfavorable for bacterial colonization and, under normal circumstances, keeps the urinary tract sterile (43,73). Gregory et al. (43) observed that large numbers of bacteria introduced into the bladders of dogs were rapidly eliminated from the urinary tract by the flow of urine. Even when bacteria were continuously instilled into the bladder over a period of 2 to 3 months, the hydrokinetic forces of the urinary tract helped prevent bacterial colonization (43).

All mucosal surfaces are exposed to the hydrokinetic forces of fluid flow (40). In the gastrointestinal tract, the fluid flow is aided by the rhythmic peristaltic movements of the tract. Loosely attached bacteria are constantly dislodged and eliminated from the mucosa (67). The mucus flow and the ciliary action of columnar epithelial cells play important roles in eliminating microorganisms from the respiratory tract (67). Microorganisms reaching the lower respiratory tract are entrapped in the mucus and are borne upward by ciliary action from the lungs through the trachea to the back of the throat. The mucus, with the entrapped organisms, is then eliminated from the respiratory tract by the combination of coughing and swallowing (67). The importance of the mucociliary "escalator" becomes most evident when it becomes impaired; the greater vulnerability of cigarette smokers and alcoholics to respiratory bacterial infections is well recognized. Cigarette smoke and ethanol impair the function of the mucociliary escalator (67). Certain microorganisms cause infection in the respiratory tract by adhering to and directly suppressing ciliary action (67). *Bordetella pertussis* organisms appear to attach exclusively to the cilia on respiratory epithelial cells (105). The ability to adhere to ciliary tufts undoubtedly contributes to the unique ability of these organisms to resist removal by the mucociliary clearance mechanisms.

Desquamation

It has been observed that epithelial cells that become heavily colonized by bacteria desquamate either singly or in sheets, and the rate of desquamation is directly proportional to the microbial burden on the mucosal epithelium (40). Desquamation of epithelial cells, with adherent bacteria, is apparently a defensive mechanism against tissue invasion of microorganisms. Desquamation, together with the hydrokinetic forces, renders the mucosal surfaces highly resistant to colonization by nonadherent or slow-growing pathogens. The desquamation of mucosal cells, however, favors survival of the most adhesive populations of colonizers, which are able to continuously reattach to the newly exposed epithelial surfaces. The cyclic nature of this process creates a strong selective pressure that tends to magnify the differences in the adhesive capabilities of various strains and species of bacteria. Thus, the most adhesive organisms establish stable colonies, whereas the less adhesive strains give rise to transient populations, and the nonadhesive organisms fail to gain any foothold at all (40,91).

Microbial Interference

The indigenous microflora inhabiting a given site on the mucosa often interfere with colonization by other microorganisms of the same or different species. Several mechanisms are thought to be involved. These include production of antibacterial factors, nutritional competition, and selective physicochemical alterations of the local environments (91). Microbial interference could also be the result of competition among bacteria for specific attachment sites on the mucosa, or it may be related to stearic hindrance by the initial colonizer (9,91).

Bibel et al. (10) recently examined the binding of a number of strains of *S. aureus*, *Corynebacterium*, and *P. aeruginosa* to nasal mucosal cells. A series of parallel adherence experiments was carried out whereby bacterial strains were incubated alone, in simultaneous mixtures, and in succession with epithelial cells (10). Interestingly, the sequence in which different bacteria were presented to the epithelial cells strongly influenced which bacteria adhered to the epithelial cells; irrespective of which strains or species of bacteria were first exposed to the buccal cells, the adherence of the initially added bacteria interfered with binding of any subsequently added bacteria. Although secondary adherence was substantially reduced, it was not completely eliminated. In certain instances, a secondary strain displaying higher binding activity was able to displace the adherent primary strains to a limited degree (10). These *in vitro* studies lend credence to the idea that nonpathogenic bacterial colonizers hinder secondary colonization by potentially pathogenic microorganisms *in vivo* (9,98).

Although primary colonization may prevent potential pathogens from attaching to the mucosal cell surfaces, the primary colonizers may themselves serve as substrates for the attachment of selected bacterial species. Thus, certain primary colonizers may actually foster rather than hinder secondary colonization. There are several examples of the same or different species of bacteria binding to each other (22,28,53). Intraspecies attachment has been observed in *Bacteroides*, which appear to bind to each other by a fibrous material (108). Type 1 fimbriae of *E. coli* have been demonstrated to mediate interbacterial attachment when grown in broth (28). A good example of interspecies attachment is seen in the interaction of *S. sanguis* or *S. mitis* with the oral pathogens *Actinomyces viscosus* and *Actinomyces naeslundii*, respectively (22,30). Studies of oral ecology have shown that the first colonizers of the freshly cleaned tooth surface are the oral streptococci, including *S. sanguis* and *S. mitis* (30,41). The *Actinomyces* that arrive as secondary colonizers may bind to buccal epithelium and other available sites on oral tissues. In addition, however, these organisms may also bind to the streptococci already adherent (22,30,41). The ability of *Actinomyces* to bind to streptococci obviously increases the number of surface habitats available to the organism and is an important determinant of its success as a colonizer of the oral cavity.

Mucus as a Physical Barrier

Mucus is a viscous fluid that is produced and secreted by goblet cells and mucus glands present in various locations on mucosal surfaces (37). The mucus forms a protective, waterproof coat over the entire mucosal surface. In addition to lubricating the mucosal surface, the mucus protects the underlying cells from sudden changes in osmotic pressure (37,66). In addition, the mucus coat physically covers the glycoprotein and glycolipid receptors for several bacterial adhesins and toxins and thereby prevents adhesion of the respective bacteria (37). Parsons et al. (76) demonstrated the importance of mucus in reducing bacterial attachment to mucosal cells in the urinary tract. Removal of the mucus coat on the surface of bladder epithelial cells by mild acid treatment markedly increased the ability of the bladder cells to bind cells of *E. coli* (76). Recoating the acid-treated and mucus-free cells with heparin or a synthetic glycosaminoglycan (sodium pantosan polysulfate) restored the barrier against bacterial attachment to a level similar to that originally formed by the bladder mucus (76–78).

A number of pathogens, such as *V. cholerae*, possess virulence determinants that facilitate their penetration through the mucus coat to the surface of the underlying epithelial cells (35,52). Flagellated vibrios swim through cleavage planes in the mucus coat, whereas nonmotile vibrios are unable to penetrate this barrier and therefore lack virulence (35,52,53). Several pathogens possess enzymes that degrade mucus; a variety of oral and intestinal microorganisms elaborate neuraminidase, which cleaves sialic acid residues, whereas others produce glycosidases, which attack the oligosaccharide residues of mucus (37,50). Degeneration of the mucus coat enables bacteria to reach the mucosal epithelium, and the products of mucus degradation provide nutrients that further facilitate bacterial colonization. Thus, although the mucus clearly provides an important natural barrier, it alone is not sufficient to prevent the adherence of certain bacteria that have developed appropriate means to penetrate the barrier.

SPECIFIC NONIMMUNE DEFENSES AGAINST BACTERIAL ADHERENCE

Exogenous Lectins

Lectins, which are carbohydrate-binding proteins, are present in the diet and may inhibit adhesion of bacteria to mucosal surfaces of the gastrointestinal tract by competing with bacteria for receptors (34). Jones reported that a variety of lectins with specificities for different sugar compounds inhibited adhesion of *E. coli* to epithelial cell brush-border membranes (52). This inhibition was attributed to stearic hindrance, because the same degree of inhibition was observed with different lectins. Brady et al. (12) demonstrated that wheat germ agglutinin, a lectin specific for *N*-acetylglucosamine, could be detected in the feces of human subjects consuming a diet containing this lectin. They speculated that ingestion of such plant lectins, which have the potential to interact with a wide variety of cell membranes, may alter mucosal cell surfaces or bacterial cell functions in the gastrointestinal tract. Gibbons and Dankers observed lectinlike activities in several commonly ingested fruits, vegetables, and seeds. Pretreatment of saliva-coated artificial tooth pellicles with some of these extracts markedly reduced subsequent adsorption of *S. mutans* and *S. sanguis* (38,39). Dietary lectins, such as wheat germ agglutinin and peanut agglutinin, remained associated with oral tissues for long periods after consumption of small quantities of raw wheat germ or raw peanuts and influenced association of microorganisms with oral tissue (38,39).

Analogues of Host-Cell Receptors

The mucosal surfaces are constantly bathed in mucus and other secretions that are rich in glycoproteins and glycolipids that are analogous to mucosal cell receptors for bacterial adhesins (37,44). These soluble receptor analogues provide an alternate binding site for bacterial attachment, resulting in reduced bacterial association with mucosal epithelial cells. The binding of bacteria to soluble receptors in mucosal secretions often results in aggregation of bacteria and facilitates their early removal by the prevailing hydrokinetic forces (37,44,45). The protective impact of some of these mucosal components in preventing bacterial attachment to mucosal cells and concomitantly inducing bacterial aggregation is becoming increasingly apparent (41,74). Rosan et al. (86,87) compared the bacterial aggregating capability of saliva obtained from individuals highly susceptible to dental caries with saliva from caries-resistant individuals; they found that the capacity of saliva from the latter group to agglutinate *S. mutans* was much higher than that of saliva from the former group.

Several receptor analogues have been isolated from mucosal secretions and biochemically characterized (41,46,107). Some have been found to consist of blood-group-reactive glycoproteins with the capacity to block binding of oral streptococci to buccal epithelial cells (37,41,46). One such blood-group-reactive compound, a high-molecular-weight sulfated glycoprotein, aggregates *S. sanguis* but not *S. mutans*; the glycoprotein appears to bind specifically to the lipoteichoic acid adhesin of *S. sanguis* (46,47) The receptive moiety on the glycoprotein has not yet been identified, although McBride and Gisslow (65) have reported that sialic acid serves as a receptor for attachment and aggregation of *S. sanguis* in saliva (65). Sialic acid residues also have been implicated as receptors for the adhesins of mucoid and nonmucoid *P. aeruginosa* (82). This deduction was based on the observation that the binding of *P. aeruginosa* to tracheal epithelium was inhibitable by rat tracheal and bovine submaxillary mucin (82). In an attempt to identify the active inhibitor in these mucins, Ramphal and Pyle examined the inhibitory effects of several simple sugars known to be present in mucin (82). Only *N*-acetylneuraminic acid inhibited the reaction, suggesting that sialic acid residues in mucin as well as in tracheal epithelial cells served as receptors for attachment of these pathogens (82).

Tamm-Horsfall protein is a glycoprotein present in urinary mucin that has a high affinity for type 1 fimbriae of *E. coli* (74,98). Orskov et al. (74) have discovered that type 1 fimbriae of *E. coli* bind specifically to and are agglutinated by the mannose residues of Tamm-Horsfall protein. By this mechanism, type 1 fimbriated *E. coli* may well become entrapped in urinary mucin and thereby be rapidly eliminated in the urine flow. Alternatively, the entrapped *E. coli* may serve as a reservoir of bacteria capable of repopulating uroepithelial cells as they are exposed during desquamation of old cells.

The concept that some of these soluble bacterial receptors in mucus secretions foster rather than hinder bacterial colonization is further strengthened by experimental studies of oral bacteria. Several salivary components adsorb to teeth surfaces to form a pellicle, which in turn serves as receptor site for the attachment of various oral species of bacteria (41). Several such receptor compounds that promote bacterial colonization have been described in the oral cavity (37,41). Because of their strong negative charge, salivary mucins adsorb avidly to teeth and are common constituents of the tooth pellicle (37,41). Hydrolysates of pellicles have a high content of acidic amino acids, suggesting that acidic proteins and peptides are selectively involved in pellicle formation (41). Contrary to previous observations (40,41), Rosan et al. (87) recently demonstrated that the salivary components mediating the adherence of bacteria to tooth pellicles were distinct from components involved in bacterial aggregation. Adsorption of salivary aggregating constituents by bacteria appears to have little effect on the ability of the residual saliva to promote adherence; conversely, adsorption of salivary adherence factors to artificial tooth surfaces does not affect the aggregating properties of residual saliva (87). Thus, the balance in the relative concentration of salivary aggregating factors and pellicle-forming components might be critical modulating factors in determining the susceptibility of the host to bacterial colonization. Indeed, it has been observed that the ratio of salivary aggregating factors to pellicle-forming components in caries-resistant individuals is higher than in caries-susceptible individuals (86).

One glycoprotein that may also play an important modulatory role in determining colonization of mucosal surfaces of the oral cavity is fibronectin. This large glycoprotein isolated from human plasma has been demonstrated to bind to *S. aureus* and to several species of streptococci (21). Furthermore, immobilized fibronectin molecules on the surfaces of buccal epithelial cells serve as receptors for attachment of group A streptococci, while hampering adhesion of Gram-negative bacteria (2,97,109,110). Fibronectin is able to aggregate several species of cariogenic streptococci, and when adsorbed to artifical tooth pellicles, it enhances the attachment of these organisms (6). Because fibronectin is found in soluble form in the saliva (6,96), this glycoprotein may play an important modulatory role in the bacterial ecology of the oral cavity.

Human milk is apparently replete with receptor analogues that are in part responsible for its bacterial antiadhesive properties (44,98). Holmgren et al. (49) showed that agglutination of erythrocytes by *E. coli* and *V. cholerae* was inhibited by milk. Moreover, the antiadhesive activity was found to be associated with a fraction of milk other than the immunoglobulins. Milk similarly inhibited adhesion of *S. pneumoniae* to human epithelial cells (98). Because the milk from an IgA-deficient mother displayed equal inhibitory activities, it was concluded that the activity resided in a fraction other than sIgA (44). Svanborg-Eden et al. (98) have reported the presence in human milk of certain oligosaccharides that act as analogues of the neolacto-series glycolipids, which are thought to serve as the receptors on pharyngeal cells for the binding of *S. pneumoniae*. The presence of these antiadhesive receptor analogues in human milk may account for the clinical observation that otitis media caused by *S. penumoniae* occurs at a lower frequency in breast-fed infants than in formula-fed infants (20,25,44).

SPECIFIC IMMUNE DEFENSES AGAINST BACTERIAL ADHERENCE

Role of sIgA

In addition to the nonimmune antiadhesive defenses, specific immunological mechanisms contribute extensively to the host's defense against bacterial adhesion. Specific antibodies secreted into the mucosa block the colonization of several pathogens. The immunoglobulin that predominates in the mucosal secretions falls in the IgA class. Consequently, the effect of these antibodies on bacterial adherence has been the subject of considerable interest (44,45,66). One of the earliest demonstrations that sIgA is antiadhesive for certain bacteria was reported by Williams and Gibbons (106). Because sIgA lacked bactericidal, complement-dependent bacterial lysis, and opsonic effects, these workers examined the effect of sIgA on the adherence of bacteria to mucosal epithelial cells (106). They found that only those strains that were agglutinated by the antibody could be inhibited by the sIgA from adhering to epithelial cells. These observations have now been confirmed by others (13,40,56,64).

Secretory IgA in the gastrointestinal tract appears to prevent attachment of *V. cholerae* organisms and their enterotoxin molecules to the mucosa of the gastrointestinal tract and thereby to protect experimental animals and humans from infection (48). Increased secretions of antiadhesive antibodies have been observed in mucosal secretions during *Neisseria gonorrhoeae* infections (104). Genital secretions collected from several patients infected with *N. gonorrhoeae* were able to inhibit attachment of the infecting strain to epithelial cells (103). The antigenic specificity of the immunoglobulins present in these secretions was determined to be directed at the adhesins of the pathogen (104). High levels of antibody in urine and serum were detected in patients with pyelonephritis (83,99). These antibodies reacted specifically with the fimbriae of *E. coli* and blocked *in vitro* attachment of the patient's own strain of *E. coli* to human epithelial cells (99).

Local production of sIgA antibodies occurs when immunocompetent cells on the mucosal surface are stimulated by the bacterial adhesins (66). The degree of the immune response depends on the degree of tissue contact by the microorganism. Specific immunologic responses are evoked only after extensive tissue contact, followed by some degree of invasion (48). Paradoxically, the adhesive properties of the bacteria apparently foster an effective immune response by the host. Most of the IgA secreted onto mucosal surfaces is produced locally by plasma cells that lie just beneath the mucosa (45,48,66). In some cases, IgA antibodies may originate from serum. For example, IgA has been demonstrated to be transported from serum via hepatocytes into bile in rats (62).

An important source of sIgA in the gastrointestinal tract of suckling infants is maternal colostrum and milk (44). Human colostrum contains 60 times more sIgA than normal unstimulated whole saliva (13). By comparing IgA levels in the saliva of adults and infants, Hanson et al. (44) deduced that infants are slow in the development of IgA immune responses. Hence, IgA antibodies in the mother's milk may be important in protecting the infant against various gastrointestinal as well as upper respiratory tract infections. This notion is supported by the observation that breast-fed infants have less gastrointestinal and upper respiratory tract infections than non-breast-fed infants (20,25). Human milk is replete with antibodies with specificities against a variety of microorganisms and virulence factors (44). Antibodies directed against several adhesive fimbriae of pathogenic *E. coli* have been found in human milk (44,98). The protective effect of maternal antifimbrial IgA and IgG antibodies in conferring immunity to suckling neonates was first demonstrated in farm animals (88). When purified fimbrial vaccines were administered at various doses and routes to pregnant farm animals, the vaccinated mothers developed high antifimbrial antibody levels in the colostrum that imparted protection against enteropathogenic *E. coli* infections to their suckling offspring (51,88).

IgA Proteases and Their Inhibitors

A number of pathogens counter the action of IgA antibodies on mucosal surfaces by elaborating extracellular enzymes that specifically cleave and inactivate the IgA antibody molecules (66). These proteases are specific for the IgA_1 subclass and cleave the immunoglobulin at an internal prolyl-threonyl or prolyl-seryl peptide bond in the heavy chain to yield intact Fab and Fc fragments (57). Human antibodies of the IgA_2 subclass are resistant to cleavage, because the primary structure of the heavy chain has a characteristic deletion in the hinge region of 13 amino acids including the protease-susceptible peptide bonds (57). These IgA_1-subclass-specific proteases are elaborated by pathogenic microorganisms such as *S. sanguis, S. pneumoniae, H. influenzae, Neisseria meningitidis,* and *N. gonorrhoeae* (57,69). In contrast to the pathogenic *Neisseria*, other nonpathogenic species of *Neisseria* that colonize mucosal surfaces do not appear to produce these enzymes (57,66). This observation suggests that the expression of IgA proteases is probably an important virulence mechanism that enables pathogenic bacteria to neutralize host immune responses.

An intriguing and complicating aspect of the IgA–parasite interaction has recently come to light. Apparently, in order to counter the activity of IgA proteases, the host develops specific protease-neutralizing antibodies; the neutralizing antibodies are themselves apparently resistant to the hydrolytic cleavage by the proteases (42). These IgA-protease-neutralizing antibodies are of the IgA and IgG class and have been found in human colostrum and serum (42). When IgA proteases obtained from *N. gonorrhoeae, N. meningitidis,* and *S. sanguis* are exposed to human colostral IgA, their functional activities are neutralized. The amount of IgA-protease-specific antibodies in the colostrum varies considerably from individual to individual (42).

In general, higher serum levels of anti-IgA-protease antibodies are detected in patients recovering from infections caused by IgA-protease-producing pathogens such as *N. gonorrhoeae* than in noninfected individuals (42). The mechanism by which the antibodies neutralize the IgA protease activity remains to be clarified. Preliminary studies suggest a specific antibody–antigen reaction, the activity of the inhibiting IgA antibody residing in the Fab region of the antibody molecule (42).

Antibodies Directed Against the Mucosal Receptors

Because active receptor analogues for several bacterial adhesins are composed of simple sugars, antibodies directed against these sugars potentially may block the binding of bacteria to host-cell receptors. The presence of antibodies directed at simple sugars has been reported in human serum (11,60). Gartner recently isolated antibodies from human serum that are directed specifically against glucose, galactose, and mannose residues (T. K. Gartner, *personal communication*). Most of these antibodies belong to the IgG class. It remains to be determined if such sugar-specific antibodies are present in mucosal secretions. It is quite conceivable that such antibodies, if present, may interfere with bacterial adherence to mucosal surfaces by binding to the receptors. Preliminary studies in our laboratory (S. N. Abraham and E. H. Beachey, *unpublished observation*) suggest that the mannose-specific, but not the galactose-specific, human IgG antibodies inhibit binding of type 1 fimbriated *E. coli* to buccal epithelial cells. That such mannose-receptor-specific antibodies might be protective *in vivo* was recently demonstrated in our laboratory, where mice passively immunized with a D-mannose-specific monoclonal antibody were protected against pyelonephritis when challenged with a pathogenic type 1 fimbriated *E. coli*. In contrast, mice immunized with monoclonal antibodies directed specifically against *N*-acetylgalactosamine residues were not protected (1).

PREVENTION OF BACTERIAL ADHERENCE

Antiadhesive Vaccines

With the recognition of adherence as a prerequisite for bacterial infection, interest has centered around finding an effective way to prevent bacterial adhesion on mucosal surfaces. Several laboratories have examined the use of different adhesins as vaccines, with the idea that antibodies that are evoked in the host would not only prevent attachment of bacteria at the mucosal surface but also enhance phagocytosis once tissue invasion has occurred (15–17,68).

One of the earliest fimbrial vaccines to be tested was the K88 antigen isolated from *E. coli* causing diarrhea in young pigs (88). Immunization was undertaken by inoculating purified fimbrial preparations into the posterior mammary glands of gilts approximately 11 weeks before parturition, followed by a subcutaneous booster dose 10 days before parturition. The piglets of vaccinated and unvaccinated control sows were orally inoculated with K88-positive *E. coli* at birth before suckling. Although all piglets demonstrated clinical symptoms of infection, piglets from vaccinated gilts had markedly less severe symptoms, and their mortality after 72 hr was significantly lower than that of the control piglets (88). Only 4 of 31 vaccinated piglets died, whereas 20 of 29 of the nonvaccinated controls succumbed to infection. No differences were detected in the bacteriostatic and bactericidal activities in the serum and mammary secretions of vaccinated and unvaccinated gilts. Nevertheless, anti-K88 antibodies were detected in the serum, colostrum, and milk of vaccinated gilts, but not in the unvaccinated gilts. The K88-specific antibodies were found to block adhesion of the related *E. coli* to epithelial cells. The logical conclusion was that the ingestion of K88-specific antibodies in maternal colostrum and milk protected the suckling piglets by preventing adhesion and colonization (88). Similar trials were conducted with purified K99 fimbriae of *E. coli*, which causes diarrhea in lambs and calves. In each case, vaccination of the mothers resulted in protection of the suckling offspring (51,68).

Protection against *E. coli*-induced ascending pyelonephritis in rats using purified type 1 fimbriae as vaccine was demonstrated by Silverblatt et al. (94). Only 3 of 16 rats immunized intramuscularly with purified type 1 fimbriae showed kidney infections after intravesicular challenge with type 1 fimbriated *E. coli*. In contrast, 10 of 15 nonimmunized rats showed such infections. Furthermore, the numbers of colonizing bacteria in the infected kidneys of immunized animals were significantly lower than in the kidneys of unvaccinated controls. Vaccination with purified p-fimbriae protected monkeys against experimental *E. coli*-induced pyelonephritis, and this protection was correlated with the presence of p-fimbriae-specific antibodies in the urine of vaccinated monkeys (85). In our laboratories we recently showed that a monoclonal antibody directed against a quaternary structural epitope of type 1 fimbriae prevented the attachment of type 1 fimbriated *E. coli* to eukaryotic cells (3). Passive adminstration of the antibody to mice protected them against ascending pyelonephritis induced by type 1 fimbriated *E. coli* instilled into their bladders (1).

The promising results obtained from these animal studies have encouraged vaccine trials in humans (15–17,63,68). Purified gonococcal fimbriae were employed to vaccinate humans against *N. gonorrhoeae* infections. The vaccine evoked high levels of antifimbrial antibodies that enhanced the phagocytosis of the homologous infecting strain (15–17). In most cases, protection was acquired against only the homologous strains, with little or no protection against heterologous strains possessing antigenically cross-reactive fimbriae (15–17). In another vaccine trial in humans, Levine et al. (63) observed that although parenteral administration of type 1 fimbriae isolated from *E. coli* evoked high serum levels of antifimbrial antibodies, it failed to protect against colonization of the gastrointestinal tract.

Thus, successful use of fimbrial vaccines has been hindered by their limited protective effect. The lack of protective activity is due, at least in part, to a high level of antigenic heterogeneity among fimbriae exhibiting the same binding specificity. Gonococcal fimbriae represent one of the best examples of antigenic heterogeneity of adhesion molecules. Extensive serological studies by Brinton et al. (16) have demonstrated the existence of hundreds of gonococcal fimbrial serotypes.

The fimbriae and the outer membrane proteins (particularly OMP2) of the gono-cocci have a tremendous tendency to vary, and multiple antigenic shifts are common during *in vitro* culturing as well as during natural infections (15,16). Evidence for such variation in natural infections was recently provided by close examination of *N. gonorrheae* cultured from the urethra in male patients and from the cervix and urethra in female contacts (27,111). Although the same strain was isolated from a given group, it was noted that the molecular weights of the outer membrane proteins and the fimbriae varied considerably among different individuals in the group (27,111). Furthermore, antibodies evoked to a particular fimbrial variant showed limited cross-reactivity with other variants produced by the same strain (111). No particular relationship was seen between the expression of proteins of different molecular weights and the host site of isolation (27,111). Such intrastrain variations in surface proteins may be related to phase variation in the adhesive properties of the strain. Such alterations may permit variants to selectively colonize different mucosal surfaces. *In vivo* variations of surface antigens may also be a manifestation of the host's immune response directed toward specific epitopes. Such immune pressures may further enhance the evolution or selection of new antigenic variants.

Despite the antigenic heterogeneity seen in the gonococcal fimbriae, peptide mapping of the fimbrial subunits has revealed considerable structural similarities between fimbrial variants (17,92). Amino acid sequence analyses of peptide frag-ments obtained by cyanogen bromide cleavage of fimbrial subunits have revealed that most of the variation occurs in the primary structure of the COOH-terminal region of the subunit molecule and that the variation does not extend to the binding moiety of the fimbriae (92). According to Schoolnick et al. (92), the binding moiety of the gonococcal fimbrial resides in the NH_2-terminal region of the fimbrial subunit and apparently is conserved.

Considerable antigenic heterogeneity has also been observed among the p-fim-briae and type 1 fimbriae of *E. coli*; a great number of serotypes can be predicted from past serological studies (3,31,59,75). Several antigenetically distinct types of p-fimbriae are expressed simultaneously by the same strain (59,75). By sequential absorption studies employing specific fimbrial antisera, Rhen et al. (84) distin-guished up to three distinct antigenic subpopulations in a single culture of p-fimbriated *E. coli*, each subpopulation expressing predominantly one antigenic type of fimbriae. Moreover, important ecological implications have been raised by the simultaneous expression of several antigenetically distinct fimbriae not only in the same species but also in different species in the same family. For example, the amino acid sequences of several type 1 fimbriae obtained from different species of *Enterobacteriaceae* were recently compared by Fader et al. (31). They observed variability similar to that previously observed for gonococcal fimbriae. The hom-ologies among the amino acid sequences of various type 1 fimbriae were as high as 79%. Yet no antigenic cross-reactivity was observed (31). These authors spec-ulated that the antigenic heterogeneity was a result of differences in tertiary struc-tural conformation (31).

Thus, the existence of multiple variants for the adhesins has been a seemingly insurmountable problem in the development of a "broad-spectrum" antiadhesive vaccine. Even the use of a polyvalent vaccine may be of limited value in view of the rapid antigenic variation that appears to occur *in vivo*. If, however, a fimbrial region that bears the host-cell receptor binding moiety (which appears to be conserved on all fimbriae demonstrating the same receptor specificity) can be identified, a vaccine prepared from this region, either by cleaving the natural protein or by chemically synthesizing the peptide, may serve as an ideal candidate to provide broad protection against many different strains. Such a peptide vaccine should display the receptor binding domain to the host's immune system in a more concentrated and effective manner and thereby evoke higher titers of the functionally relevant antibodies. Recently, Schoolnick et al. (92) used a cyanogen-bromide-derived fragment of the gonococcal fimbrial subunit, previously determined to contain the binding domain, to raise antibodies that displayed broad bacterial adhesion-inhibitory activity not only against the homologous strain but also against other gonococcal strains with serologically unrelated fimbriae. Research along these lines may eventually lead to the discovery of a broad-spectrum antiadhesive vaccine.

Another reason for the apparent lack of protection observed with the use of gonococcal and other fimbrial preparations in humans is that antifimbrial antibody levels in local mucosal secretions have been either nondetectable or present at very low levels, even though serum antibody levels have been high (17). Current lines of research are now directed toward raising the duration and height of mucosal immune responses by presenting the purified fimbriae to the mucosal surfaces (17). Similar local immunization studies were previously undertaken by Pierce et al. (80,81) to enhance the mucosal IgA response against cholera toxin in the gut. Having shown that the antitoxin is protective, these workers examined the local IgA response after a variety of immunization schedules. The highest response was obtained by primary subcutaneous injection followed by oral boosting (80,81).

Unlike active immunization, which involved stimulation of antibody production in the host, passive transfer of antiadhesive antibodies provides immediate immunity and is not dependent on immunocompetence of the host. Passive immunization with fimbriae-specific antibodies may be particularly useful when employed in high-risk populations such as neonates and immunologically compromised patients. Although the potential value of passive immunization has been clearly demonstrated in protecting neonates from gastrointestinal infection, its applications at other mucosal sites has certain limitations. These limitations concern delivery of antibodies to a particular site and at concentrations sufficient to be effective in the relatively short life-span of the administered antibodies. In our laboratory we observed that antiadhesive monoclonal antibodies introduced intravenously into mice were not detectable in the serum after 24 hr. When the same antibodies were instilled intraperitoneally, high serum levels of antibody were detectable after 24 hr; furthermore, antibodies instilled in this fashion were protective against *E. coli*-induced pyelonephritis (*vide supra*).

Dietary Lectins

A promising strategy for nonimmunologic intervention in the adherence of harmful bacteria to the gastrointestinal tract may lie in the use of specific lectins in the diet. Basic foodstuffs could be enriched with plant and animal lectins that would compete with potential bacterial pathogens for receptor sites on mucosal epithelial cells. Excessive intake of lectins, however, may not be advisable, as the ecology of the indigenous flora of the digestive and respiratory tracts might be upset (23). It is probable that a controlled and well-balanced diet plays a central role in maintaining a proper balance between the indigenous bacteria and potential pathogens on our mucosal surfaces.

Receptor Analogues

The idea that colonization by a bacterial pathogen might be prevented by application of a receptor analogue to mucosal surfaces was first investigated by Aronson et al. (5). They reasoned that because D-mannose and its derivatives act as receptor analogues for many strains of E. coli, instillation of this sugar into the urinary bladder of mice should prevent colonization by organisms that adhere to epithelial cells in a mannose-sensitive manner. To test this possibility, α-methylmannoside was instilled along with E. coli into the bladders of mice. Control mice received organisms suspended in α-methylglucoside or phosphate-buffered saline rather than α-methylmannoside. Only 20% of the mice instilled with α-methylmannoside were colonized, whereas 70% of the controls were colonized (5). Similar studies using synthetic analogues of the glycolipid receptor for the p-fimbriae of E. coli were performed to prevent p-fimbriated E. coli-induced urinary tract infections (100). These receptor analogues similarly were able to inhibit bacterial adherence to epithelial cells and to protect mice against infection (98,100).

These studies indicate that bacterial colonization can be prevented by direct application of the receptor analogues to the mucosal surface. However, it is also becoming clear that the type of receptor analogue applied to the mucosal surfaces is extremely important. In some instances, synthetic receptor analogues become incorporated into cell membranes of host cells, and bacterial adherence is thereby enhanced rather than inhibited. One of the main limitations of the use of receptor analogues is the problem of targeting the analogues to a particular mucosal surface. To prevent urinary tract infections, Svanborg-Eden et al. (99) recently proposed oral administration of glycolipid analogues linked to a carrier protein. Such oral administration of a receptor analogue is directed toward elimination of p-fimbriated bacteria from the gastrointestinal tract. This, in turn, would eliminate the source of bacterial colonization of the periurethral region that ultimately results in ascending pyelonephritis. It is theoretically possible that receptor analogues absorbed through the alimentary canal may eventually even reach other mucosal surfaces (99).

Antiadhesive Antibiotics

During the course of chemotherapy for infectious diseases, various antibiotics may intermittently reach the colonized mucosal surfaces. Classically, antibiotics are thought to exert their therapeutic effects either by killing the organism or inhibiting its growth. Recent studies indicate an additional mechanism of action; sublethal concentrations of antibiotics may exert antiadhesive effects by affecting the synthesis and expression of bacterial adhesins.

Alkan and Beachey (4) found that sublethal concentrations of penicillin G induced resting group A streptococci to release large amounts of lipoteichoic acid, the adhesin that binds the organism to epithelial cells. Furthermore, it was shown that the loss of cellular lipoteichoic acid was paralleled by loss of adhering capacity (4). Thus, penicillin, in addition to its known lethal action on growing bacteria, may influence the virulence of resting-phase bacteria by causing them to lose their adhesins. In contrast, neither penicillin nor streptomycin had any effect on the adherence of *E. coli* in the resting phase; however, both antibiotics caused growing organisms to lose adhering ability (70). Similar results have been reported by Svanborg-Eden et al. (101), who employed subinhibitory concentrations of ampicillin and amoxicillin in studies of the adherence of p-fimbriated uropathogenic *E. coli*. Recently, Kristiansen et al. (58) showed that subinhibitory concentrations of lincomycin markedly decreased fimbriation and adherence of *N. meningitidis* even though the test organisms were highly resistant to the lethal effects of the drug. Oral lincomycin administered to healthy carriers of meningococci markedly decreased meningococcal counts in the pharyngeal secretions; in one instance the strain was completely eradicated from the secretions (58).

SUMMARY AND CONCLUSIONS

Pathogenic bacteria adhere to mucosal surfaces in a highly specific manner in order to avoid being swept away in the flow of fluid constantly bathing these surfaces. A number of different adhesin–receptor systems have been described for various bacterial pathogens. The mucosal surfaces of the healthy host are virtually impermeable to the attack of virulent bacteria. A number of nonspecific factors, such as fluid flow, peristalsis, coughing, sneezing, and mucus secretions, form a physical barrier against attachment of all except the most virulent bacteria. Specific factors such as soluble lectins, receptor analogues, and immunoglobulins bind to the bacterial adhesins and thereby competitively inhibit binding to host cells. Some bacteria have developed specific proteases that destroy the antiadhesive properties of certain immunoglobulins, especially IgA. The host, in turn, has developed antibodies that neutralize certain of these bacterial proteases. Elucidation of the molecular mechanisms of the bacterial adherence process has offered new approaches to prevention of serious bacterial infections. Much progress has been made in attempts to direct therapeutic modalities against the initial mucosal adherence step of the infectious process. These modalities include application of purified receptors or receptor analogues to susceptible mucosal surfaces, local and systemic immunization with purified bacterial adhesins, and chemotherapy with antibiotics that exert an antiadhesive effect either by causing the organism to lose their adhesins or by preventing the synthesis or expression of adhesins. The choice of antiadhesive approach for a particular infection must take into consideration the populations at risk. If the population is small and the risk is limited to finite periods of exposure, chemotherapeutic measures to reestablish the mucosal barriers may be the most desirable. If, on the other hand, the population is large and exposure to potential pathogens is continuous, immunoprophylaxis with antiadhesive vaccines may provide long-lasting protection against adhesion of pathogenic bacteria to susceptible mucosal surfaces.

ACKNOWLEDGMENTS

We thank Dr. G. D. Christensen for valuable suggestions and critical review of the manuscript. The expert secretarial assistance of Johnnie Smith and Connie Carrier is gratefully acknowledged. The research work of the authors is supported by research funds from the U.S. Veterans Administration and by research grants AI-13550 and AI-10085 from the National Institutes of Health.

REFERENCES

1. Abraham, S. N., Babu, J. P., Giampapa, C., Hasty, D. L., Simpson, W. A., and Beachey, E. H. (1984): Protection against ascending pyelonephritis with bacterial adhesin-specific or host cell receptor specific monoclonal antibody. In: *Abstracts of the 84th Annual Meeting of the American Society for Microbiology*, p. 33. Am. Soc. Microbiol., Washington, D.C.
2. Abraham, S. N., Beachey, E. H., and Simpson, W. A. (1983): Adherence of *Streptococcus pyogenes*, *Escherichia coli*, and *Pseudomonas aeruginosa* to fibronectin coated and uncoated epithelial cells. *Infect. Immun.*, 41:1261–1268.
3. Abraham, S. N., Hasty, D. L., Simpson, W. A., and Beachey, E. H. (1983): Antiadhesive properties of a quaternary structure specific hydridoma antibody against type 1 fimbriae of *Escherichia coli*. *J. Exp. Med.*, 158:1114–1128.
4. Alkan, M. L., and Beachey, E. H. (1978): Excretion of lipoteichoic acid by group A streptococci: Influence of penicillin on excretion and loss of ability to adhere to human oral epithelial cells. *J. Clin. Invest.*, 61:671–677.
5. Aronson, M., Medalia, O., Schori, L., et al. (1979): Prevention of colonization of the urinary tract of mice with *Escherichia coli* by blocking of bacterial adherence with methyl-alpha-D-mannopyranoside. *J. Infect. Dis.*, 139:329–332.
6. Babu, J. P., Simpson, W. A., Courtney, H. S., and Beachey, E. H. (1983): Interaction of human plasma fibronectin with cariogenic and noncariogenic oral streptococci. *Infect. Immun.*, 41:162–168.
7. Beachey, E. H. (editor) (1980): *Bacterial Adherence, Receptor Recognition, Series B, Vol. 6*. Chapman & Hall, London.
8. Beachey, E. H. (1981): Bacterial adherence: Adhesion receptor interactions mediating the attachment of bacteria to mucosal surfaces. *J. Infect. Dis.*, 143:325–345.
9. Bibel, D. J. (1982): Bacterial interference, bacteriotherapy and bacterioprophylaxis. In: *Bacterial Interference*, edited by R. Aly and H. R. Shinefield, pp. 1–12. CRC Press, Boca Raton, Fla.
10. Bibel, J. D., Aly, R., Bayles, et al. (1983): Competitive adherence as a mechanism of bacterial interference. *Can. J. Microbiol.*, 29:700–703.
11. Bird, G. W., and Roy, T. C. (1980): Human serum antibodies to melibiose and other carbohydrates. *Vox Sang.*, 38:169–171.
12. Brady, P. G., Vannier, A. M., and Banwell, J. G. (1978): Identification of dietary lectins, wheat germ agglutinin in human intestinal contents. *Gastroenterology*, 75:236–239.
13. Brandtzaeg, P., Gjellauger, I., and Gjeruldsen, S. T. (1970): Human secretory immunoglobulins.

I. Salivary secretions from individuals with normal or low levels of serum immunoglobulins. *Scand. J. Haematol. [Suppl.]*, 12:1–83.

14. Brinton, C. D. (1965): The structure, function, synthesis and DNA and RNA transport in gram-negative bacteria. *Ann. N.Y. Acad. Sci.*, 27:1003–1054.

15. Brinton, C. C., Fusco, P., To, A., and To, S. (1977): The piliation phase syndrome and the uses of purified pili in disease control. *Proc. 13th U.S.–Japan Conf. Cholera*, pp. 34–70. National Institutes of Health, Bethesda.

16. Brinton, C. C., Wood, S. W., Brown, A., et al. (1982): The development of a neisserial pilus vaccine for gonorrhea and meningococcal meningitis. In: *Bacterial Vaccines, Seminars in Infectious Disease, Vol. IV*, edited by L. Weinstein and B. N. Fields, pp. 140–159. Thieme-Stratton, New York.

17. Buchanan, T. M., Siegel, M. S., Chen, K. C., and Pearce, W. A. (1982): Development of a vaccine to prevent gonorrhea. In: *Bacterial Vaccines, Seminars in Infectious Disease, Vol. IV*, edited by L. Weinstein and B. N. Fields, pp. 160–164. Thieme-Stratton, New York.

18. Burrows, W., and Havens, I. (1948): Studies on immunity to asiatic cholera. V. The absorption of immune globulin from the bowel and its excretion in urine and faeces of experimental animals and human volunteers. *J. Infect. Dis.*, 82:231–250.

19. Carruthers, M. M., and Kabat, W. G. (1983): Mediators of staphylococcal adherence to mucosal cells by lipoteichoic acid. *Infect. Immun.*, 40:444–446.

20. Chandra, R. K. (1979): Prospective studies of the effect of breast feeding on incidence of infection and allergy. *Acta Paediatr. Scand.*, 68:691–694.

21. Christensen, G. D., Simpson, W. A., and Beachey, E. H. (1984): Microbial adherence in infection. In: *Principles and Practice of Infectious Disease*, edited by G. L. Mandell, R. C. Douglas, and J. E. Bennet, pp. 6–23. Wiley, New York.

22. Cisar, J. O., Kolenbrander, P. E., and McIntire, F. (1979): Specificity of coaggregation reactions between human oral streptococci and strains of *Actinomyces viscosus* or *Actinomyces naeslundii*. *Infect. Immun.*, 24:742–752.

23. Costerton, J. W., and Banwell, J. G. (1984): Pathogenic colonization of the rat intestine mediated by exogenous lectin (phytohemagglutinin). In: *Abstracts of the 84th Annual Meeting of the American Society for Microbiology*, p. 18. Am. Soc. Microbiol., Washington, D.C.

24. Courtney, H. C., Simpson, W. A., and Beachey, E. H. (1983): Binding of streptococcal lipoteichoic acid to fatty-acid binding sites on human plasma fibronectin. *J. Bacteriol.*, 153:763–768.

25. Cunningham, S. S. (1979): Morbidity in breast fed and artifically fed infants. *J. Pediatr.*, 95:685–689.

26. Davis, C. P., Avots-Avotins, A. E., and Fader, R. C. (1981): Evidence for a bladder cell glycolipid receptor for *Escherichia coli* and the effect of neuraminic acid and colominic acid on adherence. *Infect. Immun.*, 34:944–948.

27. Duckworth, M., Jackson, D., Zak, K., and Heckels, J. E. (1983): Structural variation in pili expressed during gonococcal infections. *J. Gen. Microbiol.*, 129:1593–1596.

28. Duguid, J. P., and Old, D. C. (1980): Adhesive properties of Enterobacteriaceae. In: *Bacterial Adherence, Receptor and Recognition Series B, Vol. 6*, edited by E. H. Beachey, pp. 184–217. Chapman & Hall, London.

29. Eisenstein, B. (1981): Phase variation of type 1 fimbriae in *Escherichia coli* is under transcriptional control. *Science*, 214:337–339.

30. Ellen, R. P., and Balcerzak-Raczkowski, I. B. (1977): Interbacterial aggregation of *Actinomyces naeslundi* and dental plaque streptococci. *J. Peridont. Res.*, 12:11–20.

31. Fader, R. C., Duffy, L. D., Davies, C. P., and Kurosky, A. (1982): Purification and chemical characterization of type 1 pili isolated from *Klebsiella pneumoniae*. *J. Biol. Chem.*, 257:3301–3305.

32. Faris, A., Lindahl, M., and Wadstrom, T. (1980): GM$_2$-like glycoconjugates as possible eryth-rocyte receptor for the CFA/1 and K99 haemagglutinins of enterotoxigenic *Escherichia coli*. *F.E.M.S. Microbiol. Lett.*, 7:265–269.

33. Firon, N., Ofek, I., and Sharon, N. (1982): Interaction of mannose containing oligosaccharides with the fimbrial lectin of *Escherichia coli*. *Biochem. Biophys. Res. Commun.*, 105:1426–1432.

34. Freter, R. (1980): Prospects for preventing the association of harmful bacteria with host mucosal surfaces. In: *Bacterial Adherence, Receptor and Recognition, Series B, Vol. 6*, edited by E. H. Beachey, pp. 439–458. Chapman & Hall, London.

35. Freter, R. (1981): Mechanisms of association of bacteria with mucosal surfaces. In: *Adhesion and Microorganisms Pathogenicity*, pp. 36–47. Pitman Medical, London.
36. Gaastra, W., and DeGraaf, F. K. (1982): Host specific fimbrial adhesins of noninvasive enterotoxigenic *Escherichia coli* strains. *Microbiol. Rev.*, 46:129–134.
37. Gibbons, R. J. (1982): Review and discussion of role of mucus in mucosal defense. In: *Recent Advances in Mucosal Immunity*, edited by W. Strober, L. A. Hanson, and K. W. Sell, pp. 343–351. Raven Press, New York.
38. Gibbons, R. J., and Dankers, I. (1981): Lectin-like constituents of foods which react with components of serum, saliva, and *Streptococcus mutans*. *Appl. Environ. Microbiol.*, 41:880–888.
39. Gibbons, R. J., and Dankers, I. (1983): Association of food lectins with human oral epithelial cells *in vivo*. *Arch. Oral Biol.*, 28:561–566.
40. Gibbons, R. J., and Van Houte, J. (1975): Bacterial adherence in oral microbiology. *Annu. Rev. Microbiol.*, 29:19–44.
41. Gibbons, R. J., and Van Houte, J. (1980): Bacterial adherence and the formation of dental plaque. In: *Bacterial Adherence, Receptor and Recognition, Series B, Vol. 6*, edited by E. H. Beachey, pp. 60–104. Chapman & Hall, London.
42. Gilbert, J. V., Plaut, A. G., and Longmaid, B. (1983): Inhibition of bacterial IgA proteases by human secretory IgA and serum. *Ann. N.Y. Acad. Sci.*, 409:625–634.
43. Gregory, J. C., Wein, A. J., Sansone, T. C., and Murphy, J. J. (1971): Bladder resistance to infection. *J. Urol.*, 105:220–222.
44. Hanson, L. A., Ahlstedt, S., Andersson, B., Carlsson, B., et al. (1983): Mucosal immunity. *Ann. N.Y. Acad. Sci.*, 409:1–21.
45. Hanson, L. A., and Brandtzaeg, P. (1980): The mucosal defense system. In: *Immunological Disorders in Infants and Children*, edited by E. Stiehm, pp. 137–164. W. B. Saunders, Philadelphia.
46. Hogg, S. D., and Embery, G. (1979): The isolation and partial characterization of a sulphated glycoprotein from human whole saliva which aggregated strains of *Streptococcus sanguis* but not *Streptococcus mutans*. *Arch. Oral. Biol.*, 24:791–797.
47. Hogg, S. D., and Embery, G. (1982): Blood group reactive glycoprotein from human saliva interacts with lipoteichoic acid on the surface of *Streptococcus sanguis* cells. *Arch. Oral Biol.*, 27:261–268.
48. Holmgren, J., and Svennerholm, A.-M. (1983): Cholera and the immune system. *Prog. Allergy*, 33:106–119.
49. Holmgren, J., Svennerholm, A.-M., and Ahren, C. (1981): Nonimmunoglobulin fraction of human milk inhibits bacterial adhesion (haemagglutination) and enterotoxin binding of *Escherichia coli* and *Vibrio cholera*. *Infect. Immun.*, 33:136–141.
50. Hoskins, L. C., and Boulding, E. T. (1976): Degradation of blood group antigens in human colon ecosystems. I. *In vitro* production of ABH blood group degrading enzymes by enteric bacteria. *J. Clin. Invest.*, 57:63–73.
51. Isaacson, R. E., Dean, E. A., Morgan, R. L., and Moon, H. W. (1980): Immunization of suckling pigs against enterotoxigenic *Escherichia coli* induced diarrheal disease by vaccinating dams with purified K99 or 987 pili: Antibody production in response to vaccination. *Infect. Immun.*, 29:824–826.
52. Jones, G. W. (1977): The attachment of bacteria to the surface of animal cells. In: *Microbial Interactions*, edited by J. L. Reissig, pp. 139–176. Chapman & Hall, London.
53. Jones, G. W., and Isaacson, R. E. (1983): Proteinaceous bacterial adhesins and their receptors. *C.R.C. Crit. Rev. Microbiol.*, 10:229–260.
54. Kallenius, G., Mollby, R., Svenson, S. B., et al. (1980): The Pk antigen as receptor for the haemagglutination of pyelonephritogenic *Escherichia coli*. *F.E.M.S. Microbiol. Lett.*, 7:297–302.
55. Kallenius, G., Svenson, S. B., Mollby, R., and Winberg, J. (1981): Structure of carbohydrate part of receptor on human uroepithelial cells for pyelonephritogenic *Escherichia coli*. *Lancet*, 2:604–606.
56. Kilian, M., Roland, K., and Mestecky, J. (1981): Interference of secretory immunoglobulin A with sorption of oral bacteria to hydroxyapatite. *Infect. Immun.*, 31:942–951.
57. Kilian, M., Thomsen, B., Peterson, T. E., and Bleeg, H. S. (1983): Occurrence and nature of bacterial IgA proteases. *Ann. N.Y. Acad. Sci.*, 409:612–624.
58. Kristiansen, B.-E., Rustad, L., Spanne, O., and Bjorvatn, B. (1983): Effect of subminimal

inhibitory concentrations of antimicrobial agents on the piliation and adherence of *Neisseria meningitidis*. *Antimicrob. Agents Chemother.*, 24:731–734.

59. Korhonen, T. K., Vaisanen, V., Saxin, H., Hultberg, H., and Svensson, S. B. (1982): P antigen recognizing fimbriae from human uropathogenic *Escherichia coli* strains. *Infect. Immun.*, 37:286–291.

60. Lalezari, P., Jiang, A. F., and Kumar, M. (1981): Antibodies to mono and disaccharides in normal donors: Structural definition of antigenic determinants. *Clin. Res.*, 29:547A (abstract).

61. Leffler, H., and Svanborg-Eden, C. (1980): Chemical identification of a glycospingolipid receptor for *Escherichia coli* attaching to human urinary tract cells and agglutinating human erythrocytes. *F.E.M.S. Microbiol. Lett.*, 8:127–134.

62. Lemaitre-Coelho, I., Jackson, G. D., and Vaeuman, J. P. (1978): High levels of secretory IgA and free secretory components in the serum of rats with bile duct obstruction. *J. Exp. Med.*, 147:934–939.

63. Levine, M. M., Blak, R. E., Brinton, C. C., Clements, M. L., et al. (1983): Reactogenicity, immunogenicity and efficacy of *Escherichia coli* type 1 somatic pili parenteral vaccine in man. *Scand. J. Infect. Dis. [Suppl.]*, 33:83–95.

64. Liljemark, W. F., Bloomquist, C. G., and Ofstehage, J. C. (1979): Aggregation and adherence of *Streptococcus sanguis*: Role of human salivary immunoglobulin A. *Infect. Immun.*, 26:1104–1110.

65. McBride, B. C., and Gisslow, M. T. (1977): Role of sialic acid in saliva induced aggregation of *Streptococcus sanguis*. *Infect. Immun.*, 18:35–40.

66. McNabb, P. C., and Tomasi, T. B. (1981): Host defense mechanisms at mucosal surfaces. *Annu. Rev. Microbiol.*, 138:976–983.

67. Mims, C. A. (1982): *The Pathogenesis of Infectious Disease*. Academic Press, New York.

68. Moon, H. W., and Runnels, P. L. (1981): Prospects for development of a vaccine against diarrhea caused by *Escherichia coli*. In: *Acute Enteric Infections in Children*, edited by T. Holme, J. Holmgren, M. H. Merson, and R. Mollby, pp. 477–491. Elseview/North-Holland, Amsterdam.

69. Mulks, M. H., Kornfield, S. J., and Plaut, A. G. (1980): Specific proteolysis of human IgA by *Streptococcus penumoniae* and *Haemophilus influenzae*. *J. Infect. Dis.*, 141:450–455.

70. Ofek, I., and Beachey, E. H. (1980): General concepts and principles of bacterial adherence. In: *Bacterial Adherence, Receptor and Recognition, Series B, Vol. 6*, edited by E. H. Beachey, pp. 1–29. Chapman & Hall, London.

71. Ofek, I., Beachey, E. H., Eyal, F., and Morrison, J. C. (1977): Postnatal development of binding of streptococci and lipoteichoic acid by oral mucosal cells of humans. *J. Infect. Dis.*, 135:267–274.

72. Ofek, I., Simpson, W. A., and Beachey, E. H. (1982): The formation of molecular complexes between a structurally-defined M protein and acylated and deacylated lipoteichoic acid of *Streptococcus pyogenes*. *J. Bacteriol.*, 149:426–433.

73. Orikasa, S., and Hinman, F. (1977): Reaction of the vesical wall to bacterial penetration. *Invest. Urol.*, 15:185–193.

74. Orskov, I., Ferenc, A., and Orskov, F. (1980): Tamm-Horsfall protein or uromucoid is the normal urinary slime that traps type 1 fimbriated *Escherichia coli*. *Lancet*, 1:887.

75. Parry, S. H., Abraham, S. N., and Sussman, M. (1983): The biological and serological properties of adhesion determinants of *Escherichia coli* isolated from urinary tract infections. In: *Immunologic Aspects of Urinary Tract Infection in Children*, edited by H. Schulte-Wisserman, pp. 113–126. Thieme, Stuttgart.

76. Parsons, C. L., Mulholland, S. G., and Anwar, H. (1979): Antibacterial activity of bladder surface mucin duplicated by exogenous glycosaminoglycan (heparin). *Infect. Immun.*, 24:552–557.

77. Parsons, C. L., Pollen, J. J., Anwar, H., et al. (1980): Antibacterial activity of bladder surface mucin duplicated in the rabbit bladder by exogenous glycosaminoglycan (sodium pantosanpolysulphate). *Infect. Immun.*, 27:876–881.

78. Parsons, C. L., Stauffer, C., and Schmitt, J. D. (1980): Bladder surface glycosaminoglycans: An efficient mechanism of environment adaptation. *Science*, 208:605–607.

79. Pearce, W. A., and Buchanan, T. M. (1980): Structure and cell membrane-binding properties of bacterial fimbriae. In: *Bacterial Adherence, Receptor and Recognition, Series B, Vol. 6*, edited by E. H. Beachey, pp. 289–344. Chapman & Hall, London.

80. Pierce, N. F., and Gowans, J. L. (1975): Cellular kinetics of intestinal immune response to cholera toxoid in rats. *J. Exp. Med.*, 142:1550–1563.

81. Pierce, N. F., and Reynolds, H. Y. (1975): Immunity to experimental cholera II: Secretory and

humoral antitoxin response, to local and systemic toxoid administration. *J. Infect. Dis.*, 131:383–389.

82. Ramphal, R., and Pyle, M. (1983): Evidence for mucins and sialic acid as receptors for *Pseudomonas aeruginosa* in the lower respiratory tract. *Infect. Immun.*, 41:339–344.

83. Rene, P., and Silverblatt, F. (1980): Serological response to *Escherichia coli* pili in pyelonephritis. In: *Current Chemotherapy and Infectious Diseases, Vol. 2*, edited by J. D. Nelson and C. Grassi, pp. 782–783. American Society for Microbiology, Washington, D.C.

84. Rhen, M., Makela, P. H., and Korhonen, T. K. (1983): P-fimbriae of *Escherichia coli* are subject to phase variation. *F.E.M.S. Microbiol. Lett.*, 19:267–271.

85. Roberts, J. A., Hardaway, K., Kaack, B., Fussel, E. H., and Baskin, G. (1984): Prevention against pyelonephritis by immunization with p-fimbriae. *J. Urol.* 131:602–608.

86. Rosan, B., Appelbaum, B., Golub, E., Malamud, D., and Mandel, I. D. (1982): Enhanced saliva mediated bacterial aggregation and decreased bacterial adhesion in caries resistant versus caries susceptible individuals. *Infect. Immun.*, 38:1056–1059.

87. Rosan, B., Malumud, D., Appelbaum, B., and Golub, E. (1982): Characteristic differences between saliva dependent aggregation and adhesion of streptococci. *Infect. Immun.*, 35:86–90.

88. Rutter, J. M., and Jones, G. W. (1973): Protection against enteric disease caused by *Escherichia coli*. A model for vaccination with a virulence determinant. *Nature*, 242:531–532.

89. Sanford, B. A., Shelokov, A., and Ramsey, M. A. (1978): Bacterial adherence to virus-infected cells: A cell culture model of bacteria superinfection. *J. Infect. Dis.*, 137:176–181.

90. Sanford, B. A., Smith, N., Shelokov, A., and Ramsey, M. A. (1980): Adherence of influenza A viruses to group B streptococci. *J. Infect. Dis.*, 141:496–506.

91. Savage, D. C. (1972): Survival on mucosal epithelia, epithelial penetration and growth in tissue of pathogenic bacteria. In: *Microbial Pathogenicity in Man and Animals, Symposia of the Society of General Microbiology*, No. XXII, pp. 25–57. Soc. General Microbiol.

92. Schoolnick, G. K., Tai, J. Y., and Gotchlich, E. (1982): The human erythrocyte binding domain of gonococcal pili. In: *Bacterial Vaccines, Seminars in Infectious Disease, Vol. IV*, edited by L. Weinstein and B. N. Fields, pp. 172–180. Thieme-Stratton, New York.

93. Sellwood, R., Gibbons, R. J., Jones, G. W., and Rutter, J. M. (1975): Adhesion of enteropathogenic *Escherichia coli* to pig intestinal brush borders: The existence of two pig phenotypes. *J. Med. Microbiol.*, 8:405–411.

94. Silverblatt, F. J., Weinstein, R., and Rene, P. (1982): Protection against experimental pyelonephritis by antibody to pili. *Scand. J. Infect. Dis. [Suppl.]*, 33:79–82.

95. Simpson, W. A., and Beachey, E. H. (1983): Adherence of group A streptococci to fibronectin on oral epithelial cells. *Infect. Immun.*, 39:275–279.

96. Simpson, W. A., Courtney, H., and Beachey, E. H. (1982): Fibronectin—a modulator for the oropharyngeal bacterial flora. In: *Microbiology*, edited by D. Schlessinger, pp. 346–347. American Society for Microbiology, Washington, D.C.

97. Sussman, M., Abraham, S. N., and Parry, S. H. (1983): Bacterial adhesion in the host-parasite relationship of urinary tract infection. In: *Immunological Aspects of Urinary Tract Infection in Children*, edited by H. Schulte-Wisserman, pp. 103–112. Thieme, Stuttgart.

98. Svanborg-Eden, C., Andersson, B., Hagberg, L., et al. (1983): Receptor analogues and antipilus antibodies as inhibitors of bacterial attachment *in vivo* and *in vitro*. *Ann. N.Y. Acad. Sci.*, 409:580–591.

99. Svanborg-Eden, C., Gasth, A., Hagberg, L., et al. (1982): Host interaction with *Escherichia coli* in the urinary tract. In: *Bacterial Vaccines, Seminars in Infectious Disease, Vol. IV*, edited by L. Weinstein and B. N. Fields, pp. 113–131. Thieme-Stratton, New York.

100. Svanborg-Eden, C., Freter, R., Hagberg, L., Hull, R., Hull, S., et al. (1982): Inhibition of experimental ascending urinary tract infection by an epithelial cell surface receptor analogue. *Nature*, 298:560–562.

101. Svanborg-Eden, C., Hagberg, L., Hanson, L. A., et al. (1981): Adhesion of *Escherichia coli* in urinary tract infection. In: *Adhesion and Microorganism Pathogenicity*, CIBA Foundation Symp. 80, pp. 161–187. Pitman Medical, London.

102. Svennerholm, A. M. (1980): Nature of protective cholera immunity. In: *Cholera and Related Diarrheas*, edited by D. Ouchterlony and J. Holmgren, pp. 171–184. Karger, Basel.

103. Tramont, E. C. (1977): Inhibition of adherence of *Neisseria gonorrhoeae* by human genital secretions. *J. Clin. Invest.*, 59:117–124.

104. Tramont, E. C., Ciak, J., Boslego, J., McChesney, D. G., Brinton, C. C., and Zollinger, W.

(1980): Antigenic specificity of antibodies in vaginal secretions during infection with *Neisseria gonorrhoeae*. *J. Infect. Dis.*, 142:23–31.

105. Tuomanen, E. I., and Hendley, J. O. (1983): Adherence of *Bordetella pertussis* to human respiratory epithelial cells. *J. Infect. Dis.*, 148:125–130.

106. Williams, R. C., and Gibbons, R. J. (1972): Inhibition of bacterial adherence by secretory immunoglobulin A: A mechanism of antigen disposal. *Science*, 77:697–699.

107. Williams, R. C., and Gibbons, R. J. (1975): Inhibition of streptococcal attachment to receptors on human buccal epithelial cells by antigenically similar salivary glycoproteins. *Infect. Immun.*, 11:711–718.

108. Wood, D. L., Holt, S. C., and Leadbetter, E. R. (1979): Ultrastructure of bacteroides species: *Bacteroids asaccharolyticus, Bacteroides fragilis, Bacteroides melaninogenicus* subspecies melaninogenicus, and β melaninogenicus subspecies infermedicus. *J. Infect. Dis.*, 139:534–546.

109. Woods, D. E., Straus, D. C., Johansson, W. G., and Bass, J. A. (1981): Role of fibronectin in the prevention of adherence of *Pseudomonas aeruginosa* to buccal cells. *J. Infect. Dis.*, 143:784–799.

110. Woods, D. E., Straus, D. E., Johansson, W. G., and Bass, J. A. (1981): Role of salivary protease activity in adherence of gram-negative bacilli to mammalian buccal epithelial cells *in vivo*. *J. Clin. Invest.*, 68:1435–1440.

111. Zak, K., Diaz, J. L., Jackson, D., and Heckels, J. E. (1984): Antigenic variation during infection with *Neisseria gonorrhoeae*: Detection of antibodies to surface proteins in sera. *J. Infect. Dis.*, 149:166–174.

Advances in Host Defense Mechanisms, Vol. 4,
edited by J. I. Gallin and A. S. Fauci.
Raven Press, New York © 1985.

Pulmonary Host Defenses: Cellular Factors

Gary W. Hunninghake, Robert B. Fick, and Kenneth M. Nugent

Pulmonary Division, Department of Medicine, Veterans Administration Hospital, and University of Iowa College of Medicine, Iowa City, Iowa 52242

Defense of the normal human lung against a variety of microorganisms is mediated, in part, by inflammatory and immune effector cells that are present in the lower respiratory tract. Evaluation of the inflammatory and immune effector cells isolated from normal adult lung by bronchoalveolar lavage has revealed that $93 \pm 5\%$ of the cells are macrophages, and $7 \pm 1\%$ are lymphocytes; less than 1% are neutrophils, eosinophils, or basophils (1–10). Because almost all of the inflammatory and immune effector cells of the normal lung are macrophages and lymphocytes, this discussion of the normal lung will focus primarily on these two types of cells.

PROPERTIES AND FUNCTIONS OF NORMAL HUMAN ALVEOLAR MACROPHAGES

Origin

Alveolar macrophages are members of the mononuclear phagocyte system (11). In this classification, tissue macrophages, monocytes, and promonocytes are considered part of a continuum in which alveolar macrophages, Kupffer cells, splenic macrophages, connective tissue "histiocytes," lymph node macrophages, osteoclasts, and microglial cells are thought to be ultimately derived from promonocytes arising in the bone marrow. Perhaps the most convincing data for this concept derive from chimeric experiments in animals in which marrow with a unique genetic marker is placed into an animal of a different genetic type, and the unique marker is later observed in various tissue macrophages (12–14). Similar data have been obtained for alveolar macrophages in humans. The chimeric experiment has been used to evaluate the sex chromosomes of alveolar macrophages in individuals receiving bone marrow transplants from histocompatible donors of the opposite sex. Such individuals are prepared for transplantation by destruction of all bone marrow of host origin by cytotoxic drugs and irradiation. Therefore, following successful transplantation with donor marrow, all of the circulating blood monocytes are of donor origin (i.e., of the opposite sex). In a classic study of the origin of the human alveolar macrophage, Thomas et al. (15), using the techniques described earlier, showed that at least some of the alveolar macrophage population is derived from marrow precursors; 3 months after transplantation, significant numbers of these cells were of donor origin (i.e., of the sex opposite that of the recipient).

Although it is reasonable to assume that originally all alveolar macrophages are derived from marrow, it is not clear that all alveolar macrophages present in the lung at any one time are directly derived from bone marrow precursors. In this regard, Golde et al. (16) have shown that human alveolar macrophages are capable of proliferating; 0.35 to 1.25% of these cells will incorporate ^{3}H-thymidine in 30 min *in vitro*. Thus, it is likely that the population of alveolar macrophages can be sustained by two mechanisms: by recruitment from peripheral blood monocytes and by local proliferation.

If local proliferation is an important mechanism for sustaining the alveolar macrophage population in humans, it is likely that these cells replicate within the alveolar interstitium. This concept follows from the morphometric studies by Barry and associates showing that approximately 6% of the cells within the alveolar interstitium are macrophages, and from the animal studies of Adamson and Bowden showing that macrophages proliferate in the interstitium and then migrate to the epithelial surface (17–19). However, the mechanisms and route by which macrophages migrate from interstitium to alveoli have not been defined in humans; presumably, these cells migrate through epithelial junctions (20). Likewise, the eventual fate of the human alveolar macrophage is not clear. Animal studies, however, suggest they either are swept up the tracheobronchial tree by the so-called mucociliary ladder or move back into the interstitium and are taken via the lymphatics to the regional lymph nodes (20).

Surface Receptors

One way in which cells interact with their environment is through receptors on their external surfaces. Human alveolar macrophages are no exception; receptors for C3b, C3d, and the Fc portion of IgG and IgE have been identified (Fig. 1) (21–25). Human alveolar macrophages, as well as other phagocytic cells, do not have receptors for IgM; however, they may indirectly interact with this immunoglobulin class through C3b generated by IgM antibody-antigen complexes. Macrophages that also lack receptors for IgA, and IgA immune complexes (such as secretory IgA-coated microorganisms) are apparently not recognized by these cells (26).

In general, interaction of the alveolar macrophage with a particulate via the macrophage's IgG Fc or C3b receptor will lead to phagocytosis of the particulate. However, in some instances, particulates coated with C3b are not ingested by these cells; for example, human alveolar macrophages will not phagocytize erythrocytes coated with IgM and C3b, but will ingest IgG-coated erythrocytes (22,27). Such experiments also suggest that macrophage IgG and C3b receptors can act independently. This concept is supported by studies in which rabbit alveolar macrophages "loaded" with latex particles were shown to have decreased IgG, but not C3b, receptors (21).

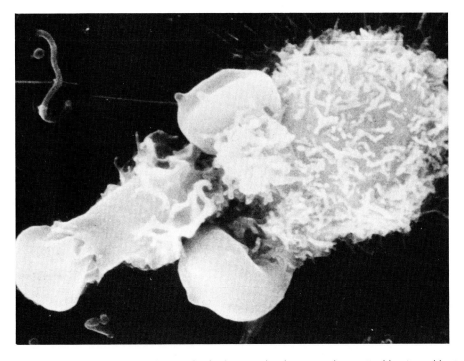

FIG. 1. Scanning electron micrograph of a human alveolar macrophage attaching to and ingesting IgG-coated ox erythrocytes. ×5,000. (Courtesy of Dr. O. Kawanami.)

As with other cells of the mononuclear phagocytic system, it is likely that alveolar macrophages possess receptors for glucocorticoids, β-adrenergic agonists, antiprotease-protease complexes, lysosomal glycosidases, and lactoferrin (28–34). As yet, there are few data concerning such receptors on human alveolar macrophages.

Interactions with Microorganisms

One of the functions usually ascribed to alveolar macrophages is keeping the lower respiratory tract sterile by engulfing and killing microorganisms. Although most studies of this process have been carried out using animal alveolar macrophages, it appears from the human data available that few, if any, species differences exist. Human alveolar macrophages can ingest bacteria, fungi, and viruses (2,27,35,36). These cells are also capable of inactivating viable staphylococci and inhibiting the growth of certain viruses (e.g., herpes simplex), but not others (e.g., cytomegalovirus) (37).

Optimal ingestion of microorganisms by macrophages is mediated by opsonins such as immunoglobulins or complement (Fig. 2) (22,26,38). IgG acts as an opsonin by attaching to the microorganism through its antigen-combining site and to the alveolar macrophage through its Fc receptor. C3b can also act as an opsonin for

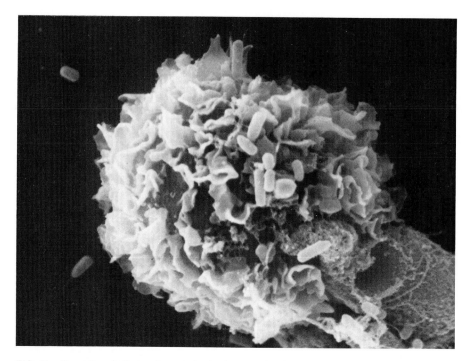

FIG. 2. Scanning electron micrograph of a human alveolar macrophage attaching to and ingesting IgG-coated *P. aeruginosa.* ×8,500.

human macrophages, either by coating the microorganism alone or by associating with IgM or IgG that has already interacted with the infectious agent (22).

When the human alveolar macrophage ingests microorganisms, it becomes activated, as manifested by increased oxygen uptake, more rapid glucose utilization, increased production of superoxide anion and hydrogen peroxide, and release of various enzymes and the alveolar macrophage-derived chemotactic factor for neutrophils (27,35,39). Presumably, the alveolar macrophage, like other macrophages, utilizes the release of reactive oxygen species and lysosomal enzymes to kill the microorganisms. The release of the alveolar-macrophage-derived chemotactic factor results in the migration of neutrophils to the lung; these newly recruited cells assist the macrophage in killing microorganisms. Some organisms, such as *Mycobacterium tuberculosis*, are not killed by the macrophages until they have been activated by T-cell-derived lymphokines (40–49). These lymphokines activate macrophages to release increased amounts of reactive oxygen species and lysosomal enzymes that then enable the cell to kill the organism. For optimal function as phagocytic cells, human alveolar macrophages depend on both glycolysis and cytochrome electron transport (38). Oxygen is not a mandatory requirement; macrophages cultured in a nitrogen atmosphere for 1 hr will still ingest microorganisms, as will macrophages incubated in a low-oxygen environment (38). The partial pressure of

CO_2 in the environment (with constant pH) seems to have little effect on macrophage function (38).

Interactions with Noninfectious Agents

Macrophages interact with a variety of noninfectious agents that may reach the alveolar surface; in many instances these agents are endocytosed by phagocytosis or pinocytosis (2,27,51). As with infectious materials, optimal phagocytosis of noninfectious agents is mediated by opsonins. However, macrophages can attach and phagocytize without opsonins; presumably, such attachment is mediated by charge interactions between the particle and the outer surface of the macrophage (50). Most of the information in this area is derived from animal studies. *In vitro*, human alveolar macrophages interact with inorganic particulates such as asbestos and Sepharose 4B (27,52). There is also evidence that such interactions occur *in vivo*, because individuals who have been exposed to various inorganic dusts have these same particulates within their alveolar macrophages (53–56).

As with the ingestion of microorganisms, phagocytosis of noninfectious particulates causes a general activation of macrophages (12). In addition, ingested particulates may injure the macrophage and eventually cause cell death (50). This process has been widely studied in animal macrophages in relation to silica, and it has also been shown to operate for human alveolar macrophages that have ingested large concentrations of asbestos (52). Injury of alveolar macrophages by inorganic particulates may impair the ability of individuals exposed to silica to adequately kill microorganisms that reach the lower respiratory tract.

Human alveolar macrophages also can ingest materials by pinocytosis (51). This process is energy-dependent and does not require serum factors in normal individuals. Presumably, pinocytosis is used by macrophages to engulf soluble substances or very small particles (<0.1 μm). For example, alveolar proteinosis is a disorder associated with accumulation of lipids and proteins within the alveoli; macrophages lavaged from individuals with this disorder have large vacuoles containing lipid and other materials, probably endocytosed by pinocytosis (57,58). These macrophages have markedly impaired ability to kill microorganisms (59).

Accessory Cells in Inflammatory and Immune Reactions

There is increasing evidence that the alveolar macrophage plays a central role in pulmonary immune processes (3). These immune responses can result in the production of specific antibodies or a cellular immune response to an infectious agent, thereby augmenting pulmonary host defenses against a microorganism. To function as accessory cells in immune responses, alveolar macrophages must physically interact with lymphocytes and present a specific antigen to these cells (60–64). They must also express Ia antigens and release interleukin-1 (IL-1). There is evidence that human alveolar macrophages physically interact with lymphocytes (Fig. 3) and are capable of functioning as accessory cells for optimal lymphocyte responses to antigens and mitogens and in mixed lymphocyte cultures (65–67). A

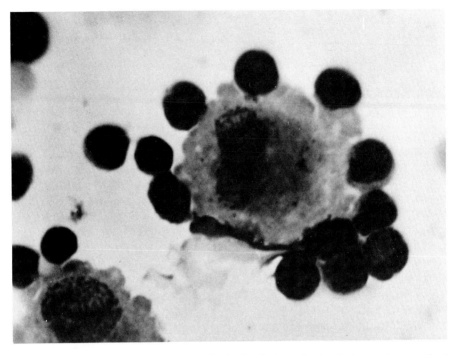

FIG. 3. A cytocentrifuge preparation of cells obtained by bronchoalveolar lavage from a patient with sarcoidosis. Several lung lymphocytes have attached to (rosetted with) an alveolar macrophage. Modified Wright-Giemsa stain. × 1,000.

large proportion of these cells also express Ia antigens (both HLA-DR and HLA-DS antigens), and they can be stimulated to release IL-1 (68–70). Thus, these cells appear to be able to function as accessory cells in immune responses. In addition, human alveolar macrophages are responsive to lymphokines (71,72); these T-cell-derived mediators *(vide supra)* activate these cells to kill organisms, such as *M. tuberculosis*, that normally are not killed by these cells.

Further evidence for specific involvement of alveolar macrophages in immune responses *in vivo* comes from studies of individuals immunized with influenza virus (73). Alveolar macrophages recovered from individuals immunized by the aerosol route have elevated levels of lysosomal enzymes, suggesting that these alveolar macrophages are activated. In comparison, no macrophage activation is seen in individuals immunized by the subcutaneous route. Thus, human alveolar macrophages probably participate in immune responses involving the lung, but not necessarily in systemic immune processes that do not involve the lung.

Protection of Alveolar Structures from Protease Attack

Large amounts of proteases may be generated in the lung by inflammatory cells at sites of infection; alveolar macrophages may also protect the alveolar structures from proteolytic attack. In this context, the exact role of the alveolar macrophage is not known, but human macrophages clearly produce α_1-antiproteinase (74,75). Although some of these antiproteases are complexed with proteases, at least some functional antiproteases must be present within the macrophages, because the cytosol of human alveolar macrophages will inhibit human neutrophil elastase (76,77). In addition, it is known that human alveolar macrophages can directly bind and internalize human neutrophil elastase through a defined receptor on the macrophage surface, thus giving this cell an additional direct protective role (78).

PROPERTIES AND FUNCTIONS OF ALVEOLAR LYMPHOCYTES

Morphologic observations of normal human lung suggest that, within the alveolar structures, lymphocytes are found within the interstitium and on the epithelial surface. There is no information concerning lymphocyte traffic to and from the human lung, but it is likely that there is movement of lymphocytes to the alveolar structures from peripheral blood, bronchus-associated lymphoid tissue, and regional lymph nodes (79,80). However, even though such lymphocyte movement is likely, it is clear that in certain instances lung lymphocytes can be "compartmentalized" from the peripheral circulation. For example, evaluations of lung and blood lymphocytes of normal individuals with positive skin tests for *M. tuberculosis* have demonstrated that cells from both sites are sensitized to *M. tuberculosis* antigens (73). In comparison, influenza virus preferentially sensitizes lung lymphocytes when administered via an aerosol, whereas immunization via the subcutaneous route preferentially sensitizes blood lymphocytes.

In normals, the types of lymphocytes found within the alveolar structures are similar to those of blood. Using surface-marker criteria, approximately 73% of alveolar lymphocytes are T cells, and 7% are B cells (1,3,5). The remaining 19% of alveolar lymphocytes do not react with conventional reagents and hence are classified as "null" cells within the lung; with more sensitive techniques, a significant number of such cells have now been identified as T lymphocytes.

The subtypes of alveolar T and B lymphocytes are also similar to those found in peripheral blood. For T lymphocytes, approximately half express OKT-4 or Leu-3a surface antigens (a marker that has been associated with helper/inducer T cells), and 15 to 30% express OKT-8 or Leu-2a surface antigens (a marker that has been associated with suppressor/cytotoxic T cells) (81). The mean ratio of helper T cells to suppressor T cells in the lung is approximately 1.8:1, similar to that found in peripheral blood. The subpopulations of lung T cells may change dramatically, especially in the presence of granulomatous lung diseases (81).

The majority of lung B lymphocytes have stable surface immunoglobulins of the IgM and IgD classes, and a much lower proportion have IgG or IgA on their surfaces (3). In addition, lung B lymphocytes have receptors for complement, probably the C3b fragment (82,83). These findings are consistent with observations made on peripheral blood lymphocytes.

Normally, approximately 0.1 to 0.3% of B lymphocytes within the lung actively secrete immunoglobulins, including IgG, IgM, IgA, and IgE (3). A higher proportion of lung B cells secrete IgA than either IgG or IgM. In addition, a higher percentage of lung B lymphocytes secrete IgA than do blood B cells. These observations are consistent with the concept that IgA is a secretory immunoglobulin localized to the respiratory tract, gut, and glandular structures. The numbers of immunoglobulin-secreting cells in the lung are markedly increased in the presence of a chronic interstitial or infectious process.

There is increasing evidence that human lung lymphocytes function in a way similar to that of peripheral blood lymphocytes. Lung lymphocytes respond to mitogens and antigens and respond in the mixed lymphocyte reaction (10,66,83,84). Human lung lymphocytes have also been shown to produce lymphokines when activated, including macrophage migration-inhibition factor, leukocyte inhibitory factor, IL-2, interferon, and monocyte chemotactic factor (1,2,73,84–87). Lung T cells isolated from patients with active granulomatous lung disorders are actively secreting these lymphokines (1,2,73,84–87). There is some evidence that lung lymphocytes respond less intensely to mitogens than do peripheral blood lymphocytes (83), but it is not clear whether this is an intrinsic property of lung lymphocytes or whether the responses of these cells were suppressed by the macrophages that were also present in these cell suspensions.

Thus, the cellular defenses of the normal lung are due primarily to the presence of alveolar macrophages and lymphocytes. Both cell types possess a wide array of functional processes that are used to protect the lung against invading microorganisms.

BACTERIAL INFECTIONS

To produce pneumonia, bacteria must reach the distal respiratory tract and multiply. The bacteria usually enter through the airway or by hematogenous spread. Only the first mechanism will be addressed, because the latter mechanism results from infection in an extrapulmonary site.

Entry of microorganisms via the airways can occur by inhalation or by aspiration of fluids from the oropharynx. Only small numbers of bacteria are normally present in inspired air. Therefore, the likelihood of significant numbers of bacteria reaching the distal airways by this method is quite small. The hypothesis that inhalation of aerosolized bacteria is an unlikely source of infection is further substantiated by animal experiments. When *Streptococcus pneumoniae* are aerosolized into normal mice, as many as 10^6 organisms may be distributed throughout the lungs, but within 4 hr more than 90% of the bacteria will be killed, and no pneumonia results (88,89). However, if the same number of bacteria are introduced as a bolus via the trachea, the bacteria rapidly multiply and produce lobar pneumonia, with death from overwhelming infection within 48 hr. Aspiration of oropharyngeal secretions during sleep is a frequent occurrence, even in normal individuals (90). These secretions may deliver large numbers of organisms to the distal respiratory tract. These observations suggest that aspiration of secretions from the oropharynx is the most common mode of entry for bacteria causing pneumonia in individuals with normal pulmonary host defenses. Both inhalation and aspiration of bacteria can be important in individuals with compromised pulmonary host defenses.

The type of bacteria that are aspirated into the lung likely is determined by the bacterial flora of the oropharynx. Large numbers of bacteria can be cultured from upper respiratory tract secretions without clinical evidence of disease (91–93). Potentially pathogenic organisms, including S. pneumoniae, Streptococcus pyogenes, Staphylococcus aureus, and Haemophilus influenzae, are present in the secretions of as many as one-third of healthy individuals. It is not clear whether community-acquired pneumonias are caused by strains that have been long-term residents of the upper tract or principally by strains recently acquired by the host. The relationship between colonization and pneumonia has been shown more clearly among hospitalized patients. In only a small percentage of normal individuals is the respiratory tract colonized by Gram-negative enteric bacilli, but most seriously ill patients become colonized with these organisms within 4 to 5 days of entering the hospital (94,95). The risk of subsequent pneumonia is increased 10-fold among such colonized patients, as compared with noncolonized patients with similar illnesses. In this situation, newly acquired organisms appear to cause the greatest risk.

CELLULAR DEFENSES OF THE LUNG

When bacteria are deposited in the lung, either they are eliminated or they multiply, resulting in a pulmonary infection. The capacity of the lung to eliminate bacteria is determined by (a) extracellular factors (described in detail in another chapter), (b) the size of the inoculum of bacteria, (c) the virulence of the bacteria, and (d) the adequacy of the cellular host defense mechanisms.

The effect of the size of the inoculum on the clearance of bacteria from the lung has been shown in various animal studies. For example, the clearance of Pseudomonas aeruginosa from the lungs of mice is dose-dependent, in that a small inoculum is partially cleared from the lung in 4 hr, whereas a larger inoculum leads to marked proliferation of organisms in the same time interval (96). In addition, clearance of the less virulent organism S. aureus is also dependent on the size of the inoculum; the largest doses cause pneumonia and death of the animals (96,97). Although similar studies have not been performed in humans, these studies suggest that the normal lung is capable of clearing small inocula of bacteria, whereas even the normal pulmonary host defenses can be overcome by larger inocula of bacteria.

Clearance of bacteria from the lung is determined not only by the size of the inoculum but also by the type (virulence) of bacteria that are present. For example, a much smaller inoculum of P. aeruginosa is required to cause pulmonary infection and death in mice, as compared with Klebsiella pneumoniae (96). Both organisms are much more virulent than S. aureus. These observations are consistent with clinical observations that have demonstrated marked differences in virulences of various strains of bacteria in humans.

The nature of the phagocytic response to bacteria deposited in the lung also appears to depend on the size of the inoculum and the virulence of the bacteria.

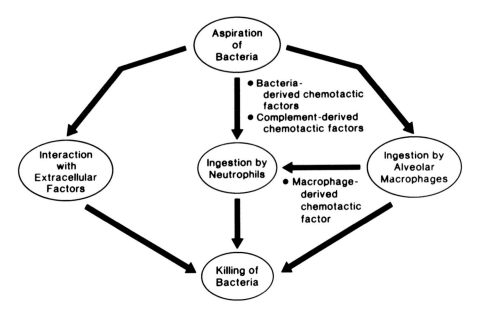

FIG. 4. Pulmonary host defenses against bacteria. Bacteria that are aspirated from the upper airways into the lower respiratory tract are killed by a variety of extracellular factors (described in another chapter), by neutrophils that have migrated from blood into the lung, and/or by resident alveolar macrophages. Neutrophils are attracted to the lung by chemotactic factors derived from bacteria, the complement cascade, and/or alveolar macrophages.

In animal models, relatively nonvirulent bacteria such as *S. aureus* usually are cleared from the lung by alveolar macrophages and extracellular factors (96–99). Neutrophils are recruited to the lung to assist in killing the organisms only following deposition of very large inocula (96,97). In contrast, neutrophils are routinely present in the lung following deposition of relatively small numbers of Gram-negative bacteria (96). Consistent with these findings is the observation that neutropenia does not impair the clearance of *S. aureus* in these models, but it severely impairs the clearance of *K. pneumoniae* and *P. aeruginosa* (96). These observations suggest that resident alveolar macrophages are adequate to clear small numbers of relatively avirulent bacteria, but neutrophils are required to clear larger numbers of more virulent organisms.

A number of factors probably trigger the recruitment of neutrophils to the lung during bacterial infections (Fig. 4). A number of bacteria, themselves, release factors chemotactic for neutrophils (100,101). In addition, a variety of bacteria are also capable of activating the complement cascade (102). As a result of this activation, complement-derived chemotactic factors, such as $C5a_{des-arg}$, are generated that are potent neutrophil chemoattractants. Alveolar macrophages, themselves, also release potent chemoattractants for neutrophils following ingestion of bacteria (103–106). One of these chemotactic factors is a protein with a molecular mass of

10,000 to 15,000 daltons, and the other factor is a lipid with a molecular mass of 400 to 600 daltons.

VIRAL INFECTIONS

Although the lung is an important site of viral infections, little is known about the pulmonary host defenses against these agents in humans. From other studies, however, it is known that the host's antiviral immune response is frequently mediated both by the production of antibodies and by cell-mediated mechanisms. These antibody and cell-mediated processes are not always distinct, and they frequently interact to contain the viral process. For example, antibody can exert an antiviral effect on its own or can mediate its effect in conjunction with complement, K cells, or macrophages. An important cellular mechanism involves T cells, which can lyse virus-infected cells directly or secondarily through the release of mediators (i.e., lymphokines such as interferon) that activate other cells such as macrophages or natural killer cells (NK cells). Thus, in most infections, antibody and cell-mediated mechanisms operate together. However, for certain viruses, particularly those that spread from cell to cell and express viral antigen in the host membrane, cell-mediated immunity appears to be of major importance. On the other hand, antiviral antibody appears to play a major role in neutralizing free virus in extracellular fluid.

B cells appears to play an important role in antiviral responses in the lung by responding to viral challenge with the production of antibody. Viral antibody can be IgG, IgA, or IgM. All three types of antibody can be produced locally in the lung (107–111). IgA antibody is particularly important on mucosal surfaces, where it plays a major role in resistance to infection by neutralizing virus and preventing its adherence to the mucous membrane (112–114). The main type of antibody in respiratory secretions is secretory IgA (107–110). For example, immunity to influenza can be shown to be related to the titer of IgA antibody in nasal or bronchial secretions (107–109). A correlation between the presence of secretory IgA and protection against viral infection has also been shown for several other viruses, including parainfluenza type I, rhinovirus type 1B, respiratory syncytial virus, and poliovirus (110). Furthermore, it appears that the production of secretory IgA is a local phenomenon occurring only at sites directly stimulated by viral antigen. For example, aerosol vaccination with influenza virus stimulates only a production of nasal and bronchial antibody (107–111).

The role of T cells in viral infections, including those that infect the lung, is clearly demonstrated in T-cell deficiency states, in which a variety of recurring and sometimes fatal viral infections occur. Patients with T-cell deficiency states usually have normal responses to most pyogenic bacterial infections, but they are particularly susceptible to viruses and infections with intracellular organisms (115–118). Children with T-cell deficiency develop an atypical and serious form of measles, with massive virus replication in the lung, often leading to giant-cell pneumonia and death (119). Severe generalized infections (frequently involving the lung) with herpesviruses are also common in T-cell deficiency states, as well as in patients receiving immunosuppressive therapy, which decreases cellular immunity (120–126). These observations suggest that T cells are essential for recovery from a variety of viral infections.

T cells can inhibit viral replication by a number of mechanisms. They can lyse virus-infected cells (127–130). Because this can occur as early as 1 to 2 hr after infection, before viral replication occurs, this mechanism can be of major importance in limiting the spread of infection *in vivo*. As noted earlier, immune T cells can also act by secreting lymphokines that activate macrophages that can ingest and destroy virus particles. These lymphokines, especially interferon, can also protect adjacent uninfected cells from the virus and can also activate NK cells (131–134). The NK cells can then further inhibit virus growth.

Although virus-specific cytotoxic T cells have been demonstrated in various animal models, the presence of these cells has not yet been shown in the human lung. However, it is likely that these T cells are also present in the human lung, for the following reasons: Human lung T cells have been shown to be capable of responding to a wide variety of other antigens *in vitro* (10,66,83,84). A large portion of the T cells in the human lung express OKT-8 or Leu-2a surface antigens; virus-specific cytotoxic T cells usually express these surface antigens (81). Most important, viral infections, which frequently occur in individuals with T-cell deficiency disorders, rarely cause severe lung disease in nonimmunosuppressed normal individuals. Furthermore, it has also been shown that human lung T cells can release a variety of lymphokines, including interferon, following activation by antigens or mitogens (1,2,73,84–87). Thus, it is likely that these cells play a major role in controlling viral infections in the human lung.

Antibody-dependent cellular cytotoxicity (ADCC) (mediated by K cells) has been demonstrated in several different systems *in vitro* (135–137). However, in contrast to the situation with T cells, the value of K cells in defense against virus infection is less clear. ADCC appears to be a very efficient system of cell lysis, requiring very small amounts of antibody (compared with the amounts required for antibody- and complement-dependent lysis of virus-infected cells). The K cell has no immunological specificity; this is conferred by the antibody coating the target cell. The role of K cells *in vivo*, however, is difficult to establish. One family with a K-cell deficiency has been described (138); all of these subjects are healthy, and there is no past history of serious illness. These observations suggest that K-cell activity may not be crucial to contain viral infections, especially if other antiviral mechanisms are intact.

NK cells may play a role in viral infections by killing virus-infected cells by an antibody-independent mechanism (131,139,140). Cells susceptible to lysis by NK cells include virus-transformed cells, cells persistently infected with virus, and certain tumor cells (132,133,141,142). Although these phenomena are demonstrable *in vitro*, the role of these cells has not been well defined *in vivo*. NK-cell activity is absent in severe combined immunodeficiency disease, but these individuals also have severe defects in T-cell functions (143). The beige mouse is an animal model of NK-cell deficiency (144). The susceptibility of these animals to viral infections has not been systemically evaluated. However, they do appear to have a lower natural resistance to virus-induced tumors (145). The beige mouse appears to be an animal homologue of the human Chediak-Higashi syndrome. Patients with this disorder also exhibit a deficiency of NK cells (146). This rare autosomal-recessive disease is characterized by partial albinism, giant lysosomal granules in most granule-containing cells, and increased susceptibility to infections, especially bacterial infections (147). The microbicidal defect appears to be due to the slow degranulation of the giant primary granules of phagocytic cells, thereby delaying the killing of ingested bacteria (148,149). This disease is also characterized by a lymphomalike infiltration in the liver, spleen, nerves, and other tissues (147). However, it is unclear if this lymphohistiocytic infiltration of tissues is related in any way to a low-grade viral process or to the defect in NK-cell activity.

It has been difficult to demonstrate the presence of K cells and NK cells in the lung. In animal models and in studies of human lung cells, the functional activities of both of these types of cells appear to be severely depressed (150,151). However, it is not clear if these cells are not present in the lung or if the functional expression of these cells is depressed by alveolar macrophages. In the studies that have been reported to date, alveolar macrophages have been present in cell suspensions isolated from the lung. It has been demonstrated that alveolar macrophages can suppress the activities of both K cells and NK cells *in vitro* (152). Recent studies using monoclonal antibodies specific for NK cells have shown that these cells are present in the lung, but the cells do not express functional activity (G. W. Hunninghake, *unpublished data*). These observations suggest that the normal lung may not be deficient in K cells or NK cells, but that the activity of these cells is simply suppressed *in vitro* by alveolar macrophages.

An important factor inducing NK activity is stimulation of these cells by interferon (131–134). Interferon induces NK-cell activity when added to the assay or when induced by viruses in cultures. Because interferon is produced *in vivo* during viral infections, activation of NK cells by this lymphokine may play an important role in the host's ability to limit viral infections. Interferon also has broad direct antiviral effects that include inhibition of viral infection in susceptible cells. Both human lung T cells and alveolar macrophages can release interferon following activation *in vitro* (87). In addition, it has also been shown in patients with collagen vascular disorders and sarcoidosis that these cells are stimulated to release interferon *in vivo* (87). These observations suggest that this important mediator is released locally during viral infections of the lung and plays an important role in recovery from these infections. In addition, as noted earlier, alveolar macrophages can also directly inactivate certain viruses (37). In summary, the antiviral defenses of the lung depend on extracellular and cellular factors that interact to contain the viral infection.

GRANULOMATOUS LUNG INFECTIONS

The presence of granulomata is a prominent feature of a wide variety of lung infections, especially those caused by certain mycobacteria, fungi, or helminths (153–156). Granulomata are focal collections of inflammatory cells characterized primarily by the presence of cells derived from mononuclear phagocytes, i.e., macrophages, epithelioid cells, and multinucleated giant cells (155,157). These "hypersensitivity" or immune granulomata are characterized not only by focal collections of mononuclear phagocytes but also by prominent collections of T lymphocytes at the periphery (155,157). Thus, these granulomatous infections are characterized by an intense interaction between mononuclear phagocytes and T lymphocytes in the lung.

Although granulomata are the characteristic pathological feature of these lung diseases, it is now clear from a variety of studies that the initial lesion in these disorders is an alveolitis, i.e., a collection of mononuclear cells in the alveolar structures (153,154). The alveolitis appears to provide the appropriate environment for granuloma formation; i.e., inflammatory cells initially accumulate in the lung, and these cells are then utilized for the formation of granulomata. A number of types of cells, including neutrophils, eosinophils, basophils, mast cells, and B lymphocytes, can compose the alveolitis of these disorders; however, the most prominent types of cells present are macrophages and T lymphocytes (153–156). The prominence of these two cell types is not surprising in view of the observation that mononuclear phagocytes and T lymphocytes also compose the majority of cells that make up these granulomata. It is the presence and interaction of these two cell types in the lung that appear to be crucial for the development of the granuloma.

Mechanisms of Granuloma Formation

The initial event that triggers granuloma formation in most of these disorders is deposition of an antigenic substance in the lung. During most cellular immune responses that are initiated by antigen exposure in humans, the antigen is taken up first by a monocyte or macrophage (60–63). These monocytes/macrophages not only attempt to destroy the antigen (by mechanisms that were described earlier) but also present the antigen to specific T lymphocytes. The monocyte/macrophage that presents these antigens to T cells also displays Ia antigens on its cell surface (Ia$^+$) (60–63). In humans, monocytes/macrophages can express two types of Ia antigens: HLA-DR (which is homologous with the murine I-E determinant) and HLA-DS (which is homologous with the murine I-A determinant) (158,159). Almost all monocytes/macrophages express HLA-DR antigens, but only a portion of these cells express the HLA-DS cell surface antigen (159). This is an important observation, because only HLA-DS$^+$ monocytes/macrophages appear to be able to present antigens to specific T cells (159).

A number of lines of evidence suggest that monocytes/macrophages play a similar role in initiating the immune response in granulomatous lung infections. In humans it has been demonstrated that almost all alveolar macrophages are HLA-DR$^+$ (68).

Glazier et al. (69) have recently shown that most alveolar macrophages are also HLA-DS$^+$. In addition, alveolar macrophages from patients with active granulomatous lung disorders spontaneously release IL-1, the other macrophage product essential for T-lymphocyte activation (70).

Consistent with these observations is the finding that alveolar macrophages from both normal individuals and patients with sarcoidosis (another granulomatous lung disorder) appear to be capable of presenting common antigens to T cells (160). Furthermore, in a murine model of granuloma formation in the lung induced by parenteral injection of schistosome eggs, it has been demonstrated that nearly 80% of macrophages derived from such granulomata are I-A$^+$ (homologous to human HLA-DS$^+$) and capable of antigen presentation *in vitro* (161). Thus, the macrophages in these disorders are particularly primed to interact with T cells in order to maintain the cellular immune response and thus granuloma formation.

Once the alveolar macrophage has presented the antigen to a specific T lymphocyte and has released IL-1, various types of lung T cells respond by expressing a receptor for IL-2 and by releasing other lymphokines, including IL-2 (64,162–164). IL-2 causes appropriately primed T cells to proliferate. Furthermore, because both IL-1 and IL-2 are chemoattractants for peripheral blood T lymphocytes, these mediators can recruit additional T cells to the site of an immune response (165). Thus, IL-1 and IL-2 can increase the numbers of T lymphocytes at sites of an immune response both by attracting T cells from the circulation and by stimulating these cells to divide.

It is likely that the numbers of T cells in the lungs of patients with granulomatous lung diseases are increased by a similar mechanism. Much of this information has been obtained from studies of patients with sarcoidosis. In this regard, supernatants of unstimulated bronchoalveolar cells from patients with active pulmonary sarcoidosis contain IL-1 (70), IL-2 (85,86), and substance(s) with chemotactic activity for blood T cells (166). The IL-1 is released by the sarcoid alveolar macrophages, and IL-2 is released by the sarcoid alveolar T cells. The chemotactic activity is due to the presence of both IL-1 and IL-2 in the supernatants. Similar support for this pulmonary sequestration of T cells is found in an animal model of hypersensitivity pneumonitis following inhalational challenge with a fungal antigen (167).

The activated lung T lymphocytes in patients with granulomatous lung disease not only release mediators that increase their own cell numbers but also release monocyte chemotactic factor (2,168–170), a lymphokine that attracts monocytes to the lung. This is a crucial feature of granuloma formation, because granulomata are composed primarily of macrophages, epithelioid cells, and multinucleated giant cells, all cells that are ultimately derived from blood monocytes (155). Similar results have been reported in a murine model of pulmonary hypersensitivity granuloma formation (168).

The lung T lymphocyte also releases other lymphokines, such as migration-inhibition factor (MIF) and various macrophage-activating factors, that interact with monocytes/macrophages to form the structure we recognize as a granuloma. This has been shown to be the case in various animal models of granulomatous lung disease (168–170), and in both hypersensitivity pneumonitis (171) and sarcoidosis (84), lung T cells have been found to be spontaneously releasing MIF.

The granuloma provides a site at which very resistant organisms can be "walled off" from noninfected areas of lung and, most important, an environment in which these organisms can be killed (40,155,157). As noted earlier, normal macrophages will not kill mycobacterial or fungal organisms unless they have been activated. In the granulomata, macrophages are highly activated and release large amounts of reactive oxygen species and digestive enzymes that are toxic to these organisms. If the organisms are low in number, the granulomatous response is entirely beneficial. However, if the numbers of organisms are high, the reaction is frequently detrimental. Macrophages and the surrounding tissue die, undergoing caseous necrosis.

Modulation of Disease Activity

Both the quantity and the physical characteristics of the antigen deposited in the lung influence disease activity in many of the granulomatous lung infections. Many of the antigens that trigger a granulomatous process resist degradation by inflammatory cells. Thus, in diseases such as tuberculosis and pulmonary fungal infections, the persistence of antigen in the lung is the primary stimulus for active disease (155,156). The disease usually remains active until either the antigen is removed or the antigen load is markedly decreased.

Deposition of antigen in the lung, however, does not always lead to the same type or degree of immune response in all individuals similarly exposed. The immune response is determined by the amount and duration of antigen exposure, but it is also influenced by the competence of the exposed individual's immune system. For example, individuals in whom cellular immunity is depressed, either because of an underlying disease or because of immunosuppressive therapy, remove viable organisms from the lower respiratory tract in a less efficient fashion and tend to have more severe and progressive disease (172–175).

Another variable that likely helps determine the immune response in the lung is the genetic background of the individual in whom the disease develops. In this regard, it has been demonstrated in an animal model that deposition of tuberculous organisms in the lower respiratory tract results in variable responses in animals of different genetic backgrounds (176). In some mice, for example, deposition of BCG into the lower respiratory tract results in a minor granulomatous response. In other mice, deposition of the same numbers of organisms leads to a marked granulomatous response. Although it is much more difficult to determine if genetic factors are important in these diseases in humans, it is likely that they play a significant role in determining the severity of the disease process.

Although it is likely that the process of granuloma formation is influenced by the type and duration of exposure to antigen and the genetic background and immune status of the individual with the disorder, it is also clear that the process of granuloma formation is modulated by the presence of regulatory T lymphocytes. It has been demonstrated in a number of animal models that helper T lymphocytes are prominent early in the process of granuloma formation, but later, during a time of diminishing granuloma size, suppressor T cells predominate (169,177). Presumably these suppressor T lymphocytes dampen or modulate the disease process.

There is also evidence in patients with granulomatous lung disorders that disease activity is modulated by suppressor T lymphocytes. In patients with sarcoidosis, for example, the lung T lymphocytes of patients with active disease are characterized by marked increases in the numbers of helper T cells (81,86). In normal individuals, the ratio of helper to suppressor T cells in both blood and lung is approximately 1.8:1. In patients with active sarcoidosis, this ratio can be as high as 5:1 to 20:1. In marked contrast, the T lymphocytes that are present at sites of disease in patients with inactive or stable lung disease are primarily suppressor T lymphocytes, and the ratio of helper to suppressor T cells is decreased (81,86).

SUMMARY

These studies demonstrate that the human lung has a potent cellular armamentarium that is used to contain a variety of pulmonary infections. This hypothesis is supported by the observation that severe and prolonged pulmonary infections are unusual in normal individuals. Although many of these cellular processes are poorly understood, our knowledge in this area is expanding at a rapid rate. These studies should increase our knowledge of the pathogenesis of these disorders and also improve our therapy for these disorders.

REFERENCES

1. Hunninghake, G. W., Fulmer, J. D., Young, R. C., Gadek, J. E., and Crystal, R. G. (1979): Localization of the immune response in sarcoidosis. *Am. Rev. Respir. Dis.*, 120:49–57.
2. Hunninghake, G. W., Gadek, J. E., Young, R. C., Kawanami, O., Ferrans, V. J., and Crystal, R. G. (1980): Maintenance of granuloma formation in pulmonary sarcoidosis by T-lymphocytes within the lung. *N. Engl. J. Med.*, 302:594–598.
3. Hunninghake, G. W., Gadek, J. E., Kawanami, O., Ferrans, V. J., and Crystal, R. G. (1979): Inflammatory and immune processes in the human lung in health and disease: Evaluation by bronchoalveolar lavage. *Am. J. Pathol.*, 97:149–206.
4. Hunninghake, G. W., Gadek, J. E., Szapiel, S. V., Strumpf, I. J., Kawanami, O., Ferrans, V. J., and Crystal, R. G. (1980): The human alveolar macrophage. In: *Methods in Cell Biology, Vol. 21A,* edited by C. Harris, B. F. Trump, and G. D. Stonder, pp. 95–112. Academic Press, New York.
5. Hunninghake, G. W., Kawanami, O., Ferrans, V. J., Young, R. C., Jr., Roberts, W. C., and Crystal, R. G. (1981): Characterization of the inflammatory and immune effector cells in the lung parenchyma of patients with interstitial lung disease. *Am. Rev. Respir. Dis.*, 123:407–412.
6. Reynolds, H. Y., and Newball, H. H. (1976): Fluid and cellular milieu of the human respiratory tract. In: *Immunologic and Infectious Reactions in the Lung. Vol. I,* edited by C. H. Kirkpatrick and H. Y. Reynolds, pp. 3–27. Marcel Dekker, New York.
7. Reynolds, H. Y., and Newball, H. H. (1974): Analysis of proteins and respiratory cells obtained from human lungs by bronchial lavage. *J. Lab. Clin.*, 84:559–573.
8. Low, R. B., David, G. S., and Giancola, M. S. (1978): Biochemical analyses of bronchoalveolar lavage fluids of healthy human volunteer smokers and nonsmokers. *Am. Rev. Respir. Dis.*, 118:863–875.
9. Reynolds, H. Y. (1979): The importance of lymphocytes in pulmonary health and disease. *Lung,* 155:225–242.
10. Daniele, R. P., Dauber, J. H., Altose, M. D., Rowlands, D. T., and Gorenberg, D. J. (1977):

Lymphocyte studies in asymptomatic cigarette smokers. A comparison between lung and peripheral blood. *Am. Rev. Respir. Dis.*, 116:997–1005.

11. Langevoort, H. C., Cohn, Z. A., Hirsch, J. G., Humphrey, J. H., Spector, W. G., and van Furth, R. (1970): The nomenclature of mononuclear phagocytic cells. In: *Proposal for a New Classification, Mononuclear Phagocytes*, edited by R. Van Furth, pp. 1–6. F. A. Davis, Philadelphia.

12. Brain, J. D., Golde, D. W., Green, G. M., Massaro, D. J., Valberg, P. A., Ward, P. A., and Werb, Z. (1978): Biologic potential of pulmonary macrophages. *Am. Rev. Respir. Dis.*, 118:435–443.

13. Cline, M. J., Lehrer, R. I., Territo, M. C., and Golde, D. W. (1978): Monocytes and macrophages: Functions and disease. *Ann. Intern. Med.*, 88:78–88.

14. Golde, D. W. (1977): Kinetics and function of the human alveolar macrophage. *J. Reticuloendothel. Soc.*, 22:223–230.

15. Thomas, E. D., Ramberg, R. E., Sale, G. E., Sparkes, R. S., and Golde, D. W. (1976): Direct evidence for a bone marrow origin of the alveolar macrophage in man. *Science*, 192:1016–1017.

16. Golde, D. W., Byers, L. A., and Finley, T. N. (1974): Proliferative capacity of alveolar macrophage. *Nature*, 247:373–375.

17. Barry, B. E., Crapo, J. D., Gehr, P., Bachofen, M., and Weibel, E. R. (1979): Population characteristics of the cells in normal human lung. *Am. Rev. Respir. Dis.*, 119:287A.

18. Adamson, I. Y. R., and Bowden, D. H. (1979): Role of monocytes and interstitial cells in the generation of alveolar macrophages. *F.A.S.E.B.*, 38:1205.

19. Bowden, D. H., and Adamson, I. Y. R. (1972): The pulmonary interstitial cell as immediate precursor of the alveolar macrophage. *Am. J. Pathol.*, 68:521–536.

20. Brian, J. D., Sorkin, S. P., and Godleski, J. L. (1977): Quantification, origin, and fate of pulmonary macrophages. In: *Respiratory Defense Mechanisms, Vol. 5, Part 2*, edtied by J. D. Brain, D. R. Proctor, and L. M. Reed, pp. 849–892. Marcel Dekker, New York.

21. Daughaday, C. C., and Douglas, S. D. (1976): Membrane receptors on rabbit and human pulmonary alveolar macrophages. *J. Reticuloendothel. Soc.*, 19:37–45.

22. Reynolds, H. Y., Atkinson, J. P., Newball, H. H., and Frank, M. M. (1975): Receptors for immunoglobulin and complement on human alveolar macrophages. *J. Immunol.*, 114:1813–1819.

23. Warr, G. A., and Martin, R. R. (1977): Immune receptors of human alveolar macrophages. Comparison between cigarette smokers and nonsmokers. *J. Reticuloendothel. Soc.*, 22:181–187.

24. Joseph, M., Tonnel, A., Torpier, G., and Capron, A. (1983): Involvement of immunoglobulin E in the secretory processes of alveolar macrophages from asthmatic patients. *J. Clin. Invest.*, 71:221–230.

25. Speigelberg, H. L., Boltz-Nitulescu, G., Plummer, J. M., and Melewicz, F. M. (1983): Characterization of the IgE Fc receptors on monocytes and macrophages. *Fed. Proc.*, 72:124–128.

26. Reynolds, H. Y., Kazmierowski, J. A., and Newball, H. H. (1975): Specificity of opsonic antibodies to enhance phagocytosis of *Pseudomonas aeruginosa* by human alveolar macrophages. *J. Clin. Invest.*, 56:376–385.

27. Hunninghake, G. W., Gadek, J. E., and Crystal, R. G. (1980): Human alveolar macrophage neutrophil chemotactic factor: Stimuli and partial characterization. *J. Clin. Invest.*, 66:473–483.

28. Werb, Z., Foley, R., and Munck, S. (1978): Interaction of glucocorticoids with macrophages. Identification of glucocorticoid receptors in monocytes and macrophages. *J. Exp. Med.*, 147:1684–1694.

29. Loscasco, J., and Daniele, R. P. (1979): Modulation of β-adrenergic receptors in alveolar macrophage membranes: The effect of phagocytosis and adherence. *Am. Rev. Respir. Dis.*, 119:74A (abstract).

30. Debanne, M. T., Bell, R., and Dolovich, J. (1975): Uptake of proteinase-α-macroglobulin complexes by macrophages. *Biochim. Biophys. Acta*, 411:295–304.

31. Dolovich, J., Debanne, M. T., and Bell, R. (1975): The role of alpha-antitrypsin and alpha-macroglobulins in the uptake of proteinase by rabbit alveolar macrophages. *Am. Rev. Respir. Dis.*, 112:521–525.

32. Stahl, P. D., Rodman, J. S., Miller, M. J., and Schlesinger, P. H. (1978): Evidence for receptor-mediated binding by glycoproteins, glycoconjugates, and lysosomal glycosidases by alveolar macrophages. *Proc. Natl. Acad. Sci. U.S.A.*, 75:1399–1403.

33. Van Snick, J. L., and Masson, P. L. (1976): The binding of human lactoferrin to mouse peritoneal cells. *J. Exp. Med.*, 144:1568–1580.

34. Van Snick, J. L., Markowetz, B., and Masson, P. L. (1977): The ingestions and digestion of human

lactoferrin by mouse peritoneal macrophages and the transfer of its iron into ferritin. *J. Exp. Med.*, 146:817–827.

35. Harris, J. O., Swenson, E. W., and Johnson, J. E., III (1970): Human alveolar macrophages: Comparison of phagocytic ability, glucose utilization, and ultrastructure in smokers and non-smokers. *J. Clin. Invest.*, 49:2086–2096.

36. Martin, R. R., and Warr, G. A. (1977): Cigarette smoking and human alveolar macrophages. *Hosp. Practice*, 86:97–104.

37. Drew, W. L., Mintz, L., Hoo, R., and Finley, T. N. (1979): Growth of herpes simplex and cytomegalovirus in cultured human alveolar macrophages. *Am. Rev. Respir. Dis.*, 119:287–291.

38. Cohen, A. B., and Cline, M. J. (1971): The human alveolar macrophages: Isolation, cultivation *in vitro*, and studies of morphologic and functional characteristics. *J. Clin. Invest.*, 50:1390–1398.

39. Hoidal, J. R., Fox, R. B., Takiff, H. E., and Repine, J. E. (1979): Alveolar macrophages (AM) from young, asymptomatic cigarette smokers (CS) and nonsmokers (NS) use equal amounts of oxygen (O_2) and glucose (1-^{14}C), but smoke AM make more superoxide anion (O_2^-). *Am. Rev. Respir. Dis.*, 119:222A (abstract).

40. Dannenberg, A.M., Jr. (1982): Pathogenesis of pulmonary tuberculosis. *Am. Rev. Respir. Dis.*, 125:25–29.

41. Bates, J. H. (1982): Susceptibility and resistance. *Am. Rev. Respir. Dis.*, 125:20–24.

42. North, R. J. (1974): T-cell dependence of macrophage activation and mobilization during infection with *Mycobacerium tuberculosis. Infect. Immun.*, 10:66–71.

43. Dannenberg, A. M., Jr., Ando, M., and Shima, K. (1972): Macrophage accumulation, division, maturation, and digestive and microbicidal capacities in tuberculous lesions. *J. Immunol.*, 109:1109–1121.

44. Dannenberg, A. M., Jr., and Ando, M., Shima, K., and Tsuda, T. (1973): Macrophage turnover and activation in tuberculous granulomata. In: *Mononuclear Phagocytes in Immunity, Infection and Pathology*, edited by R. Van Furth, p. 959. Blackwell, Oxford.

45. Dannenberg, A.M., Jr. (1975): Macrophages in inflammation and infection. *N. Engl. J. Med.*, 293:489–493.

46. Mitchison, D. A., Selkon, J. B., and Lloyd, J. (1963): Virulence in the guinea-pig, susceptibility to hydrogen peroxide, and catalase activity of isoniazid-sensitive tubercle bacilli from South Indian and British patients. *J. Pathol. Bacteriol.*, 86:377–386.

47. Armstrong, J. A., and Hart, P. D. (1975): Phagosome-lysosome interactions in cultured macrophages infected with virulent tubercle bacilli. *J. Exp. Med.*, 142:1–16.

48. Jackett, P. S., Aber, V. R., and Lowrie, D. B. (1978): Virulence of *Mycobacterium tuberculosis* and susceptibility to peroxidative killing systems. *J. Gen. Microbiol.*, 107:273–278.

49. Jackett, P. S., Aber, V. R., and Lowrie, D. B. (1980): The susceptibility of strains of *Mycobacterium tuberculosis* to catalase-mediated peroxidative killing. *J. Gen. Microbiol.*, 121:381–386.

50. Allison, A. C. (1977): Mechansisms of macrophage damage in relation to the pathogenesis of some lung diseases. In: *Respiration Defense Mechanisms, Vol. 5, Part 2*, edited by J. D. Brain, D. R. Proctor, and L. M. Reed, pp. 1075–1102. Marcel Dekker, New York.

51. Yeager, H., Jr., Zimmet, S. M., and Schwartz, S. L. (1974): Pinocytosis of human alveolar macrophages. Comparison of smokers and nonsmokers. *J. Clin. Invest.*, 54:247–251.

52. McLemore, T. L., Corson, M. A., Martin, R. R., Arnott, M., Jenkins, W. T., Brinkley, B. R., Mace, M. L., Snodgrass, D. R., and Wray, N. P. (1979): Cytototoxicity and AHH enzyme induction in human pulmonary macrophages and lymphocytes cultured with asbestos. *Am. Rev. Respir. Dis.*, 119:229A (abstract).

53. Abraham, J. L., and Brambilla, C. (1979): Particle size for differentiation between inhalation and injection pulmonary talcosis. *Am. Rev. Respir. Dis.*, 119:196A (abstract).

54. Brambilla, C., Abraham, J. L., Brambilla, E., Venirschke, K., and Bloor, C. (1979): Comparative pathology of silicate pneumoconiosis. *Am. J. Pathol.*, 96:149–170.

55. Abraham, J. L. (1978): Recent advances in pneumoconiosis: The pathologist's role in etiologic diagnosis. In: *The Lung*, edited by W. M. Thurlbeck and M. R. Abell, pp. 96–137. Williams & Wilkins, Baltimore.

56. McCuen, D., and Abraham, J. L. (1972): Particulate concentration in pulmonary alveolar proteinosis. *Environ. Res.*, 17:334–339.

57. Hook, G. E. R., Bell, D. Y., Gilmore, L. B., Nadeau, D., Reasor, M. J., and Talley, F. A. (1978): Composition of bronchoalveolar lavage effluents from patients with pulmonary alveolar proteinosis. *Lab. Invest.*, 39:342–357.

58. Golde, D. W., Territo, M., Finley, T. N., and Cline, M. J. (1976): Defective lung macrophages in pulmonary alveolar proteinosis. *Ann. Intern. Med.*, 85:304–309.

59. Nugent, K. M., and Pesanti, E. L. (1983): Macrophage function in pulmonary alveolar proteinosis. *Am. Rev. Respir. Dis.*, 127:780–781.

60. Shevach, E. M., and Rosenthal, A. S. (1973): Function of macrophages in antigen recognition by guinea pig T lymphocytes: II. Role of the macrophage in the regulation of genetic control of the immune response. *J. Exp. Med.*, 138:1213–1229.

61. Unanue, E. R. (1980): Cooperation between mononuclear phagocytes and lymphocytes in immunity. *N. Engl. J. Med.*, 303:977–985.

62. Rosenthal, A. S. (1980): Regulation of the immune response: Role of the macrophage. *N. Engl. J. Med.*, 303:1153–1156.

63. Unanue, E. R. (1981): Symbiotic relationships between macrophages and lymphocytes. *Adv. Exp. Med. Biol.*, 155:49–63.

64. Oppenheim, J. J., Stadler, B. M., and Mathieson, B. (1982): Lymphokines: Their role in lymphocyte responses. Properties of interleukin-1. *Fed. Proc.*, 4:257–262.

65. Lussier, L. M., Chandler, D. K. F., Sybert, A., and Yaeger, H. (1978): Human alveolar macrophages: Antigen-independent binding of lymphocytes. *J. Appl. Physiol.*, 45:933–938.

66. Laughter, A. H., Martin, R. R., and Twomey, J. R. (1977): Lymphoproliferative responses to antigens mediated by human pulmonary alveolar macrophages. *J. Lab. Clin. Med.*, 89:1326–1332.

67. Toews, G. B., Vial, W. C., Dunn, M. M., Guzzetta, P., Nunez, G., Stastny, P., and Lipscomb, M. F. (1984): The accessory cell function of human alveolar macrophages in specific T cell proliferation. *J. Immunol.*, 132:181–186.

68. Mason, R., Austyn, J., Brodsky, F., and Gordon, S. (1982): Monoclonal antimacrophage antibodies: Human pulmonary macrophages express HLA-DR (Ia-like) antigens in culture. *Am. Rev. Respir. Dis.*, 125:586–593.

69. Glazier, A. J., Jr., Monick, M., and Hunninghake, G. W. (1984): Human alveolar macrophages express HLA-DS as well as HLA-DR antigens. *(Submitted)*.

70. Hunninghake, G. W. (1984): Correlation of interleukin-1 release by alveolar macrophages with disease activity in pulmonary sarcoidosis. *Am. Rev. Respir. Dis.*, 129:569–572.

71. Warr, G. A., and Martin, R. R. (1973): Responses of human pulmonary macrophages to migration inhibition factor. *Am. Rev. Respir. Dis.*, 108:371–373.

72. Bartfeld, H., and Atoynatan, T. (1970): Cellular immunity: Activity and properties of human migration inhibitory factor. *Int. Arch. Allergy Appl. Immunol.*, 38:549–553.

73. Jurgensen, P. F., Olsen, G. N., Johnson, J. E., III, Swenson, E. W., Ayoub, E. M., Henney, C. S., and Waldman, R. H. (1973): Immune response of the human respiratory tract: II. Cell-mediated immunity in the lower respiratory tract to tuberculin and mumps and influenza viruses. *J. Infect. Dis.*, 128:730–735.

74. Cohen, A. B. (1973): Interrelationships between the human alveolar macrophage and alpha-1-antitrypsin. *J. Clin. Invest.*, 52:2793–2799.

75. Olsen, G. N., Harris, J. O., Castle, J. R., Waldman, R. H., and Karmgard, H. J. (1975): Alpha-1-antitrypsin content in the serum, alveolar macrophages, and alveolar lavage fluid of smoking and nonsmoking normal subjects. *J. Clin. Invest.*, 55:527–530.

76. Harris, J. O., and Goldblatt, J. (1976): Properties of alveolar alpha-1-antitrypsin in man. *Clin. Res.*, 24:385A (abstract).

77. Blondin, J., Rosenbert, R., and Janoff, A. (1972): An inhibitor in human lung macrophages active against human neutrophil elastase. *Am. Rev. Respir. Dis.*, 106:477–479.

78. Campbell, E. J., White, R. R., Senior, R. M., Rodriguez, F. J., and Kuhn, C. (1979): Receptor-mediated binding and internalization of leukocyte elastase by alveolar macrophages *in vitro. J. Clin. Invest.*,   .

79. Bienenstock, J., Clancy, R. L., and Perey, D. Y. (1976): Bronchus associated lymphoid tissue (BALT): Its relationship to mucosal immunity. In: *Immunologic and Infectious Reactions in the Lung, Vol. 1*, edited by C. H. Kirkpatrick and H. Y. Reynolds, pp. 29–58. Marcel Dekker, New York.

80. Daniele, R. P., Beacham, C. H., and Gorenberg, D. J. (1977): The bronchoalveolar lymphocyte: Studies on the life history and lymphocyte traffic from blood to the lung. *Cell. Immunol.*, 31:48–54.

81. Hunninghake, G. W., and Crystal, R. G. (1981): Pulmonary sarcoidosis: A disorder mediated by excess helper T-lymphocyte at sites of disease activity. *N. Engl. J. Med.*, 305:429–434.

82. Warr, G. A., Martin, K. K., Holleman, C. L., and Criswell, B. S. (1976): Classification of bronchial lymphoctyes from smokers and nonsmokers. *Am. Rev. Respir. Dis.*, 113:96–100.

83. Daniele, R. P., Altose, M. D., and Rowlands, D. T., Jr. (1975): Immunocompetent cells from the lower respiratory tract of normal human lungs. *J. Clin. Invest.*, 56:986–995.

84. Hunninghake, G. W., Keogh, B. A., Line, B. R., Gadek, J. E., Kawanami, O., Ferrans, V. J., and Crystal, R. G. (1981): Pulmonary sarcoidosis: Pathogenesis and therapy. In: *Basic and Clinical Aspects of Granulomatous Disease*, edited by D. Boros and T. Yoshida, pp. 275–290. Elsevier/North-Holland, Amsterdam.

85. Pinkston, P., Bitterman, P. B., and Crystal, R. G. (1983): Spontaneous release of interleukin-2 by lung T-lymphocytes in active pulmonary sarcoidosis. *N. Engl. J. Med.*, 308:793–800.

86. Hunninghake, G. W., Bedell, G. H., Zavala, D. C., Monick, M.,and Brady, M. (1983): Role of interleukin-2 release by lung T-cells in active pulmonary sarcoidosis. *Am. Rev. Respir. Dis.*, 128:634–638.

87. Nugent, K., Monick, M., and Hunninghake, G. W. (1983): Alveolar macrophages from patients with sarcoidosis spontaneously secrete interferon. *(submitted)*.

88. Ansfield, M. J., Woods, D. E., and Johanson, W. G., Jr. (1977): Lung bacterial clearance in murine pneumococcal pneumonia. *Infect. Immun.*, 17:195–201.

89. Johanson, W. G., Pierce, A. K., and Sanford, J. P. (1974): Bacterial growth *in vivo*: An important determinant of pulmonary clearance of *Diplococcus pneumoniae* in rats. *J. Clin. Invest.*, 53:1320–1329.

90. Huxley, E. J., Viroslav, J., Gray, W. R., and Pierce, A. K. (1978): Pharyngeal aspiration in normal adults and patients with depressed consciousness. *Am. J. Med.*, 64:564–572.

91. Ostrom, C. A., Wolochow, H., and James, H. A. (1958): Studies on the experimental epidemiology of respiratory disease: IX. Recovery of airborne bacteria from the oral cavity of humans: The effect of dosage on recovery. *J. Infect. Dis.*, 102:251–256.

92. Meyers, C. E., James, H. A., and Zippin, C. (1961): The recovery of aerosolized bacteria from humans: I. Effects of varying exposure, sampling times, and subject variability. *Arch. Environ. Health*, 2:384–389.

93. Kraus, F. W., and Guston, C. (1973): Individual constancy of numbers among the oral flora. *J. Bacteriol.*, 71:703–711.

94. Johanson, W. G., Pierce, A. K., Sanford, J. P., and Thomas, G. D. (1972): Nosocomial respiratory infections with Gram-negative bacilli. *Ann. Intern. Med.*, 77:701–712.

95. Johanson, W. G., Pierce, A. K., and Sanford, J. P. (1969): Changing pharyngeal bacterial flora of hospitalized patients. *N. Engl. J. Med.*, 281:1137–1144.

96. Rehm, S. R., Gross, G. N., and Pierce, A. K. (1980): Early bacterial clearance from murine lungs: Species-dependent phagocyte response. *J. Clin. Invest.*, 66:194–199.

97. Onofrio, J. M., Toews, G. B., Lipscomb, M. F., and Pierce, A. K. (1983): Granulocyte-alveolar macrophages interaction in the pulmonary clearance of *Staphylococcus aureus*. *Am. Rev. Respir. Dis.*, 127:335–341.

98. Nugent, K. M., and Pesanti, E. L. (1982): Nonphagocytic clearance of *Staphylococcus aureus* from murine lungs. *Infect. Immun.*, 36:1185–1191.

99. DeMaria, T. F., and Kapral, F. A. (1978): Pulmonary infection of mice with *Staphylococcus aureus*. *Infect. Immun.*, 21:114–123.

100. Ward, P. A., Lepow, I. H., and Newman, L. J. (1968): Bacterial factors chemotactic for polymophonuclear leukocytes. *Am. J. Pathol.*, 52:725–736.

101. Schiffman, E., Showell, H., Corcoran, B., Smith, E., Ward, P. A., Tempel, T., and Becker, E. L. (1974): Isolation and characterization of the bacterial chemotactic factor. *Fed. Proc.*, 33:631.

102. Gallin, J. I., Clark, R. A., and Frank, M. M. (1975): Kinetic analysis of chemotactic factor generation in human serum via activation of the classical and alternate complement pathways. *Clin. Immunol. Immunopathol.*, 3:334–346.

103. Hunninghake, G. W., Gallin, J. I., and Fauci, A. S. (1978): Immunological reactivity of the lung. VI. The *in vitro* and *in vivo* generation of a neutrophil chemotactic factor by alveolar macrophages. *Am. Rev. Respir. Dis.*, 117:15–23.

104. Hunninghake, G. W., Gadek, J. E., and Crystal, R. G. (1980): Human alveolar macrophage neutrophil chemotactic factor: Stimuli and partial characterization. *J. Clin. Invest.*, 66:473–483.

105. Hunninghake, G. W., Gadek, J. E., Lawley, T. J., and Crystal, R. G. (1981): Mechanisms of neutrophil accumulation in the lungs of patients with idiopathic pulmonary fibrosis. *J. Clin. Invest.*, 68:259–269.

106. Kazmierowski, J. A., Gallin, J. I., and Reynolds, H. Y. (1977): Mechanism for the inflammatory response in primate lungs. Demonstration and partial characterization of an alveolar macrophage-derived chemotactic factor with preferential activity for polymorphonuclear leukocytes. *J. Clin. Invest.*, 59:273–281.

107. Waldman, R. H., and Coggins, W. J. (1972): Influenza immunization: Field trial on a university campus. *J. Infect. Dis.*, 126:242–248.

108. Waldman, R. H., Kasel, J. A., Fulk, R. V., Togo, Y., Hornick, R. B., Heiner, G. G., Dawkins, A.T., and Mann, J. J. (1968): Influenza antibody in human respiratory secretions after subcutaneous or respiratory immunization with inactivated virus. *Nature*, 218:594–597.

109. Waldman, R. H., Mann, J. J., and Small, P. A. (1969): Immunization against influenza: Prevention of illness in man by aerosolized inactivated vaccine. *J.A.M.A.*, 207:520–525.

110. Ewan, P. W. (1976): Immunological defense mechanisms against respiratory disease. In: *Advanced Medicine, Vol. 12*, edited by D. K. Peters, pp. 74–83. Pitman Medical, San Francisco.

111. Mann, J. J., Waldman, R. H., Togo, Y., Heiner, G. G., Dawkins, A. T., and Kasel, J. A. (1968): Antibody response in respiratory secretions of volunteers inoculated with live and dead influenza virus. *J. Immunol.*, 100:726–731.

112. Ogra, P. L., and Karzon, D. T. (1969): Distribution of poliovirus antibody in serum nasopharynx and alimentary tract following segmental immunization of lower alimentary tract with poliovaccine. *J. Immunol.*, 102:1423–1431.

113. Ogra, P. L., and Karzon, D. T. (1969): Poliovirus antibody response in serum and nasal secretions following intranasal inoculation with inactivated polio-vaccine. *J. Immunol.*, 102:15–19.

114. Livray, M. (1968): Immunoglobulin response in serum and secretions after immunization with live and inactivated poliovaccine and natural infection. *N. Engl. J. Med.*, 279:893–896.

115. Wollinsky, J. S., Dan, P. C., Buimovici-Klein, E., Medwick, J., Berg, B. O., Lang, P. B., and Coopers, L. Z. (1979): Progressive rubella panencephalitis: Immunovirological studies and results of inoprinosine therapy. *Clin. Exp. Immunol.*, 35:397–401.

116. Purtilo, D. T., DeFlorio, D., Hutt, L. M., Bhawan, J., Yang, J. P. S., Otto, R., and Edwards, W. (1977): Variable phenotypic expression of an X-linked recessive lymphoproliferative syndrome. *N. Engl. J. Med.*, 297:1077–1081.

117. Notkins, A. L. (1973): Immunological defense and injury in vital infections: The role of the inflammatory response. *Adv. Biosciences*, 12:367–378.

118. Cooper, M. D., Chase, H. P., Lowman, J. T., Krivit, W., and Good, R. A. (1968): Wiskott-Aldrich syndrome. An immunological deficiency disease involving the afferent limb of immunity. *Am. J. Med.*, 44:499–506.

119. Perrin, L. H., Tishon, A., and Oldstone, M. B. A. (1977): Immunologic injury in measles virus infection. *J. Immunol.*, 118:282–287.

120. Korsager, B., Spencer, E. S., and Mordhorst, C.-H. (1975): Herpesvirus hominis infections in renal transplant recipients. *Scand. J. Infect. Dis.*, 7:11–18.

121. Rand, K. H., Rasmussen, L. E., Pollard, R. B., Arvin, A., and Merigan, T. C. (1977): Cellular immunity and herpes virus infections in cardiac-transplant patients. *N. Engl. J. Med.*, 296:1372–1375.

122. Montgomerie, J. Z., Becroft, D. M. O., Croxson, M. C., Doak, P. B., and North, J. D. K. (1969): Herpes simplex virus infection after renal transplantation. *Lancet*, 2:867–870.

123. Ho, M., Suwansirikul, S., Dowling, J. N., Youngblood, I. A., and Armstrong, J. A. (1975): The transplanted kidney as a source of cytomegalovirus infection. *N. Engl. J. Med.*, 293:1109–1112.

124. Henson, D., Siegel, S. E., Fuccillo, D. A., Matthew, W., and Levine, A. S. (1972): Cytomegalovirus infections during acute childhood leukemia. *J. Infect. Dis.*, 126:469–474.

125. Crawford, D. J., Thomas, J. A., Janossy, G., Sweny, P., Fernando, O. N., Moorhead, J. F., and Thompson, J. H. (1980): Epstein-Barr virus nuclear antigen positive lymphoma after cyclosporin A treatment in patient with renal allograft. *Lancet*, 1:1355–1358.

126. Bird, A. G., McLachlan, S. M., and Britton, S. (1981): Cyclosporin A promotes spontaneous outgrowth *in vitro* of Epstein-Barr virus-induced B-cell lines. *Nature*, 289:294–296.

127. Biddison, W. E., and Shaw, S. (1979): Differences in HLA antigen recognition by human influenza virus-immune cytotoxic T cells. *J. Immunol.*, 122:1705–1707.

128. Blanden, R. V., Doherty, P. C., Dunlop, M. B. C., Gardner, I. D., and Zinkernagel, R. M. (1975): Gene required for cytotoxicity against virus-infected target cells in K and D regions of H-2 complex. *Nature*, 254:269–271.

129. Brunner, K. T., MacDonald, H. R., and Cerottini, J. C. (1980): Antigenic specificity of the

cytolytic T lymphocyte (CTL) response to murine sarcoma virus-induced tumours. *J. Immunol.*, 124:1627–1631.

130. Doherty, P. C., and Zinkernagel, R. M. (1975): H-2 compatibility is required for T-cell-mediated lysis of target cells infected with lymphocytic choriomeningitis virus. *J. Exp. Med.*, 141:502–507.

131. Herberman, R. B., Djeu, J. Y., Kay, H. D., Ortaldo, J. R., Riccardi, C., Bonnard, G. D., Holden, H. T., Fagnani, R., Santoni, A., and Puccetti, P. (1979): Natural killer cells: Characteristics and regulation of activity. *Immunol. Rev.*, 44:43–58.

132. Santoli, D., and Koprowsky, H. (1979): Mechanisms of activation of human natural killer cells against tumor and virus infected cells. *Immunol. Rev.*, 44:125–132.

133. Santoli, D., Trinchieri, G., and Koprowski, H. (1978): Cell-mediated cytotoxicity in humans against virus-infected target cells. II. Interferon induction and activation of natural killer cells. *J. Immunol.*, 121:532–538.

134. Trinchieri, G., and Santoli, D. (1978): Antiviral activity induced by culturing lymphocytes with tumor-derived or virus-transformed cells. Enhancement of human natural killer cell activity by interferon and antagonistic inhibition of susceptibility of target cells to lysis. *J. Exp. Med.*, 147:1314–1318.

135. Scott, R., de Landazuri, M. O., Gardner, P. S., and Owen, J. J. T. (1977): Human antibody-dependent cell-mediated cytotoxicity against target cells infected with respiratory syncytial virus. *Clin. Exp. Immunol.*, 28:19–24.

136. Shore, S. L., Black, C. M., Melewicz, F. M., Wood, P. A., and Nahmias, A. J. (1976): Antibody-dependent cell-mediated cytotoxicity to target cells infected with type I and type 2 herpes simplex virus. *J. Immunol.*, 116:194–198.

137. Jondal, M. (1976): Antibody-dependent cellular cytotoxicity (ADCC) against Epstein-Barr virus-determined membrane antigens. I. Reactivity in sera from normal persons and from patients with acute infections mononucleosis. *Clin. Exp. Immunol.*, 25:1–6.

138. Portaro, J. K., Zighelboim, J., and Fahey, J. L. (1978): Hereditary deficiency of K cells in a normal subject. *Clin. Immunol. Immunopathol.*, 11:458–462.

139. Ortaldo, J. R., Bonnard, G. D., McDermott, R. P., Kind, P. H., and Herberman, R. B. (1979): Cytotoxicity from cultured cells: Analysis of precursors involved in generation of human cells mediation natural and antibody-dependent cell-mediated cytotoxicity. *J. Immunol.*, 122:1489–1494.

140. Kaplan, J., and Calleqaert, D. M. (1978): Expression of human T-lymphocyte antigens by natural killer cells. *J. Natl. Cancer Inst.*, 60:961–966.

141. Williams, R. M., Leifer, J., and Moore, M. J. (1977): Hybrid effect in natural cell-mediated cytotoxicity of SV40-transformed fibroblasts by rat spleen cells. *Transplantation*, 23:283–286.

142. Minato, N., Bloom, B. R., Jones, C., Holland, J., and Reid, L. M. (1979): Mechanisms of rejection of virus persistently infected tumour cells by athymic nude mice. *J. Exp. Med.*, 149:1117–1121.

143. Koren, H. S., Amost, D. B., and Buckley, R. H. (1978): Natural killing in immunodeficient patients. *J. Immunol.*, 120:796–801.

144. Roder, J., and Duwe, A. (1979): The beige mutation in the mouse selectively impairs natural killer cell function. *Nature*, 278:451–453.

145. Karre, K., Klein, G. O., Kiessling, R., Klein, G., and Roder, J. C. (1980): Low natural *in vivo* resistance to syngeneic leukemias in natural killer-deficient mice. *Nature*, 284:624–627.

146. Roder, J. C., Haliotis, T., Klein, M., Korec, S., Jett, J. R., Ortaldo, J., Herberman, R. B., Katz, P., and Fauci, A. S. (1980): A new immunodeficiency disorder in human involving NK cells. *Nature*, 284:553–556.

147. Blume, R. S., and Wolff, S. M. (1972): The Chediak-Higashi syndrome: Studies in four patients and a review of the literature. *Medicine (Baltimore)*, 51:247–286.

148. Gallin, J. (1980): Disorders of phagocyte chemotaxis. *Ann. Intern. Med.*, 92:520–532.

149. Gallin, J. I., Elin, R. J., Hubert, R. T., Fauci, A. S., Kaliner, M. A., and Wolff, S. M. (1979): Efficacy of ascorbic acid in Chediak-Higashi syndrome: Studies in humans and mice. *Blood*, 53:226–232.

150. Hunninghake, G. W., and Fauci, A. S. (1976): Immunological reactivity of the lung. II. Cytotoxic effector function of pulmonary mononuclear cell subpopulations. *Cell. Immunol.*, 26:98–104.

151. Bordignon, C., Villa, F., Vecchi, A., Biondi, A., Avallone, R., and Mantovani, A. (1982): Natural cytotoxic activity in human lungs. *Clin. Exp. Immunol.*, 47:437–441.

152. Bordignon, C., Villa, R., Allavena, P., Introna, M., Biondi, A., Avallone, R., and Mantavani,

A. (1982): Inhibition of natural killer activity by human bronchoalveolar macrophages. *J. Immunol.*, 129:587–591.

153. Hunninghake, G. W., and Gadek, J. E. (1982): Immunological aspects of chronic non-infectious pulmonary diseases of the lower respiratory tract in man. *Clin. Immunol. Rev.*, 1:337–374.

154. Hunninghake, G. W., and Moseley, P. L. (1984): Immunological abnormalities of chronic noninfectious pulmonary diseases. In: *Immunology of the Lung and Upper Respiratory Tract*, edited by J. Bienstock, pp. 345–364. McGraw-Hill, New York.

155. Boros, D. L. (1978): Granulomatous inflammation. *Prog. Allergy*, 24:183–267.

156. Lurie, M. B. (1964): *Resistance to Tuberculosis: Experimental Studies in Native Acquired Defensive Mechanisms.* Harvard University Press, Cambridge.

157. Adams, D. O. (1976): The granulomatous inflammatory process. A review. *Am. J. Pathol.*, 84:164–191.

158. Goyert, S. M., Shively, J. E., and Silver, J. (1982): Biochemical characterization of a second family of human Ia molecules, HLA-DS, equivalent to murine I-A subregion molecules. *J. Exp. Med.*, 156:550–566.

159. Gonwa, T. A., Picker, L. J., Raff, H. V., Goyert, S. M., Silver, J., and Stobo, J. D. (1983): Antigen-presenting capabilities of human monocytes correlates with their expression of HLA-DS, an Ia determinant distinct from HLA-DR. *J. Immunol.*, 130:706–711.

160. Venet, A. R., Hunninghake, G. W., and Crystal, R. G. (1982): Antigen presentation by human alveolar macrophages: Evaluation in normals and interstitial lung diseases. *Am. Rev. Respir. Dis.*, 125:178A.

161. Stadecker, M. J., Wyler, D. J., and Wright, J. A. (1982): Ia antigen expression and antigen-presenting function by macrophages isolated from hypersensitivity granulomas. *J. Immunol.*, 128:2739–2744.

162. Gillis, S., and Watson, J. (1980): Biochemical and biological characterization of lymphocyte regulatory molecules. V. Identification of an interleukin-2-producing human leukemia T-cell line. *J. Exp. Med.*, 152:1709–1719.

163. Mier, J. W., and Gallo, R. C. (1980): Purification and some characteristics of human T-cell growth factor from phytohemagglutinin-stimulated lymphocyte-conditioned media. *Proc. Natl. Acad. Sci. U.S.A.*, 77:6134–6138.

164. Smith, K. A. (1980): T-cell growth factor. *Immunol. Rev.*, 51:337–357.

165. Hunninghake, G. W., and Monick, M. (1983): Interleukin-2 (IL-2) is a chemotactic factor for human T-lymphocytes. *(submitted)*.

166. Hunninghake, G. W., and Monick, M. (1983): Mechanism of T-lymphocyte redistribution in sarcoid. *Clin. Res.*, 31:512A.

167. Ratajczak, H. V., Richards, D. W., and Richerson, H. B. (1980): Systemic and local lymphocyte responses in experimental hypersensitivity pneumonitis. *Am. Rev. Respir. Dis.*, 122:761–768.

168. Carrick, L., Jr., and Boros, D. L. (1980): The artificial granuloma: I. *In vitro* lymphokine production by pulmonary artificial hypersensitivity granulomas. *Clin. Immunol. Immunopathol.*, 17:415–426.

169. Yoshida, T. (1980): Role of lymphokines in the induction and maintenance of the granuloma. In: *Basic and Clinical Aspects of Granulomatous Diseases*, edited by D. L. Boros and T. Yoshida, pp. 81–96. Elsevier/North-Holland, Amsterdam.

170. Boros, D. L. (1981): The role of lymphokines in granulomatous inflammation. *Lymphokines*, 3:257–281.

171. Schuyler, M. R., Thigpen, T. P., and Salvaggio, J. E. (1978): Local pulmonary immunity in pigeon breeder's disease: A case study. *Ann. Intern. Med.*, 88:355–358.

172. Hunninghake, G. W., and Fauci, A. S. (1977): Immunologic reactivity of the lung. III. Effects of corticosteroids on alveolar macrophage cytotoxic effector cell function. *J. Immunol.*, 118:146–150.

173. Hunninghake, G. W., and Fauci, A. S. (1976): Immunologic reactivity of the lung. IV. Effects of cyclophosphamide on alveolar macrophages cytotoxic effector function. *Clin. Exp. Immunol.*, 27:555–559.

174. Green, G. M., Jakab, G. J., Low, R. B., and Davis, G. S. (1977): Defense mechanisms of the respiratory membranes. *Am. Rev. Respir. Dis.*, 115:479–514.

175. Pennington, J. E. (1978): Differential effects of cyclophosphamide and cortisone acetate on bronchoalveolar phagocytic cell populations. *Am. Rev. Respir. Dis.*, 118:319–324.

176. More, V. L., Mondloch, V. M., Pedersen, G. M., Schrier, D. J., and Allen, E. M. (1981): Strain

variation in BCG-induced chronic pulmonary inflammation in mice: Control by a cyclophospha-mide-sensitive thymus-derived suppressor cell. *J. Immunol.*, 127:339–342.

177. Wellhausen, J., Chensue, S. W., and Boros, D. L. (1980): Modulation of granulomatous hypersen-sitivity: Analysis by adoptive transfer of effector and suppressor T-lymphocytes involved in granulomatous inflammation in murine schistosomiasis. In: *Basic and Clinical Aspects of Gran-ulomatous Diseases*, edited by D. L. Boros and T. Yoshida, pp. 219–234. Elsevier/North-Holland, Amsterdam.

Advances in Host Defense Mechanisms, Vol. 4,
edited by J. I. Gallin and A. S. Fauci.
Raven Press, New York © 1985.

Pulmonary Host Defenses: Humoral Immune Components

John A. Rankin and Herbert Y. Reynolds

Pulmonary Section, Department of Internal Medicine, Yale University School of Medicine, New Haven, Connecticut 06510

To maintain host viability and at the same time perform their primary function of oxygenation and carbon dioxide elimination, the lungs must cope effectively with exposure to the vast array of elements other than oxygen found in inspired air. Viruses, bacteria, fungi, noxious gases, and particulate matter are but a few of the foreign materials that can gain entry to the lungs in the 12,000 liters of air inspired by the resting adult each day. Consequently, the respiratory tract contains impressive host defenses that clearly work efficiently, considering the burden of exposure versus the rarity of respiratory illness.

Part of these defenses begin at the point of air intake in the nares and extend to the level of oxygen uptake on the alveolar surface. One classification divides them into two broad groups: surveillance mechanisms and augmenting mechanisms (1,2). Included in the surveillance mechanisms are anatomic barriers and airway angulation, mucociliary clearance, reflex mechanisms such as cough and bronchoconstriction, local immunoglobulin (secretory IgA), other immunoglobulins (IgG, IgM, and IgE), iron-containing proteins (transferrin), alternate-pathway components, surfactant, and alveolar macrophages. All of these function in a largely mechanical fashion, or activation can occur with nonspecific stimuli, with the exception of immunoglobulins that have specific antibody activity. These surveillance mechanisms do not depend on the prior immune status of the host, and they usually suffice to maintain airway sterility and integrity. When these mechanisms prove insufficient or fail, augmenting mechanisms come into play. These include initiation of immune responses such as humoral and cellular reactions and generation of an inflammatory response that includes the influx of polymorphonuclear granulocytes, eosinophils, and possibly lymphocytes.

Our review will concentrate on one facet of pulmonary host defense mechanisms: the humoral components. The role of humoral factors in immunity is related generally to agglutinative action and to augmenting phagocytic function through opsonization of particles and bacteria. Antimicrobial activity can be generated by humoral components and complement to cause cell lysis. However, it is difficult to dissect such a specific role, because the various lung host defense mechanisms work in concert, and the functions of individual immune components frequently overlap. Nevertheless, a detailed discussion of humoral immunity alone has an advantage, because it permits examination of a very specific area—a careful, in-depth look at an individual tree without attempting to view the entire forest.

Despite continuing investigation into humoral immune components of the respiratory tract, our knowledge in this area remains incomplete. Therefore, two of our objectives will be to describe and discuss the humoral components of the respiratory tract and to highlight those areas in which information is particularly lacking and research is needed. Much of our current understanding of this area is based on animal research and has not been tested in humans. However, for this review, human data will be discussed whenever possible. Moreover, emphasis will be on humoral components present in normal lungs, not on abnormalities found in disease.

Humoral components of the immune system of the respiratory tract may reside in any or all of four locations: the fluid lining the epithelial surface of the respiratory tract, the mucosa and submucosa, the bronchus-associated lymphoid tissue, and the interstitium. Each of these locations will be examined individually.

RESPIRATORY MUCOSAL SURFACE AND STRUCTURE

It is impossible to present a thorough review of the many cells composing the mucosa and its substratum layers (3) or to discuss the regional changes in this surface as it spans from nares to alveoli, but general concepts should be recalled when sampling methods to obtain secretions are evaluated or when individual protein values are measured in this dynamic and complex fluid mixture (4). The surface epithelium varies along the airways. Stratified squamous epithelium present in the nares undergoes transition to a pseudostratified, columnar, ciliated, mucus-secreting epithelium over the nasal turbinates that continues into the posterior pharynx. In the oropharynx, squamous epithelium again is present, covering the buccal surfaces and extending to cover the epiglottis, glottis, and part of the larynx. In the upper trachea, the ciliated pseudostratified epithelium returns, interspersed with globlet cells and effluent openings from bronchial glands, and extends down to the respiratory bronchioles. However, toward the periphery of the airways, the epithelial layer gradually becomes thinner and less stratified, and cells assume a more cuboidal shape; cilia are shorter. In the terminal air sacs and over the alveolar surface, the cell layer flattens and blends to a single layer of epithelium (type 1 pneumocytes) interspersed with type 2 pneumocytes. This layer supports various free-moving, detachable phagocytic cells and lymphocytes present on the alveolar surface.

In the transitional zone of the respiratory bronchioles, different secretory cells are present, such as clara cells, for globlet cells and mucus glands disappear as the alveolar surface is reached. Lymphocytes and plasma cells are distributed in the submucosa and lamina propria areas of the larger conducting airways and nasal passages where the thick, pseudostratified, ciliated columnar epithelium exists, but these cells may have different relative locations to the airway surface as the epithelium attenuates in the alveolar areas. Surface lymphocytes, for example, appear.

Emphasis is usually placed on the secretory apparatus of the mucosal surface, i.e., mucus production by bronchial glands and globlet cells, serous and clara-cell secretion, local immunoglobulin production, transudation of proteins from the vascular space, and surfactant secretion by type 2 cells; but the equally important phenomenon of fluid absorption from the mucosa is overlooked. Absorptive mechanisms are less obvious and generally have been investigated less, but they appear to be as complex as the secretory ones. Clearance of fluid and senescent cells and phospholipids from the alveolar surface by macrophages is an example. Mucociliary clearance is not operant here, and coughing is ineffective for cleansing this portion of the airways. Lymphatic drainage, which begins in the region of the respiratory bronchioles, remains poorly charted in the lungs. Among the mucosal lining cells are brush cells with apical border microvilli that are shorter than the cilia on epithelial cells and so remain submerged in the periciliary sol fluid. These cells appear to be constructed for absorbing fluid, similar to such cells found in the gut, gallbladder, and paranasal sinuses. Although brush cells are not numerous in the mucosa, they are located at all levels along the airways. The integrity of the apical junctions joining epithelial cells is likewise crucial to overall fluid absorption, as these can be affected by irritation from inhaled smoke or other airborne pollutants and by immediate allergic injury that can occur with antigen-antibody reactions. Finally, autonomic nervous control that regulates humidification and heat exchange of the mucosal surface is a factor in conserving fluid balance, especially in the nose and trachea in normals (5). Thus, sampling respiratory lining secretions and accurately quantifying a particular immunologic component in relation to others present in the specimen are dependent on general homeostatic fluid balance along the airways and the status of local irritation, and so forth, at the mucosal site.

Actual physical diffusion or local penetration of immunoglobulins, for example, may be linked with other features of the respiratory mucosa. Restricting transudation of plasma components into the alveolar space is the semipermeable blood-air interface composed of the capillary endothelium, interstitial space, and alveolar epithelium. This barrier in normal lungs prevents appreciable entry into alveolar lining secretions of globular proteins larger than 150,000 daltons, so that albumin-size proteins and those that range in size up to immunoglobulin G can be found in reasonable amounts. For local secretion of proteins, the thickness of the stratified epithelial surface separating the lamina propria and basement membrane from the luminal surface of the airway might be a significant factor. To facilitate secretion of dimeric IgA, epithelial cells have developed secretory component, but the role of this glycoprotein moiety seems selective and generally not usable for other immunoglobulins (IgM or IgE). This fact is not resolved, for we were surprised to find secretory component attached to IgM in canine airway secretions (6). Moreover, mast cell or macrophage mediators, perhaps leukotrienes released with antigen stimulation (or by calcium flux, as shown with ionophore stimulation of in vitro cultured cells), may alter local mucosal permeability. The actual thickness of the

TABLE 1. *Nasal wash proteins from normals*

	Total protein	Albumin	IgG	IgA	FSC
Nonsmokers (N = 31)	220[a]	29	7.9	23	2.2
Cigarette smokers (N = 35)	199	11	3.1	24	2.7

[a]Mean values in micrograms per milliliter; fluid volume ~10 ml of nasal wash.

epithelial surface varies with the estrus cycle in female animals, and this could contribute to changes in protein penetration, but this has not been probed to our knowledge. Certain immunoglobulins originate from several sources in the airways, and the final concentration in respiratory secretions is a composite value. IgG is an illustration, as it can diffuse from the plasma space across the blood-air barrier; some is secreted locally by submucosally located plasma cells, and intraalveolar lymphocytes can release IgG directly into the alveolar lumen.

In summary, measurements of humoral immune components (immunoglobulin antibodies, perhaps complement fragments, such "nonimmune" opsonins as fibronectin and surfactant, and iron-containing proteins with antimicrobial activity) require an overall awareness about how these things arrive in airway secretions, what mechanisms clear or degrade them (i.e., bacteria-derived proteases that can degrade secretory IgA), and regional changes in the respiratory tract that can alter relative concentrations, such as those found for secretory IgA/IgG values in upper versus lower respiratory fluids.

NASAL SECRETIONS

In normals, washing the mucosa of the nose with small aliquots of saline that are drained anteriorly from the nasal passages will provide a protein-dilute specimen that can be concentrated and analyzed for content of immunoglobulins. Several reports have provided this kind of information (4). For a group of normals, representative values can be found (Table 1).

For nonsmokers, albumin constitutes approximately 13% of the total protein content, IgA approximately 10%, and IgG approximately 3.5%, and there is a small but detectable quantity of free secretory component (FSC). Despite comparable recoveries of total protein in specimens from smokers, albumin accounted for a smaller (~5%) amount of the protein in the specimens; IgG constituted 1.6%, whereas IgA (12%) and FSC were comparable to those for nonsmokers. Such results suggest that possible irritant effects of smoke inhalation in the nose may not promote a wholesale influx of low-molecular-weight protein onto the nasal surface in the form of albumin, nor does immunoglobulin secretion seem to be affected, although IgG is slightly lower.

PAROTID AND OROPHARYNGEAL SECRETIONS

Parotid fluid can be collected without contamination of other mouth secretions by fitting a small suction cup around the parotid duct orifice (Stensen's duct) and allowing fluid to drain through a plastic tube into a container. Acid stimulation (sour-ball candy) is usually required to produce a sustained flow of fluid (~ 1 ml/min). Other secretions recovered in the floor of the mouth around the base of the tongue reflect salivary gland output. Minute amounts of fluid can be aspirated from the gum-tooth margins and represent gingival specimens. Because of the selective recovery of parotid fluid, it has been a common source for analyzing external secretory body fluids and is included along with such other well-characterized secretions from the lacrimal glands, breasts, gut, and gallbladder (7). Whether it is representative of airway secretions obtained from the nose and lower respiratory tract is questionable, but parotid fluid is convenient for analysis of IgA and FSC content (8).

Parotid fluid is usually acellular, except for rare squamous buccal epithelial cells that are abraded from the cheek mucosa by the collection cup. The total protein in the usual 20-ml sample of parotid fluid that has been concentrated 10-fold is approximately 1.5 mg. Albumin accounts for approximately 10% of this protein, IgA for 12 to 15%, and IgG for less than 0.05%. In parotid saliva samples that were not concentrated, the mean value ($\pm$ SEM) for IgA was 72 ± 3.5 µg/ml, and the mean value for FSC was 218 ± 65 ng/ml (8). Double radioimmunoassay methods were used for these measurements. Parotid fluid contains IgA in both the dimeric secretory form and 7S monomer, which indicates that some IgA is not synthesized in the gland but may diffuse from serum. All salivary gland secretions in the oropharynx contain mostly IgA and relatively little IgG. In contrast, crevicular fluid obtained from the gingival surfaces is rich in total protein and IgG, but contains little IgA. It more closely resembles an ultrafiltrate of plasma than the dilute fluids produced by the secretory glands.

TRACHEOBRONCHIAL FLUIDS

Secretions from the trachea and major bronchi at the root of the lungs have not been analyzed precisely, because the sampling methods used have not limited or isolated specimens to these mucosal areas. Airway lavage through a rigid or flexible bronchoscope cannot control the distal limit of the fluid. Alternatively, direct application of absorbent material to the bronchial mucosa usually does not yield sufficient liquid to permit satisfactory elution and recovery of fluid either, especially from normals who have received some atropine medication before bronchoscopy. Perhaps the most representative bronchial samples have been obtained unwittingly by tracheobronchial lavages performed with very small volumes of fluid (5–10 ml) in patients and patient controls who yielded small recovery of lavage fluid (1.0–2.5-ml samples). Results of several studies are summarized in Table 2 (9–11).

Cells were not analyzed in the samples. Keimowitz (9) made tracheobronchial washings in patients without lung disease, but undergoing general anesthesia that

TABLE 2. *Protein and immunoglobulin concentrations in bronchial washings*

Study	n	TP[a] (mg/dl)	Albumin/TP (%)	IgG/TP (%)	IgA/TP (%)	IgG/albumin ratio[b]	IgA/ albumin ratio[b]	IgG/K (%)	IgA/K[c] (%)	Ref.
Controls	12	ND[d]	ND	ND	ND	0.39	0.73			9
Controls	8[e]	60.0 ± 8.5	15 ± 3.5	6.7 ± 1.9	7.5 ± 1.3					10
COPD[f]	9	56.0 ± 7.0	14 ± 2.4	4.0 ± 0.9	4.5 ± 1.4					10
Controls	20	ND	ND					1.96 ± 0.76	1.75 ± 0.72	11
Uninvolved lung	48	ND	ND					2.07 ± 1.13	2.01 ± 0.84	11

[a]TP, total protein.
[b]Ratio: milligrams Ig to milligrams albumin.
[c]Concentration of IgG or IgA (mg/ml) as a fraction of the concentration of potassium (mEq/liter) in the washing.
[d]ND, not determined.
[e]Several patients in each group had a washing in each mainstem bronchus, and each washing was analyzed separately; thus, there were more samples than patients.
[f]COPD, chronic obstructive pulmonary disease.

required intubation. Through a catheter located at the level of the carina, 10 ml of saline were instilled, with recovery of approximately 1 ml. This specimen was concentrated fivefold, and albumin, β_{2A}-globulin (IgA), and γ_2-globulin (IgG) were measured by radial immunoprecipitation. The IgG ratio to albumin in the lung specimen was similar to that in serum, whereas the IgA ratio was approximately nine times greater than in serum (0.73 vs. 0.08), indicating a local excess of IgA. Falk et al. (10) expressed albumin and immunoglobulin values in bronchial specimens as a percentage of total protein; IgG and IgA were found in comparable proportions. Because total protein measurements were poorly reproducible, the potassium contents in the specimens were used by Mandell et al. (11) as a denominator to express IgG and IgA ratios. Serum values were not measured for comparisons. The relative amounts of IgG and IgA were the same, both in samples from normals and in samples from bronchi uninvolved with disease. Thus, two studies (10,11) found that in the major bronchi of middle-aged adults (age range 31–67 years), IgG and IgA were recovered from the mucosa in virtually equal amounts. Molecular characterization of IgA was not attempted, but presumably it would be principally secretory IgA (S-IgA) in the absence of overt irritation or inflammation of the airways.

Wiggins et al. (12) have performed the most detailed study in humans (mean age 62 years for 33 patients) attempting to segregate fluid in various areas of the lower respiratory tract. Patients with chronic bronchitis and expectoration underwent fiberoptic bronchoscopy, during which tracheal fluid was aspirated off the mucosa from the vocal cords to the carina; a small bronchial lavage (5–10 ml saline) was made in a mainstem bronchus, followed by a bronchoalveolar lavage. Albumin, α_1-antichymotrypsin, and IgA were quantified in the airway fluids and compared with values in the sol phase of sputum and in serum. Progressive dilution of the proteins was found in the peripheral airway fluids, but when ratios were normalized against serum albumin, high values for IgA and α_1-antichymotrypsin indicated that local secretion of these occurred along the airways. Of interest, the protein profile in sputum was similar to the protein profiles in the selective alveolar lining fluid (sampled by lung lavage).

ALVEOLAR LINING FLUID

Inhaled gases, microbes, and other particulates first make contact with the lower respiratory tract when they are deposited on the fluid lining the epithelial surface. Since the introduction of bronchoalveolar lavage (BAL) to sample the proteinaceous and cellular components of this lung lining fluid some 10 years ago, our understanding of lung immunologic events both in normal individuals and in patients with numerous lung diseases has increased dramatically. BAL provides a means for dissecting out specific immune mechanisms at the cellular level, something not previously so easy in studies of intact animals and in humans. Because this procedure has been important in advancing lung immunology in humans, a brief discussion of how it is performed and how the data obtained are expressed will be given.

TABLE 3. *Humoral components of pulmonary host defenses in lower airway and alveolar lining fluids, as sampled by bronchoalveolar lavage*

Immunoglobulins	Free secretory component
IgA	Complement components
11S dimeric, bound secretory	Properdin B, C1q, C4,
component, J chain (>90%)	C3, C6
7S monomeric (<10%)	Transferrin
IgG (IgG$_1$, IgG$_2$, IgG$_3$, IgG$_4$)	Surfactant
IgM	Fibronectin
IgE	B cells (plasma cells) producing
	IgG
	IgA
	IgM
	IgE

BAL is performed through a fiberoptic bronchoscope wedged in a segmental bronchus (13–15). Several aliquots (usually 20–50 ml of normal saline) are infused through a channel in the bronchoscope and then retrieved by application of gentle suction. Approximately 60% of the instillate is recovered from normal individuals. Lung lining fluid and cells lying within this fluid in the airways and alveoli distal to the tip of the bronchoscope are mixed together. Because the cross-sectional area of the alveoli is so much greater than that of the subtended airways, most of the retrieved fluid and cells are of alveolar origin. Because a large volume of saline is instilled, the lung lining fluid actually retrieved is diluted manyfold. Precise quantification of sol-phase material is difficult, because a completely satisfactory reference material has not yet been found that would (a) compensate for the dilution of lung lining fluid that occurs as a result of the lavage and (b) reflect air-side origin or selectivity, thus removing the possibility that plasma contaminates the sample. To date, most investigators have expressed the levels of soluble substances quantitated in BAL by making a ratio to total protein, to albumin, or to a small molecule such as potassium or urea. Albumin, because of its relatively small size (~67,000 daltons) and passive influx from plasma, has been a popular denominator for protein ratios. Different reference substances are being explored (16) but are not widely used yet.

Of the humoral components associated with pulmonary host defenses, immunoglobulins with potential specific antibody activity and complement components that can augment attachment of opsonic antibody to phagocytic cells or activate the lytic complement cascade are most important. However, evidence is accumulating that favors roles for other substances not traditionally considered part of the humoral immune system. A list of the principal humoral components of pulmonary host defenses is given in Table 3.

Of the humoral components of the immune system present in lung lining fluid, those present in greatest quantity are the immunoglobulins, in particular IgG and IgA. Numerous investigators have quantitated IgG and IgA in lung lining fluid (15,17–22). Whereas IgA clearly is predominant in the upper respiratory tract, the relative proportion of IgG increases steadily through the distal airways. In a dog model (23,24) in which secretions from a major bronchus were sampled, IgG accounted for a higher percentage of the total protein than IgA. This contrasts with a ratio of 0.1 for IgG to IgA found in dog saliva. In normal humans, all studies agree that IgG and IgA are the immunoglobulins found in largest quantity. Some studies suggest that IgA predominates to a slight degree (15,19,22), and others suggest that IgG is present in greater quantities (2,17,25). The variation between these results may be due to minor differences in specificity and/or sensitivity of the various assays used to quantitate these immunoglobulins. We can say safely that these immunoglobulins are present in approximately equal amounts in lung lining fluid. In normal adults, more than 90% of this IgA is in the dimer form (15,21,26), as is the case for IgA in other external secretions, but not in serum, where IgA is principally monomeric (7). The 11S sedimenting IgA is the typical form of immunoglobulin (S-IgA), in that it contains both secretory component and joining chain (J chain). Precipitin analysis of purified S-IgA from BAL has identified both alpha heavy-chain classes (25). However, their relative proportions remain to be analyzed.

In preliminary analyses of lung lining fluid, IgG subclasses have been detected. Using a sensitive ELISA method, we have quantitated levels of IgG_1, IgG_3, and IgG_4 in BAL from 29 volunteers (27,28). In normals, IgG_1 was by far the most abundant, and IgG_4 levels exceeded IgG_3 levels to some degree. The same pattern was found in measurements from paired serum samples.

There are at least two potential sources of immunoglobulin found in lung lining fluid: transudation from serum, and *in situ* synthesis by lung lymphocytes (plasma cells) fixed in the submucosa and interstitium or free cells in the airway lumen. The observation that IgG/albumin ratios in BAL and in serum of nonsmoking adults are about equal suggests that IgG (150,000–180,000 daltons) is able to leak from serum onto the alveolar surface (4,14,22). However, other studies indicate that serum IgG may not passively move into the lung lining fluid in appreciable amounts (29). Additional evidence exists that all immunoglobulin classes, except IgD, may be released locally into the lung lining fluid by plasma cells residing on the mucosal surface (22,30–32).

Characterization of the cellular components of BAL in normal adults shows that almost all retrieved cells are macrophages (90%), and the remainder are lymphocytes (~9%). Occasional polymorphonuclear granulocytes (1%), basophils (0.5%), and eosinophils (<0.1%) are found (2,13–15). The subtypes of lymphocytes that are in BAL fluid closely approximate those found in blood. Approximately 70% of BAL lymphocytes possess surface markers characteristic of T lymphocytes; approximately 10% are B cells, and the remainder null cells—they do not react with currently used T- and B-cell markers (2,14,33). With the use of a reverse hemolytic plaque assay, we (22) and others before us (14,30,31) have estimated that some 0.1 to 2.5% of the B cells in lung lining fluid from normal adults may actively secrete immunoglobulins, including classes IgG, IgA, IgM, and occasionally IgE. Immunoglobulin-releasing cells also have been isolated from minced cell preparations of normal lung parenchyma obtained from patients undergoing tho-racotomy for solitary pulmonary nodules (32). Because IgG-releasing cells can be detected in BAL fluid, this suggests that some IgG is released locally in the air spaces.

Specific conclusions about the sources of lung lining fluid IgA are difficult. Good evidence suggests that submucosal lymphocytes are the main site of S-IgA production (7,34–36). Presumably these cells originated in bone marrow, where large numbers of IgA-bearing cells are found (36), and from there traveled to mucosa-associated lymphoid tissue. Recent studies in animals have shown that from mucosa-associated lymphoid tissue, lymphoblasts may migrate to both bronchial and intestinal mucosa (36). When IgA is produced by local submucosal plasma cells, the molecule is in its dimeric form. From there this IgA is thought to be transported into respiratory secretions by diffusion through the basement membrane to the surfaces of columnar epithelial cells, where it combines with secretory component and is taken into the epithelial cells and secreted from them by an exocytotic mechanism into the respiratory lumen. It is not clear whether the small amount of monomeric IgA present in lung lining fluid is synthesized by IgA-secreting cells that have been detected in BAL or by passive transudation from serum, or by a combination of these two sources. Excess free secretory component not complexed to IgA can be found in lung lining fluid (21).

Immunoglobulin M is usually not found, or found in only very limited quantities, in BAL from normal persons (11,15,18–20,37,38). Using a sensitive immunofluo-rometric assay, we have found significantly greater ratios of IgM/albumin in serum than in BAL (22). This is not surprising, as the large size of IgM ($\sim 900,000$ daltons) undoubtedly limits its transudation from serum. IgM-releasing cells are present in lung lining fluid, providing evidence that at least some local production occurs, although there are significantly fewer IgM-releasing cells than cells for either IgG or IgA (14,22,30).

IgE can be found in lung lining fluid of approximately 80% of normal individuals (15,39,40) in small quantities. Similar findings have been observed in monkeys (31). Some authors consider IgE to be a secretory immunoglobulin (40,42–44) that belongs to the mucosal secretory immune system. Our data suggest that IgE in airways of nonallergic persons arrives, at least in part, by transudation from the intravascular pool (40). However, the lamina propria of the respiratory tract con-tains approximately 5% IgE-producing cells (45), and IgE-releasing cells have been found in the lung lining fluid of a few normal adults (30; J. A. Rankin, *personal observations*). The high affinity of IgE for mast cells and basophils suggests that much of lung IgE may be bound, and therefore the levels in fluids may not accurately reflect the total amount of IgE in the lung.

IgD is the one immunoglobulin that has not been detected in lung lining fluids (2,14), a surprising finding, because its molecular mass of approximately 180,000 daltons and its presence in serum (although only in very small quantities) suggest that it could pass from the intravascular pool. It is possible that a more sensitive assay, if used, might detect this immunoglobulin. The main function of IgD has not been determined. Along with IgM, it is the predominant immunoglobulin on the surfaces of human B lymphocytes.

Complement is a series of proteins activated in sequence by antibody-antigen complexes of various bacterial products and responsible for numerous host defense mechanisms. The precise quantity of complement in lung lining fluid has been difficult to determine. Levels of total complement or individual components have been quantitated on the basis of hemolytic titer assays, and it appears that complement activity is quite labile in stored and thawed BAL specimens (15,46). In addition, the catabolic studies of some of the plasma complement components studied, such as C4, C3, C5, and factor B, demonstrate that these proteins are among the more rapidly metabolized human proteins (47). Nevertheless, several components of the complement system have been identified in normal airway secretions, with both classic and alternate complement pathways being represented. In humans, classic complement pathway factor C4 has been detected occasionally (14,15,38,46), whereas alternate-pathway factor B (48) has been found consistently in normal individuals, as have two of the common pathway components, C3 and C6 (14,15,38). As was the case for lung lining fluid immunoglobulins, the predominant source or sources of complement components remain undetermined. Aside from C1q, which has an approximate molecular weight of 390,000, other complement components have molecular weights of approximately 220,000 or less (47). Therefore, the molecular weights of many of the complement components are such that some transudation from serum would be expected. However, some element of local production also is likely, because mononuclear phagocytes can secrete several complement components, such as C1, C4, C2, C3, C5, factors B and D, properdin, C3b inactivator, and β_{1H} (49), and because human lung fibroblasts synthesize C1 components (50). Moreover, recent investigations have established that human alveolar macrophages secrete C4 and C2 (51,52). Therefore, it is not surprising that studies on fresh BAL fluid immediately after recovery (not frozen) revealed reasonable complement activity (15,38). Nevertheless, it is likely that complement components are present in normal BAL fluid in proportionally small amounts, as compared with serum, and that the supply of early components of the classic pathway, C1 and C4, is limited. The fact that properdin factor B is more readily detected (48) than classic complement components suggests that the alternate pathway of activation may predominate.

Fibronectin is a 440,000-daltons glycoprotein found in plasma, interstitial connective tissue, and lung lining fluid of normal humans and patients with various lung diseases (53–58). Its principal function appears to be in the mediation of many cell-matrix interactions, and evidence suggests a likely role in tissue remodeling. Fibronectin has been demonstrated in alveolar structures by several investigators using immunofluorescence methods (53,59), and it has been isolated directly from lung parenchyma (60). Reports vary on the actual amount of fibronectin relative to albumin present in normal individuals' lung lining fluid. One report found an average of 25% of the quantities found in plasma (54), and another report found approximately equal amounts in these two fluids (58). Both lung fibroblasts

(61,62) and alveolar macrophages (63,64) may secrete this glycoprotein, suggesting that local sources are important. The relatively high molecular weight of fibronectin makes it unlikely that passive transudation from plasma is a major route for levels in air-side secretions.

Secretory component (SC) has no known intrinsic immune function that would qualify it as one of the humoral components of the respiratory tract, except for its association and binding to dimeric IgA to complete the secretory form of IgA. Much of the SC supply is bound in S-IgA. However, unbound (free) SC has been quantitated in lung lavage fluid, where it constitutes approximately 1% of total BAL protein (21). SC is synthesized by glandular epithelial cells lining the respiratory tract (7). It is of special interest because it is added to respiratory secretions selectively without an additional source from the intravascular pool.

Transferrin, an iron-binding protein with molecular mass of 90,000 daltons, is easily detected in sera of humans. Transferrin also has been detected in the lung lavage fluid of normal smoking and nonsmoking individuals (15,18). In view of the relatively low molecular weight of this protein, it is likely that passive transudation from serum is primarily responsible for its presence in lung lining fluid. To date, no published data exist on BAL transferrin levels in diseases affecting the lungs.

Whereas BAL provides a reasonable sampling of lung lining fluid cells and proteins, it does not retrieve cells from extraluminal tissue or the interstitium. Previous work defined methods for handling guinea pig lung parenchyma to isolate cells for the study of interstitial immune events, as opposed to airway-associated ones (65). With these techniques the cellular constitution of the interstitium was evaluated in three nonsmoking humans (32). For comparison, airway cells were obtained from these same individuals using BAL. Differential cell counts and enumerations of T and B cells on these respective samples were strikingly similar. Lymphocytes constituted 16% of the interstitial cells and 7% of the BAL cells. Of these lymphocytes, comparable percentages were T and B cells ($\sim$70% T cells and 10% B cells). In the same study, the authors demonstrated that in patients with sarcoidosis or idiopathic pulmonary fibrosis, BAL cell differentials and lymphocyte subset populations compared favorably with results from cellular analysis of lung biopsy specimens from these patients. Because quantities of lung tissue sufficient to perform numerous immunologic studies are difficult to obtain, it is encouraging that the more easily obtained BAL samples may give a reasonably good approximation of interstitial tissue events.

BRONCHUS-ASSOCIATED LYMPHOID TISSUE

Bronchus-associated lymphoid tissue (BALT) refers to submucosal cellular aggregates of lymphoid tissue distributed diffusely and sparsely beneath the lamina propria of the respiratory tract. Microscopically, BALT (described most extensively in the rabbit and rat) consists of one or two follicles of lymphocytes covered by an epithelium that is devoid of cilia and goblet or glandular cells and is infiltrated by lymphocytes (2,66). The major mass of lymphoid tissue lies external to the cartilage but is connected to the more superficial aggregates by a narrow neck. Most BALT cells are mononuclear, consisting mostly of lymphocytes, scattered reticulum cells, and rare macrophage-like cells. Classic germinal centers characteristic of lymph nodes are found rarely.

In contrast to the findings in lung lining fluid, peripheral blood, and lymph nodes, the majority of lymphocytes in BALT are B cells. The ratio of B to T cells in BALT is approximately 2:1 to 3:1 (2,66). When examined for the presence of heavy-chain immunoglobulins bound to the surfaces of B lymphocytes, IgA and IgM surface staining predominated. Staining of BALT cells for cytoplasmic immunoglobulin demonstrated that less than 1% of the cells accepted anti-heavy-chain antiserum, suggesting that these cells did not contain intracellular immunoglobulin and therefore were not plasma cells. In essence, BALT contains predominantly B lymphocytes not yet committed to production of an immunoglobulin class, but with the potential to do so when presented with appropriate antigen.

Additional but less well defined collections of lymphocytes can be found in more distal airways. These occur at the transition point between ciliated epithelial cells of the terminal bronchioles and the alveolar epithelial lining cells. This anatomic location may favor encounters between the lymphoid aggregates and possibly alveolar macrophages during their transit from interstitial tissue to airway lumen (67).

FUNCTIONAL ASPECTS OF HUMORAL IMMUNE COMPONENTS IN THE LUNGS

Antibody activity in the various classes of immunoglobulins is the purposeful expression of humoral immunity, i.e., specific antibody made in response to an immunizing antigen, for this promotes agglutination or clumping among microorganisms and particulates, or, by coating them, may facilitate phagocytosis. Certain antibodies can interact with the complement cascades to create lytic conditions that puncture cell membranes or to fabricate dual opsonic attachments (C3b plus IgG) that enhance phagocytic uptake. Antigen and antibodies can combine in various ratios, creating complexes that can circulate or fix in tissue, and, by secondary effects of physical size or molecular activity, may trigger other proteolytic and inflammatory pathways. Such immune complexes are usually considered an undesirable effect of excessive antibody formation or poor immunoregulation. Selective antibody activity of the humoral immune system must be distinguished from nonspecific, nonimmune responses that often are very similar in function and are increasingly difficult to classify. For example, phlogistic fragments of complement (C5a), antimicrobial activity of iron-containing proteins, opsonin action of fibronectin fragments and phospholipids (surfactant), and the role of cytophilic immunoglobulins are all parts of the humoral system, and some may work in concert with antibody molecules, but none is specifically "immune." The respiratory tract is an excellent example of the interaction of these immune and nonimmune factors in host defense.

In secretions from the nose and oropharynx, the content of immunoglobulins, especially S-IgA, represents an appreciable proportion of the total protein. Little has been reported about the base-line natural antibody activity in normal secretions. In subjects with allergic rhinitis (ragweed hayfever) anti-antigen-E ragweed antibodies are produced, predominantly in the S-IgA class, and some in the IgG class (68). With topical immunization of the nose with certain viruses, *Mycoplasma pneumoniae*, and diphtheria toxin, local antibody reactivity will develop in nasal wash specimens that is principally IgA and to a lesser degree IgG (17,69,70); these antibodies are sufficiently protective against a homologous microbial challenge, but their persistence or duration of protection is short. Even parenteral immunization has been shown to elicit specific antibodies in nasal secretions against *Salmonella typhosa*-derived endotoxin (71); however, this probably reflects diffusion of antibodies from the intravascular compartment rather than a specific humoral response in nasal mucosa. Yet this experimental result underscores the apparent dichotomy in predicting the efficacy of many vaccines now used to protect against pertussis, diphtheria, mumps, rubella, influenza, meningococcus, and pneumococcus—that parenteral immunization (intramuscular or subcutaneous routes) does elicit protection for local respiratory tract surfaces, although antigen localization in the initial immune responsive phase of antibody formation does not occur in respiratory tissue to any appreciable amount. Serum antibodies, rather than S-IgA, seem to be the active source. The ultimate circulation and localization of antibody-secreting plasma cells in respiratory mucosa that might perpetuate a local immune response are uncharted in humans, and this emphasizes how little is known about lymphocyte traffic to specific organ tissues in humans. Optimal forms of microbial antigens for use in nasal immunization have not been devised. Inactivated vaccine preparations seem inadequate, compared with live or attenuated ones, in their efficacy to elicit reproducible antibody responses. Temperature-sensitive mutants of virus or mycoplasma that have restricted growth in the nasopharynx would seem to be the best solution, but engineering stable mutants has remained an unexpectedly tough technical problem.

Similar research has been performed on the immunoreactivity of the oral cavity (immunization of glandular and lymphoid tissue) to produce antibody against cariogenic strains of streptococci and other bacteria. This work will not be reviewed. Although specific antibodies can be elicited after local immunization of animals that will reduce the incidence of caries, no practical way to manipulate such immunity in humans is available yet.

Along the conducting airways of the thoracic respiratory tract, trachea, and major bronchi, secretory immunoglobulins exist, and submucosally located plasma cells are present (72). As yet, little has been achieved in animals or humans to selectively elicit local antibody formation in this airway segment. This area is potentially of great vulnerability: to infection by aspirated microorganisms from the oronasopharynx; to the deposition of inhaled, aerosolized microbes that may impact on the mucosa because of angulation of the air stream; to noxious effects of airborne pollutants that can cause local damage to the ciliated epithelium, impairing mu-

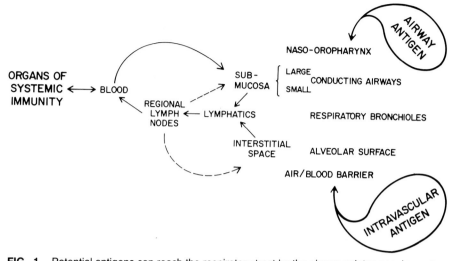

FIG. 1. Potential antigens can reach the respiratory tract by the airway or intravascular route. Inhaled or aspirated material may be localized at numerous points along the airways or may reach the alveolar surface. Intravascular antigen can be trapped in the capillary filter and might reach the lung interstitial space and lymphatic network only if the antigen alters permeability of the air-blood barrier. The regional lymph nodes of the lung appear to be an important site for processing antigen and for initiating an immune response. Some spillover into blood and recruitment of systemic organs to complete the immune response are often necessary. A major source of immune effector cells that return to respiratory tissue is blood. Whether or not local circuits exist between lymphoid tissue adjacent to the lung and airway mucosa and parenchymal sites is uncertain.

cociliary clearance or disrupting tight apical cellular junctions. Colonization of the trachea and bronchi with common respiratory flora, such as *Haemophilus* species and *Streptococcus pneumoniae*, is usual for many patients with chronic bronchitis and other degenerative forms of lung disease. Further impairment of local host defenses may result from secretion of proteolytic enzymes from these bacteria that cleave secretory IgA (specifically IgA_1) (73,74). Potentially, a lot of desirable immune manipulation could be done to enhance local antibody synthesis, induce more IgA_2-class-specific antibody, or perhaps switch to more IgG or possibly IgM. However, major obstacles exist. As we have mentioned, precise sampling of secretions from these segments of the airways is almost impossible. Selective placement and retention of antigen, even if the correct immunogenic form were known, is not addressed with most aerosol protocols and obviously is bypassed in experiments that instill antigen directly into alveoli, as will be discussed. The intricate steps of antigen absorption and processing from the mucosal surface (Fig. 1) (2) and subsequent presentation to other components of the immune apparatus, either adjacently in draining lymph nodes or in removed sites of systemic immunity, have not been dissected well in animal models or in humans.

A preliminary experiment in humans is of interest (75). Twenty-two patients with primary lung tumor scheduled for surgical ressection were selected to receive aerosol immunization with a mixture of bacterial cell wall antigens. Half of the patients were immunized (twice a day for 10 days), and the others received saline. At surgery, a portion of normal-appearing bronchial mucosa was stripped from the resected lung lobe and submitted to immunofluorescent microscopy to identify directly immunoglobulin-containing cells. On the same tissue, an indirect method (immunizing antigen reacted with antibody in tissue and then reacted with fluorescein-tagged rabbit antiserum against bacterial antigen) was used to identify type-specific antibodies in the mucosa. Of the 19 bacterial antigens in the immunizing preparation, five were assayed and included three strains of *S. pneumoniae* and *Haemophilus influenzae*, and a *Klebsiella pneumoniae* strain. In 8 immunized patients, more plasma cells were found in the submucosal glands than in controls and were identified as IgA cells; specific antibodies against the three strains of streptococci were found, but not for the Gram-negative bacteria. It may be feasible in humans to immunize the lower airways with aerosol antigens.

Studies to date have shown that of all the immunoglobulins, IgG is probably the most effective opsonin. As detailed earlier in this review, IgG is present in approximately equal amounts as S-IgA in the lung lining fluid of the lower respiratory tract in humans. All four subtypes of IgG have been detected in human lung lavage fluid from normal healthy volunteers (27,28). To identify specific Fc gamma-chain receptors on alveolar macrophages that might interact with opsonic antibody and enhance attachment, human alveolar macrophages have been examined for the presence of IgG-subclass receptors (76). Alveolar macrophages from both smoking and nonsmoking individuals possessed receptors for IgG_1, IgG_3, and IgG_4, but not for IgG_2. IgG_3 receptors were found on approximately 60% of alveolar macrophages, and IgG_1 and IgG_4 receptors were found on approximately 20% of alveolar macrophages tested within a few hours of harvesting. These observations are pertinent for understanding the function of the IgG subclasses, for IgG-subclass biologic functions (77–81) vary considerably, and opsonization can occur by several different mechanisms (82). In one mechanism, the Fab portion of antigen-specific antibody binds to an antigen, and the Fc portion of the immunoglobulin attaches to its respective Fc receptor on the macrophage membrane. Such surface binding enhances macrophage phagocytosis. Because IgG_1 reacts with receptors on blood monocytes (83), and IgG_1, IgG_3, and IgG_4 with receptors on alveolar macrophages (76), most likely IgG_1 and IgG_3, but also possibly IgG_4, subclasses would appear to be the subclasses conveying opsonic activity. IgM does not have a prominent receptor site on phagocytic cells.

An additional mechanism of opsonization involves the interaction of antigen with specific antibody, which then activates complement via the classic pathway. Of the four IgG subclasses, IgG_1 and IgG_3 fix complement (84,85). Approximately 80% of human alveolar macrophages possess C3b receptors (86). The role of complement in this mechanism appears to be a compensating one for circumstances in which only small amounts of antibody may be present. Brief mention of a study involving rabbit alveolar macrophages is enlightening with respect to this mechanism (87). In that study, alveolar macrophage phagocytosis of bacteria was good if ample amounts of specific IgG were used to preopsonize the bacteria; a complement source did not increase the efficiency. However, if subcritical amounts of antibody were used for opsonization, then complement generated by classic pathway activation could restore optimal phagocytic uptake. An individual not previously exposed to a given antigen (or exposed in the distant past) may not possess large amounts of specific antibody. On rechallenge with the antigen, a rise in antibody titer (anamnestic response) would not be expected for several days. Thus, a level of antibody insufficient to cause optimal opsonization could activate the complement system, which results in complement-mediated cell membrane attachment of the antigen, and macrophage phagocytosis proceeds.

Finally, opsonization may occur nonspecifically via the alternate complement pathway. As discussed earlier, current findings suggest that alternate-pathway complement components may have greater representation in lung lining fluid than classic-pathway components. Activation of the alternate pathway does not require antigen-antibody interaction, but instead may be triggered directly by bacterial or fungal polysaccharides, antibody-antigen complexes, or aggregated forms of immunoglobulins, including IgG, IgA, and IgE. This results in the binding of C3b to the antigen surface. Therefore, failure of phagocytosis that is dependent on complement or IgG subclasses could result in defects in host resistance that lead to infection. Indeed, patients who do mount a specific antibody response and also demonstrate a deficiency of C3 may experience recurrent bacterial infections (88–90). These observations suggest that a synergistic action between antibody and C3b receptors is crucial for normally functioning host defenses against microorganisms controlled by phagocytosis (47). In addition, the relative importance of the IgG subclasses is underscored by recent reports describing frequent sinopulmonary infections in individuals deficient in IgG_2 and/or IgG_4 (80,81,91). To date, all these reports have measured serum IgG-subclass or complement levels; nothing has been reported concerning local levels in the respiratory tract.

The potential role of other lung lining fluid immunoglobulins is less clear. When IgM has been sought, it has been found to be elevated only in patients with hypersensitivity pneumonitis (38). The reasons for this remain unclear. Human alveolar macrophages do not appear to have significant numbers of IgM receptors, but IgM can activate the classic complement pathway and therefore might act to initiate the complement-mediated opsonization discussed earlier.

Recently, new evidence has emerged implicating IgE immune-complex activation of human macrophages as an important component in humoral immune mechanisms. Several investigators, using rat (but also human) peripheral blood monocytes, have shown that IgE immune complexes, via interaction with an IgE receptor, cause these cells to become cytotoxic for certain parasites (92–94). Further studies with human alveolar macrophages have shown that approximately 10% of these cells in nonasthmatics and 15 to 20% of these cells in asthmatics possess IgE receptors (95,96). In addition, IgE-dependent activation of alveolar macrophages results in the release of lysosomal enzymes (95,96). Despite the fact that IgE antibodies are of particular importance in atopic disease, the amount of IgE present in the lower respiratory tract in individuals with atopic asthma is still unknown. It seems very likely that IgE-allergen interactions with macrophages will be found to have an important role in atopic lung diseases.

A great deal of work remains to be done on the role of S-IgA in the respiratory tract. Because IgA is more abundant in the upper respiratory tract than all other immunoglobulins, its role there may be proportionately greater. IgA can bind to antigens, preventing attachment of viruses and bacteria to the ciliated epithelium (2). In contrast, IgG antibodies, with their superior opsonizing potential, specific receptor sites on phagocytes, and ability to fix complement, might be preferable in peripheral airways and alveoli, where more aggressive destruction of particles might be desirable after they have evaded upper airway defenses. IgA receptors exist on human peripheral blood monocytes (97), and a recent report suggests that IgA activation of these cells via an IgA receptor is effective in promoting antibody-dependent cell cytotoxicity (98). Bacteria opsonized with IgA can be phagocytosed by human alveolar macrophages (99), suggesting that these cells possess IgA receptors, but definitive investigations for the presence of alveolar macrophage IgA receptors have not been reported.

Only a few studies have looked for antibody with antigen specificity in lung lavage material. In one study, antibody to influenza virus was detected in the lung washings from apparently healthy volunteers (17). Local immunization via an aerosol, in contrast to subcutaneous immunization, resulted in boosting detectable antibody activity that was found in both the IgG and IgA classes of immunoglobulin. A study from our laboratory examined lung lavage material from 2 patients with pneumocystis pneumonia and the acquired immunodeficiency syndrome (AIDS), and from normal healthy controls and patients with various interstitial lung diseases (100). Antipneumocystis and anticytomegalovirus antibodies were present in approximately equal amounts in all groups. The reason for the failure of AIDS patients to mount a more impressive antipneumocystis antibody response in the lungs is unclear, but it may relate to defects described in immunoregulation of humoral immunity in these patients (101). In one recent study, enhanced phagocytic activity of alveolar macrophages for *S. pneumoniae* was due to an opsonic serum factor in individuals who had received pneumococcal vaccine (102). Lung lavage material was not examined, but, clearly, investigations such as this, which in addition evaluated the effects of immunization on local respiratory tract antibodies, would be an important contribution.

Only a few studies have followed antigen from its site of deposition in the airways to the place where the host first mounts an immune response to it (Fig. 1). For the most part, in these studies the particulate antigen used was sheep red blood cells (SRBC), and the host studied was an animal. Investigators, appropriately, have been reluctant to instill antigen into human lungs. These animal studies are discussed briefly here because of their relevance to the topic of this review and because of the lack of human data.

When SRBC were instilled into selective parts of the lungs of dogs (103) or guinea pigs (104), antibody-forming cells (AFC) were detected in material retrieved by lung lavage within 4 to 6 days after the primary immunization. When antigen was selectively deposited in a single lobe, the resultant immune response remained localized to that lobe (105). Histologic evaluation of the various aspects of this immune response led to the conclusion that the immune cells found in the airways were recruited from the blood (108). Moreover, data have suggested that the primary blood source of these cells was the thoracic lymph nodes (106–108), not BALT or lymphoid aggregates in the distal airways. Thus, it seemed that SRBC were cleared to regional lymph nodes, probably by macrophages that stained with Prussian blue, indicating the presence of intracellular hemosiderin (106), and that, at least for this antigen, the antibody response began in this extraparenchymal location. Follow-up studies showed that chimpanzees, which immunologically more closely resemble humans than do other nonhuman primates (109,110), developed an immune response to intrapulmonary placement of SRBC that qualitatively resembled that observed in dogs (111). It is of interest that SRBC-induced recruitment appears not to be antigen-specific (108).

In summary, foreign particulate antigen (SRBC) placed in the terminal airways is cleared to regional draining lymph nodes, where an immune response is quickly mounted. Within 5 to 7 days, immune effector cells may appear in the airways after being recruited from the circulation. In these models it does not appear that a strictly airway or intrapulmonary immune circuit exists. Airway-associated lymphoid tissue is not capable of responding locally to this antigen and initiating an effector response; rather, an extrapulmonary tissue site is needed. This might not be the case for other antigens or antigenic substances deposited in the trachea and upper airways, but data relevant to these issues are sparse.

Fibronectin, transferrin, and surfactant are three substances not traditionally considered components of the humoral immune system. They are included in this review because at least indirect evidence supports a potential nonimmune opsonic role in host defense mechanisms for each of them. As research into the functional roles of these substances continues, it is likely that they will be found to be even more important in host defenses and possibly humoral immune mechanisms.

Recent evidence shows that fibronectin may be functionally important in enhancing macrophage/monocyte phagocytosis of particles (56,112). In one of these studies, fibronectin was found to enhance monocyte phagocytosis, not as a conventional opsonin, but rather by stimulating these cells to ingest opsonized particles (112). Another study reported that fragments of fibronectin, but not the intact molecule, augmented human alveolar macrophage phagocytosis of zymosan particles (56). This of particular interest because of zymosan's known ability to activate the alternate complement pathway. Additional work is clearly needed with this very interesting substance.

The bacteriostatic effects of transferrin on bacterial strains are strongly dependent on ionized iron and have been appreciated for many years (113). However, to date, virtually no studies have examined the activity of transferrin found in the lower respiratory tract. Given the bacteriostatic effects of transferrin, one might speculate that transferrin binds iron required for bacterial growth and thereby contributes to host defense. It is also possible that in the lower respiratory tract transferrin may share the synergistic bacteriostatic effects observed for S-IgA and lactoferrin in breast milk (114).

Surface-active (surfactant) materials are crucial to the normal function of the lung. Their most widely appreciated role is in reducing alveolar surface tension. Recent data suggest another potential role for this phospholipid substance, namely, facilitating alveolar macrophage killing of bacteria (115,116). In these experiments, incubation of staphylococci with surfactant enhanced rat or rabbit alveolar macrophage bactericidal activity against this organism. Similar studies using surfactant isolated from humans demonstrated that this surfactant also enhanced rat alveolar macrophage bactericidal activity (117). More recently, other investigators have shown that rat surfactant has antibacterial activity against several Gram-positive bacteria and can rapidly lyse and kill pneumococci (118). From these studies it appears that surfactant (probably a lipid component) can kill directly some bacteria. An alternative explanation for these observations is that surfactant either causes sublethal injury to bacteria (enabling them to be more easily killed by alveolar macrophages) or actually possesses an antibody-like activity with which bacteria are coated (opsonized), and alveolar macrophage phagocytosis and bactericidal activity are increased.

The role of BALT in immune reactions remains one of the most poorly understood issues in lung immunology, in part because technically the BALT system is difficult to work with, especially in comparison with Peyer's patches, with which it is frequently compared. Based primarily on studies from animals, there are some interesting but still unproven hypotheses about possible functions for BALT (119):

1. As previously stated, the BALT lymphoepithelium, which is devoid of cilia, goblet cells, and glandular cells, closely resembles that of Peyer's patches. This epithelial layer may allow special capture (it may be sticky) and selective transport of antigen (both particulate and soluble) to macrophages and lymphocytes immediately beneath the surface. Indeed, BALT appears strategically located in the trachea and bronchi to intercept aerosolized antigens that impact at branching points in the conducting airways. Thus, BALT may be a specialized tissue, where antigen deposited in the airways is sampled and processed.

2. BALT might be a repository for cells with the potential to secrete IgG and IgE, in addition to IgA; however, because plasma cells are not prominent, further B-lymphocyte differentiation outside the milieu of the BALT follicle must occur before immunoglobulin production takes place (a putative plasma-cell function). These immunoglobulin-bearing cells might migrate directly to the lamina propria along the respiratory tract and produce local antibody that coats mucosal surfaces. In this way BALT might be involved in the dissemination of mucosal immune responses to other tissue sites (26,119).

As previously stated, almost all our knowledge about BALT comes from studies with animals, in particular rabbits, chickens, and rats. There may be considerable species variability in the physical prominence of BALT and consequently the ease with which it can be identified. Unfortunately, in our experience (120) such lymphoid aggregates were difficult to locate in lung tissue from monkeys. Studies with human lungs obtained at autopsy are few (121).

SUMMARY

In conclusion, the respiratory tract is endowed with many of the components necessary for humoral immune responses. It is probable that these regional components operate, in some cases, independent of systemic immune responses. However, it would appear that local and systemic immune responses more frequently work together to maintain host viability. Indeed, elements of immune defenses work remarkably well considering the formidable exposure to ambient air and all its potentially injurious components. A single deficiency of one component of the humoral arm of immunity may predispose to recurrent respiratory tract infections, but these rarely are fatal to the host. Moreover, selective deficiencies enable us to probe the importance of individual components of respiratory tract defenses. The future is bright for continued progress in unraveling the complexity of host defense mechanisms.

ACKNOWLEDGMENTS

Dr. Rankin is a Parker B. Francis fellow of the Puritan-Bennett Foundation. Dr. Reynolds's work was supported in part by NIH grant HL-22302.

REFERENCES

1. Reynolds, H. Y. (1979): Lung host defenses: A status report. *Chest*, 75:239–242.
2. Reynolds, H. Y., and Merrill, W. W. (1981): Pulmonary immunology: Humoral and cellular immune responsiveness of the respiratory tract. In: *Current Pulmonology*, edited by D. H. Simmons, pp. 381–422. Wiley, New York.
3. Gail, D. B., and Lenfant, C. J. M. (1983): Cells of the lung: Biology and clinical implications (state of the art). *Am. Rev. Respir. Dis.*, 127:366–387.
4. Reynolds, H. Y., and Chretien, J. (1984): Respiratory tract fluids: Analysis of content and contemporary use in understanding lung diseases. *D.M.*, 30:1–103.
5. McFadden, E. R., Denison, D. M., Waller, J. E., Assoufi, B., Peacock, A., and Sopwith, J. (1982): Direct recordings of the temperatures in the tracheobronchial tree in normal man. *J. Clin. Invest.*, 69:700–705.
6. Thompson, R. E., Reynolds, H. Y. (1977): Isolation and characterization of canine secretory immunoglobulin M. *J. Immunol.*, 118:323–329.
7. Tomasi, T. B., Jr. (1972): Secretory immunoglobulins. *N. Engl. J. Med.*, 287:500–506.
8. Strober, W., Krakauer, R., Kleaveman, H. L., Reynolds, H. Y., and Nelson, D. L. (1976): Secretory IgA deficiency: A unique disorder of the IgA immune system. *N. Engl. J. Med.*, 294:351–366.
9. Keimowitz, R. I. (1964): Immunoglobulins in normal human tracheobronchial washings: A qualitative and quantitative study. *J. Lab. Clin. Med.*, 63:54–59.
10. Falk, G. A., Okinaka, A. J., and Siskin, G. W. (1972): Immunoglobulins in the bronchial washings of patients with chronic obstructive pulmonary disease. *Am. Rev. Respir. Dis.*, 105:14–21.
11. Mandell, M. A., Dvorak, K. J., Worman, L. W., et al. (1976): Immunoglobulin content in bronchial washings of patients with benign and malignant pulmonary disease. *N. Engl. J. Med.*, 295:694–698.
12. Wiggings, J., Hill, S. L., and Stockley, R. A. (1983): Lung secretion sol-phase proteins: Comparison of sputum with secretions obtained by direct sampling. *Thorax*, 38:102–107.

13. Reynolds, H. Y., and Merrill, W. W. (1982): Applied immunology of the lung. In: *Current Pulmonology*, edited by D. H. Simmons, pp. 167–188. Wiley, New York.

14. Hunninghake, G. W., Gadek, J. E., Kawanami, O., Ferrans, V., and Crystal, R. G. (1979): Inflammatory and immune processes in the human lung in health and disease: Evaluation by bronchoalveolar lavage. *Am. J. Pathol.*, 97:149–206.

15. Reynolds, H. Y., and Newball, H. H. (1974): Analysis of proteins and respiratory cells obtained from human lungs by bronchial lavage. *J. Lab. Clin. Med.*, 84:559–573.

16. Baughman, R. P., Bosken, C. H. G., Loudon, R. G., Hurtubise, P., and Wesseler, T. (1983): Quantitation of bronchoalveolar lavage with methylene blue. *Am. Rev. Respir. Dis.*, 128:266–270.

17. Waldman, R. H., Jurgensen, P. F., Olsen, G. N., Ganguly, R., and Johnson, J. E., III. (1973): Immune response of the human respiratory tract. I. Immunoglobulin levels and influenza virus vaccine antibody response. *J. Immunol.*, 111:38–41.

18. Warr, G. A., Martin, R. R., Sharp, P. M., and Rossen, R. D. (1977): Normal human bronchial immunoglobulins and proteins: Effects of cigarette smoking. *Am. Rev. Respir. Dis.*, 116:25–30.

19. Low, R. B., Davis, G. S., and Giancola, M. S. (1978): Biochemical analyses of bronchoalveolar lavage fluids of healthy human volunteer smokers and nonsmokers. *Am. Rev. Respir. Dis.*, 118:863–875.

20. Bell, D. Y., Haseman, J. A., Spock, A., McLennan, G., and Hook, G. E. R. (1981): Plasma proteins of the bronchoalveolar surface of the lungs of smokers and nonsmokers. *Am. Rev. Respir. Dis.*, 124:72–79.

21. Merrill, W. W., Goodenberger, D., Strober, W., Matthay, R. A., Naegel, G. P., and Reynolds, H. Y. (1980): Free secretory component and other proteins in human lung lavage. *Am. Rev. Respir. Dis.*, 122:156–161.

22. Rankin, J. A., Naegel, G. P., Schrader, C., Matthay, R. A., and Reynolds, H. Y. (1983): Airspace immunoglobulin production and levels in bronchoalveolar lavage fluid of normal subjects and patients with sarcoidosis. *Am. Rev. Respir. Dis.*, 127:442–448.

23. Pennington, J. E., and Reynolds, H. Y. (1973): Concentrations of gentamycin and carbenicillin in bronchial secretions. *J. Infect. Dis.*, 128:63–68.

24. Kaltreider, H. B., and Chan, M. K. L. (1976): The class-specific immunoglobulin composition of fluids obtained from various levels of the canine respiratory tract. *J. Immunol.*, 116:423–429.

25. Reynolds, H. Y., Merrill, W. W., Amento, E. P., and Naegel, G. P. (1978): Immunoglobulin A in secretions from the lower human respiratory tract. In: *Proceedings of an International Symposium on the Secretory Immune System and Caries Immunity*, edited by J. R. McGhee, J. Mestecky, and J. L. Babb, pp. 553–564. Plenum Press, New York.

26. Scrobogna, S., and Trani, S. (1979): Polymeres d'IgA dans la secretion bronchique et dans Les Liquides biologiques. *Bull. Eur. Physiopathol. Respir.*, 15:40P.

27. Merrill, W. W., Naegel, G. P., Olchowski, J., and Reynolds, H. Y. (1984): Immunoglobulin G subclasses in blood and lavage fluid of patients with hypersensitivity pneumonitis. *Clin. Res.*, 32:433A.

28. Rankin, J. A., Olchowski, J., Naegel, G. P., Merrill, W. W., and Reynolds, H. Y. (1984): IgG subclasses in bronchoalveolar lavage fluid (BAL) and serum from patients with sarcoidosis. *Abstracts of 10th International Conference on Sarcoidosis*, Baltimore, Maryland.

29. Kazmierowsky, J. A., Durbin, W. A., and Reynolds, H. Y. (1976): Kinetics of immunoglobulin transport into canine bronchial secretions. *Proc. Soc. Exp. Biol. Med.*, 152:493–498.

30. Lawrence, E. C., Blaese, R. M., Martin, R. R., and Stevens, P. M. (1978): Immunoglobulin secreting cells in normal human bronchial lavage fluids. *J. Clin. Invest.*, 62:832–835.

31. Hunninghake, G. W., and Crystal, R. G. (1981): Mechanisms of hypergammaglobulinemia in pulmonary sarcoidosis. *J. Clin. Invest.*, 67:86–92.

32. Hunninghake, G. W., Kawanami, O., Ferrans, V. J., Young, R. C., Jr., Roberts, W. C., and Crystal, R. G. (1981): Characterization of the inflammatory and immune effector cells in the lung parenchyma of patients with interstitial lung disease. *Am. Rev. Respir. Dis.*, 123:407–412.

33. Daniele, R. P., Altose, M. D., and Rowlands, D. T., Jr. (1975): Immunocompetent cells from the lower respiratory tract of normal human lungs. *J. Clin. Invest.*, 56:986–995.

34. Lamm, M. E. (1976): Cellular aspects of immunoglobulin. *Adv. Immunol.*, 22:244–259.

35. Bienenstock, J., and Befus, A. D. (1983): Some thoughts on the biologic role of immunoglobulin A. *Gastroenterology*, 84:178–185.

36. Bienenstock, J., Befus, D., McDermott, M., Mirski, S., and Rosenthal, K. (1983): Regulation of lymphoblast traffic and localization in mucosal tissues, with emphasis on IgA. *Fed. Proc.*, 42:3213–3217.

37. Valeyre, D., Saumon, G., Bladier, D., Amouroux, J., Pre, J., Battesti, J.-P., and Georges, R. (1982): The relationship between noninvasive explorations in pulmonary sarcoidosis of recent origin, as shown in bronchoalveolar lavage, serum, and pulmonary function tests. *Am. Rev. Respir. Dis.*, 126:41–45.

38. Reynolds, H. Y., Fulmer, J. D., Kazmierowski, J. A., Roberts, W. C., Frank, M. M., and Crystal, R. G. (1977): Analysis of cellular and protein content of bronchoalveolar lavage fluid from patients with idiopathic pulmonary fibrosis and chronic hypersensitivity pneumonitis. *J. Clin. Invest.*, 59:165–175.

39. Weinberger, S. E., Kelman, J. A., Elson, N. A., Young, R. C., Reynolds, H. Y., Fulmer, J. D., and Crystal, R. G. (1978): Bronchoalveolar lavage in interstitial lung disease. *Ann. Intern. Med.*, 89:459–466.

40. Merrill, W. W., Naegel, G. P., and Reynolds, H. Y. (1980): Reaginic antibody in the lung lining fluid: Analysis of normal human bronchoalveolar lavage fluid IgE and comparison to immunoglobulins G and A. *J. Lab. Clin. Med.*, 96:494–599.

41. Patterson, R., McKenna, J. M., Suszko, I. M., Solliday, N. H., Pruzansky, J. J., Roberts, M., Kehoe, T. J. (1977): Living histamine containing cells from the bronchial lumens of humans. Description and comparison of histamine content with cells of rhesus monkeys. *J. Clin. Invest.*, 59:217–225.

42. Yunginer, J. W., and Gleich, G. J. (1973): Seasonal changes in serum and nasal IgE concentrations. *J. Allergy Clin. Immunol.*, 51:174–186.

43. Tada, T., and Ishizaka, K. (1970): Distribution of gamma E forming cells in lymphoid tissue of human and monkey. *J. Immunol.*, 104:377–387.

44. Waldmann, R. H., Virchow, C., and Rowe, D. S. (1973): IgE levels in external secretions. *Int. Arch. Allergy*, 44:242–248.

45. Tomasi, T. B., Jr., and McNabb, P. C. (1980): The secretory immune system. In: *Basic and Clinical Immunology*, edited by H. H. Fundenberg, D. P. Sites, J. L. Caldwell, and J. V. Wells, pp. 240–250. Lange Medical, Los Altos, Calif.

46. Reynolds, H. Y., and Merrill, W. W. (1982): Lung immunology: The inflammatory response in lung parenchyma. In: *Current Pulmonology*, edited by D. H. Simmons, pp. 299–323. Wiley, New York.

47. Benacerraf, B., and Unanue, E. R. (1980): *Textbook of Immunology*, pp. 218–238. Williams & Wilkins, Baltimore.

48. Robertson, J., Caldwell, J. R., Castle, J. R., and Waldman, R. H. (1976): Evidence for the presence of components of the alternate (properdin) pathway of complement activation in respiratory secretions. *J. Immunol.*, 117:900–903.

49. Nathan, C. F., Murray, H. W., and Cohn, Z. A. (1980): The macrophage as an effector cell. *N. Engl. J. Med.*, 303:622–626.

50. Reid, K. B. M., and Solomon, E. (1977): Biosynthesis of the first component of complement by human fibroblasts. *Biochem. J.*, 167:647–660.

51. Cole, S., Matthews, W. J., Jr., Rossing, T. H., Gash, D. J., Lichtenberg, N. A., and Pennington, J. E. (1983): Complement biosynthesis by human bronchoalveolar macrophages. *Clin. Immunopathol.*, 27:153–159.

52. Alpert, S. E., Auerbach, H. S., Cole, S., and Colten, H. R. (1983): Macrophage maturation: Differences in complement secretion by marrow, monocyte, and tissue macrophages detected with an improved hemolytic plaque assay. *J. Immunol.*, 130:102–107.

53. Matsuda, M., Yoshida, N., Aoki, N., and Wakabayashi, K. (1978): Distribution of cold insoluble globulin in plasma and tissues. *Ann. N.Y. Acad. Sci.*, 312:74–92.

54. Rennard, S. I., and Crystal, R. G. (1981): Fibronectin in human bronchopulmonary lavage fluid: Evaluation in patients with interstitial lung disease. *J. Clin. Invest.*, 69:113–127.

55. Rudslahti, E., Engvall, E., and Hayman, E. G. (1981): Fibronectin: Current concepts of its structure and functions. *Coll. Res.*, 1:95–128.

56. Pommier, C. G., Inada, S., Fries, L. F., Takahashi, T., Frank, M., and Brown, E. J. (1983): Plasma fibronectin enhances phagocytosis of opsonized particles by human peripheral blood monocytes. *J. Exp. Med.*, 157:1844–1854.

57. Yamada, K., and Olden, K. (1978): Fibronectins—adhesive glycoproteins of cell surface and blood. *Nature*, 275:179–184.

58. Villiger, B., Broeklermann, T., Kelley, D., Heymach, G. J., McDonald, J. A. (1981): Bronchoalveolar fibronectin in smokers and nonsmokers. *Am. Rev. Respir. Dis.*, 124:652–654.

59. Stenman, S., and Vaheri, A. (1978): Distribution of a major connective tissue protein, fibronectin, in normal human tissues. *J. Exp. Med.*, 147:1054–1067.

60. Bray, B. A. (1978): Cold insoluble globulin (fibronectin) in connective tissues of adult human lung and in trophoblast basement membrane. *J. Clin. Invest.*, 62:745–752.

61. Baum, B. J., McDonald, J. A., and Crystal, R. G. (1977): Metabolic fate of major cell surface protein of normal human fibroblasts. *Biochem. Biophys. Res. Commun.*, 79:8–15.

62. Yamada, K. M., Yamada, S. S., and Pastan, I. (1977): Quantitation of a transformation-sensitive, adhesive cell surface glycoprotein. *J. Cell Biol.*, 74:649–654.

63. Villiger, B., Kelley, D. G., Kuhn, C., Englemen, W., and McDonald, J. A. (1981): Human alveolar macrophage fibronectin: Synthesis secretion and ultrastructural localization during gelatin-coated latex particle binding. *J. Cell Biol.*, 90:711–720.

64. Rennard, S. I., Bitterman, P., Hunninghake, G., Gadek, J., and Crystal, R. (1981): Alveolar macrophage fibronectin: A possible mediator of tissue remodeling in fibrotic lung disease. *Clin. Res.*, 29:267A.

65. Hunninghake, G. W., and Fauci, A. S. (1976): Immunologic reactivity in the lung. I. A guinea pig model for the study of pulmonary mononuclear cell subpopulations. *Cell. Immunol.*, 26:89–97.

66. Bienenstock, J., McDermott, M. R., and Befus, A. D. (1982): The significance of bronchus-associated lymphoid tissue. *Bull. Eur. Physiopath. Resp.*, 18:153–177.

67. Murray, J. F. (1976): *The Normal Lung: The Basis for Diagnosis and Treatment of Pulmonary Disease*, pp. 59–64. W. B. Saunders, Philadelphia.

68. Platts-Mills, T. A. E., Von Maur, R. K., Ishizaka, K., Norman, P. S., and Lichtenstein, L. M. (1976): IgA and IgG anti-ragweed antibodies in nasal secretions. *J. Clin. Invest.*, 57:1041–1050.

69. Brunner, H., Greenberg, H. B., James, W. D., Horswood, R. L., Couch, R. B., Chanock, R. M. (1973): Antibody to *Mycoplasma pneumoniae* in nasal secretions and sputa of experimentally infected human volunteers. *Infect. Immun.*, 8:612–620.

70. Newcomb, R. W., Ishizaka, K., and DeVald, B. L. (1969): Human IgG and IgA diphtheria antitoxins in serum, nasal fluids and saliva. *J. Immunol.*, 103:215–224.

71. Rossen, R. D., Wolff, S. M., and Butler, W. T. (1964): The antibody response in nasal washings and serum to *S. typhosa* endotoxin administered intravenously. *J. Immunol.*, 99:246–254.

72. Soutar, C. A. (1976): Distribution of plasma cells and other cells containing immunoglobulins in the respiratory tract of normal man and class of immunoglobulin contained therein. *Thorax*, 3:158–165.

73. Mulks, M. H., Kornfeld, S. W., and Plaut, A. G. (1980): Specific proteolysis of human IgA by *Streptococcus pneumoniae* and *Haemophilus influenzae*. *J. Infect. Dis.*, 141:450–456.

74. Kilian, M., Mestecky, J., Kulhavy, R., Tomana, M., and Butler, W. T. (1980): IgA, proteases from *Haemophilus influenzae*, *Streptococcus pneumoniae*, *Neisseria meningitidis* and *Streptococcus sanguis*: Comparative immunochemical studies. *J. Immunol.*, 124:2596–2600.

75. Latil, F., Vervloet, D., Casanova, P., Garbe, L., Fuentes, P., Wierzbicki, N., and Charpin, J. (1983): Efficacy of aerosol microbial immunization to elicit plasma cells in bronchial mucosa. *Rev. Fr. Mal. Resp.*, 11:338.

76. Naegel, G. P., Young, K. R., Jr., and Reynolds, H. Y. (1984): Receptors for human IgG subclasses on human alveolar macrophages. *Am. Rev. Respir. Dis.*, 129:413–418.

77. Morell, A., Terry, W. D., and Waldmann, T. A. (1970): Metabolic properties of IgG subclasses in man. *J. Clin. Invest.*, 49:673–680.

78. Huber, H., Douglas, S. D., Nusbacher, J., Kochwa, S., and Rosenfield, R. E. (1971): IgG subclass specificity of human monocyte receptor sites. *Nature*, 229:419–420.

79. Hay, F. C., Torrigiani, G., and Roitt, I. M. (1972): The binding of human IgG subclasses to human monocytes. *Eur. J. Immunol.*, 2:257–261.

80. Shur, P. H., Borel, H., Gelfand, E., Alper, C. A., and Rosen, F. S. (1970): Selective gamma-G globulin deficiencies in patients with recurrent pyogenic infections. *N. Engl. J. Med.*, 263:631–634.

81. Yount, W. J., Hong, R., Seligmann, M., and Kunkel, H. G. (1970): Imbalances of gammaglobulin subgroups and gene defects in patients with primary hypo-gamma-globulinemia. *J. Clin. Invest.*, 49:1957–1966.

82. Drutz, D. J., and Mills, J. (1980): Immunity and infection. In: *Basic and Clinical Immunology*, edited by H. H. Fundenberg, D. P. Sites, J. L. Caldwell, and J. V. Wells, pp. 251–273. Lange Medical, Los Altos, Calif.

83. Huber, H., Douglas, S. D., Nusbacher, J., Kochwa, S., and Rosenfield, R. E. (1971): IgG subclass specificity of human monocyte receptor sites. *Nature*, 229:419–420.
84. Kronvall, G., and Williams, R. C., Jr. (1969): Differences in anti-protein a activity among IgG subgroups. *J. Immunol.*, 103:828–833.
85. Kurlander, R. J., Rosse, W. F., and Logue, G. L. (1977): Qualitative influence of antibody and complement coating of red cells on monocyte mediated cell lysis. *J. Clin. Invest.*, 61:1309–1319.
86. Reynolds, H. Y., Atkinson, J. P., Newball, H. H., and Frank, M. M. (1975): Receptors for immunoglobulin and complement on human alveolar macrophages. *J. Immunol.*, 114:1813–1819.
87. Murphy, S. A., Schreiber, A. D., and Root, R. K. (1979): The role of antibody and complement in phagocytosis by rabbit alveolar macrophages. *J. Infect. Dis.*, 140:876–903.
88. Alper, C. A., Bloch, J. H., and Rosen, F. S. (1973): Increased susceptibility to infection in a patient with type II essential hypercatabolism of C3. *N. Engl. J. Med.*, 288:601–606.
89. Alper, C. A., Abramson, N., Johnson, R. B., Jandl, J. H., and Rosen, F. S. (1970): Increased susceptibility to infection associated with abnormalities of complement-mediated functions and of the third component of complement C3. *N. Engl. J. Med.*, 282:349–354.
90. Alper, C. A., Rosen, F. S., and Lachmann, P. J. (1972): Inactivator of the third component of complement as an inhibitor in the properdin pathway. *Proc. Natl. Acad. Sci. U.S.A.*, 69:2910–2913.
91. Beck, C. S., and Heiner, D. C. (1981): Selective immunoglobulin G4 deficiency and recurrent infections of the respiratory tract. *Am. J. Respir. Dis.*, 124:94–96.
92. Caparon, A., Dessaint, J.-P., Rousseau, R., Capron, M., and Bazin, H. (1977): Interaction between IgE complexes and macrophages in the rat: A new mechanism of macrophage activation. *Eur. J. Immunol.*, 7:315–322.
93. Joseph, M., Capron, A., Butterworth, A. E., Sturrock, R. F., and Houba, V. (1978): Cytotoxicity of human and baboon mononuclear phagocytes against schistosomula *in vitro*: Induction by immune complexes containing IgE and *Schistosoma mansonii* antigens. *Clin. Exp. Immunol.*, 33:48–56.
94. Rankin, J. A., and Askenase, P. W. (1984): The potential role of alveolar macrophages as a source of pathogenic mediators in allergic asthma. In: *Asthma: Physiology, Immunopharmacology, and Treatment*, edited by M. Lichtenstein and K. F. Austen, Academic Press, New York.
95. Joseph, M., Tonnel, A. B., Capron, A., and Dessaint, J.-P. (1981): The interaction of IgE antibody with human alveolar macrophages and its participation in the inflammatory processes of lung allery. *Agents and Actions*, 11:619–622.
96. Joseph, M., Tonnel, A. B., Torpier, G., Capron, A., Arnoux, B., and Benveniste, J. (1983): Involvement of immunoglobulin E in the secretory processes of alveolar macrophages from asthmatic patients. *J. Clin. Invest.*, 71:221–230.
97. Fanger, M. W., Shen, L., Pugh, J., and Bernier, G. M. (1980): Subpopulations of human peripheral granulocytes and monocytes express receptors for IgA. *Proc. Natl. Acad. Sci. U.S.A.*, 77:3640–3644.
98. Lowell, G. H., Smith, L. F., Griffiss, J. M., and Brandt, B. L. (1980): IgA-dependent, monocyte-mediated, antibacterial activity. *J. Exp. Med.*, 152:452–457.
99. Reynolds, H. Y., Kazmierowski, J. A., and Newball, H. H. (1975): Specificity of opsonic antibodies to enhance phagocytosis of *Pseudomonas aeruginosa* by human alveolar macrophages. *J. Clin. Invest.*, 56:376–385.
100. Rankin, J. A., Walzer, P. D., Dwyer, J. M., Schrader, C. E., Enriquez, R. E., and Merrill, W. W. (1983): Immunologic alterations in bronchoalveolar lavage fluid in the acquired immunodeficiency syndrome (AIDS). *Am. Rev. Respir. Dis.*, 128:189–194.
101. Lane, H. C., Masur, H., Edgar, L. C., Whalen, G., Rook, A. H., and Fauci, A. S. (1983): Abnormalities of B-cell activation and immunoregulation in patients with the acquired immunodeficiency syndrome. *N. Engl. J. Med.*, 309:453–458.
102. Hill, J. O., Bice, D. E., Harris, D. L., and Muggenberg, B. A. (1983): Evaluation of the pulmonary immune response by analysis of bronchoalveolar fluids obtained by serial lung lavage. *Int. Arch. Allergy Appl. Immunol.*, 72:173–177.
103. Kaltreider, H. B., Kyselka, L., and Salmon, S. E. (1974): Immunology of the lower respiratory tract. II. The plaque-forming response of canine lymphoid tissue to sheep erythrocytes after intrapulmonary or intravenous immunization. *J. Clin. Invest.*, 54:263–270.
104. Hunninghake, G. W., and Fauci, A. S. (1977): Immunologic reactivity of the lung. V. Regulatory effects of antibody on the pulmonary immune response to locally administered antigen. *J. Immunol.*, 118:1728–1733.

105. Bice, D. E., Harris, D. L., Hill, J. O., Muggenberg, B. A., and Wolff, R. K. (1980): Immune responses in the dog after localized lung immunization. *Am. Rev. Resp. Dis.*, 122:755–760.
106. Brownstein, D. G., Rebar, A. H., Bice, D. E., Muggenberg, B. A., and Hill, J. O. (1980): Immunology of the lower respiratory tract: Serial morphologic changes in the lungs and tracheobronchial lymph nodes of dogs after intrapulmonary immunization with sheep erythrocytes. *Am. J. Pathol.*, 98:499–514.
107. Bice, D. E., Harris, D. L., and Muggenberg, B. A. (1980): Regional immunologic responses following localized deposition of antigen in the lung. *Exp. Lung Res.*, 1:33–41.
108. Bice, D. E., Degen, M. A., Harris, D. L., and Muggenberg, B. A. (1982): Recruitment of antibody-forming cells in the lung after local immunization is nonspecific. *Am. Rev. Respir. Dis.*, 126:635–639.
109. Mohagheghpour, N., and Leone, C. A. (1969): An immunologic study of the relationships of nonhuman primates to man. *Comp. Biochem. Physiol.*, 31:437–452.
110. Schur, P. H., Connelly, A., and Jones, T. C. (1975): Phylogeny of complement components in nonhuman primates. *J. Immunol.*, 114:270–273.
111. Bice, D. E., Harris, D. L., Muggenberg, B. A., and Bowen, J. A. (1982): The evaluation of lung immunity in chimpanzees. *Am. Rev. Respir. Dis.*, 126:358–359.
112. Czop, J. K., McGowan, S. E., and Center, D. E. (1982): Opsonin-independent phagocytosis by human alveolar macrophages: Augmentation by human plasma fibronectin. *Am. Rev. Respir. Dis.*, 125:607–609.
113. Schade, A. L. (1960): The microbiological activity of siderophilin. In: *Protides of the Biological Fluids*, edited by H. Peeters, p. 261. Elsevier, Amsterdam.
114. Stephens, S., Dolby, J. M., Montreuil, J., and Spik, G. (1980): Differences in inhibition of the growth of commensal and enteropathogenic strains of *Escherichia coli* by lactotransferrin and secretory immunoglobulin A isolated from human milk. *Immunology*, 41:597–603.
115. Laforce, F. M., Kelly, W. J., and Huber, G. L. (1973): Inactivation of staphylococci by alveolar macrophages with preliminary observations on the importance of alveolar lining material. *Am. Rev. Respir. Dis.*, 108:784–790.
116. Laforce, F. M. (1976): Effect of alveolar lining material in the phagocytic and bactericidal activity of lung macrophages against *Staphylococcus aureus. J. Lab. Clin. Med.*, 88:691–699.
117. Juers, J. A., Rogers, R. M., McCurdy, J. B., and Cook, W. W. (1976): Enhancement of bactericidal capacity of alveolar macrophages by human alveolar lining material. *J. Clin. Invest.*, 589:271–275.
118. Coonrod, J. D., and Yoneda, K. (1983): Detection and partial characterization of antibacterial factor(s) in alveolar lining material of rats. *J. Clin. Invest.*, 71:129–141.
119. Bienenstock, J., Clancy, R. L., and Percy, D. Y. C. (1976): Bronchial associated lymphoid tissue: Its relationship to mucosal immunity. In: *Immunologic and Infectious Reactions in the Lung*, edited by C. H. Kirkpatrick and H. Y. Reynolds, pp. 29–58. Marcel Dekker, New York.
120. Moritz, E. D., Naegel, G. P., Smith, G. J. W., and Reynolds, H. Y. (1984): Bronchus-associated lymphoid tissue in a sub-human primate model of cell-mediated immunity. *Am. Rev. Respir. Dis., (in press)*.
121. Clancy, R. L., Pucci, A. A., Jelihovsky, T., and Bye, P. (1978): Immunologic "memory" for microbial antigens in lymphocytes obtained from human bronchial mucosa. *Am. Rev. Respir. Dis.*, 117:513–518.

Advances in Host Defense Mechanisms, Vol. 4,
edited by J. I. Gallin and A. S. Fauci.
Raven Press, New York © 1985.

Immunosuppression of Pulmonary Host Defenses

James E. Pennington

Infectious Disease Division, Department of Medicine, Brigham and Women's Hospital and Harvard Medical School, Boston, Massachusetts 02115

The lung is the organ most frequently involved with infection in immunosuppressed and myelosuppressed hosts, regardless of the underlying disease process (11–13,17,42,50,61). Although a number of factors may contribute to this susceptibility, the unusually large bronchoalveolar epithelial surface area exposed to potentially infectious agents in the environment offers a particularly attractive explanation (52). There has been great concern over the high mortality associated with pneumonia in immunosuppressed hosts. This has been especially noteworthy among patients receiving chemotherapy for hematologic neoplasias. Mortalities of 65% or greater have been reported for pneumonia among patients with acute leukemia (54). One report compared the mortality associated with fever and neutropenia alone and the mortality associated with fever and neutropenia plus pulmonary infiltrates (45). The mortality among those without pneumonia was 25%, compared with 62% mortality if lungs were involved.

In addition to cancer chemotherapy, the immunosuppressive regimens used for organ transplant recipients also result in life-threatening pulmonary infections. In earlier days, up to 42% of renal transplant recipients experienced pneumonia (10). More recently, this complication has been reduced to approximately 20 to 25% (22,50). However, pneumonia remains the most common cause of fatality among renal, as well as bone marrow, transplant patients (12). Even more discouraging in one report was the common occurrence of fatal secondary lung infections among renal transplant patients with primary pneumonias (50). Others have reported that at least 50% of bone marrow recipients will develop pneumonia and that one-third of these cases will be fatal (37,61). Finally, a population of patients with a condition currently known as acquired immune-deficiency syndrome (AIDS) has recently been described (13,17). Just as with drug-induced immunosuppression, the lung is the organ system most frequently involved with life-threatening infection (13,17,43). Furthermore, the mortality from pneumonias caused by opportunistic pathogens in patients with AIDS has been between 40 and 60% (43).

Impaired host defenses undoubtedly play a major role in accounting for the high mortality from pneumonia among immunosuppressed patients. However, diagnostic

TABLE 1. *Association between specific defects in host defense and specific infectious agents in the lung*

Defect	Usual condition	Pulmonary pathogens
Granulocytopenia	Cancer chemotherapy (especially hematologic neoplasias)	Gram-negative bacilli; *Staphylococcus aureus; Aspergillus; Mucor*
Cell-mediated immunity	Organ transplantation; high-dosage glucocorticosteroids; AIDS; Hodgkin's disease	Herpes-group virus (e.g., CMV); *Pneumocystis carinii; Nocardia; Cryptococcus; Legionella* sp.; mycobacteria
Hypogammaglobulinemia/dysgammaglobulinemia	Chronic lymphocytic leukemia; multiple myeloma	Pneumococci; *Haemophilus influenzae*

difficulties compound the problem of providing early and appropriate therapy. A wide array of possible causes, many requiring different therapies, confront the clinician in such a patient with pneumonia. Sputum and blood cultures are generally not diagnostic, and serologic diagnoses in the immunocompromised host are usually not possible. Although invasive diagnostic procedures may be useful in guiding therapy, procedures such as bronchoscopy, transthoracic needle aspiration, or open lung biopsy may not always be possible in these high-risk patients (11,12,42). Thus, empiric therapy often must be chosen for the immunosuppressed patient with pneumonia.

One of the most useful approaches to choosing empiric therapy for the immunocompromised patient with pneumonia is based on immunoepidemiologic observations that have been collected over the past 15 years (11,12). Taken together, these observations demonstrate clear-cut associations between the type of immune risk factor present in the host and specific infectious agents (Table 1). In addition to providing a rational means for choosing empiric therapy in a particular type of patient with pneumonia, these associations strongly suggest that discrete defects in pulmonary host defenses exist that predispose to certain pathogens and that a better understanding of the mechanisms by which these defects occur might provide insight into better methods of prevention or treatment of pneumonia. Furthermore, whereas it is now clear that specific types of immunosuppression and myelosuppression predispose to specific pulmonary pathogens, it is even more fascinating to consider that specific facets of a particular immune response are preferentially impaired by certain immunosuppressing conditions. For example, whereas corticosteroids and cyclosporin A each suppress the cell-mediated immune system, it may be that one of these agents (e.g., steroids) acts preferentially in suppressing interleukin-1 (IL-1) generation by alveolar macrophages, and the other (e.g., cyclosporin A) might preferentially affect pulmonary lymphocyte production of interleukin-2 (IL-2). Might certain facultative intracellular pathogens be associated with defective IL-1 rather than IL-2 deficiency? Whether or not such detailed analyses of the mechanisms of lung immunosuppression will reveal discrete differences such as these is speculative. However, systemic analyses suggest that such an approach to studies of pulmonary immunosuppression might be fruitful.

With these rather practical clinical points in mind, and with a clinical problem of such enormous magnitude, it is surprising that so little information is available regarding mechanisms of pulmonary immunosuppression. Although ample data exist regarding the systemic effects of various immunosuppressive and myelosuppressive drugs, the well-known dissociation between systemic and local pulmonary immune reactions (4,6,29) precludes extrapolation from systemic data to local defects in the lung. In recent years, the availability of flexible fiberoptic bronchoscopy has provided a well-tolerated method for obtaining clinical specimens for immunologic studies (26). However, relatively few such studies have been reported among immunocompromised patients.

HUMAN STUDIES

Studies to define local mechanisms of pulmonary immunosuppression in humans are hampered by two major factors. First is the known risk of bronchoscopically induced pneumonitis, even among normal volunteers. Thus, it has generally been considered too hazardous to undertake bronchoscopic lavage of immunosuppressed and myelosuppressed patients for the sole purpose of obtaining cells and fluid for laboratory investigation. Second, the usual circumstances in which bronchopulmonary lavage is carried out in these patients involve a diagnostic procedure for infiltrative lung disease, often in association with a fever. In this setting, interpretation of data demonstrating alterations in numbers or function of cells retrieved at bronchoscopy is difficult, because the acute illness or the underlying disease and therapy might affect these specimens. Thus, it is almost impossible to find clearcut data defining the effects of immunosuppressing medications on cell numbers and function in the human lung. Despite these obvious problems with human studies, a few relevant investigations have been carried out.

Two studies have been reported in which the effects of immunosuppressing and myelosuppressing drugs on human alveolar macrophages have been analyzed. In one report, Golde et al. (15) studied pulmonary cells obtained by bronchoscopic lavage in 3 patients with acute leukemia. Each patient was myelosuppressed, and in each case clinical and microbiologic evidence for intercurrent lung infection was present. Although quantitative analyses were not carried out, a qualitative assessment of alveolar macrophages revealed the capacity for ingestion of *Candida* and also revealed that Fc surface receptors were present on the macrophage membranes. Furthermore, alveolar macrophages were able to produce a colony-stimulating growth factor in tissue cultures. Although these observations suggest that chemotherapy did not abrogate certain alveolar macrophage functions, it must be pointed out that drug effects in the lung are unlikely to be all-or-nothing phenomena. Rather, quantitative analysis of lung cells, with concomitant normal controls, might provide the most sensitive method of analysis.

In a second study, carried out at the same institution, such controlled studies were described. Seven adult bone marrow transplantation patients underwent bronchoscopy, in this case without obvious intercurrent lung diseases (62). In each case, the patient's underlying disease was acute leukemia. Patients were studied only once, but the time intervals after transplantation varied widely, ranging from 2 to 11 months. Other than 3 patients receiving weekly methotrexate, no immunosuppressive drugs were given concomitant with the bronchoscopic examinations. Alveolar macrophages were evaluated for chemotaxis, phagocytosis of *Candida* (microscopic analysis), and killing activity against *Staphylococcus aureus*. Marked decreases in these functions were noted for cells obtained during the first 4 months following transplantation, a period associated with the highest risk of pneumonia. Furthermore, concomitant studies carried out with autologous blood monocytes revealed normal function among blood cells in patients with impaired alveolar macrophage function. It was concluded that local pulmonary cellular defenses are impaired for several months following bone marrow transplantation, even without concurrent drug treatments. Furthermore, it appeared that monitoring blood monocyte function would not suffice in estimating the status of lung defenses in these patients. Of some interest was that among the 5 patients found to have abnormal alveolar macrophage function, cytomegalovirus (CMV) was subsequently cultured from the lung washings of 2 patients. The role of CMV in suppressing macrophage function could not be ascertained.

Even less information is available regarding humoral immune status in the immunosuppressed human lung. In one study, a group of 28 patients with unilateral carcinoma of the lung underwent bilateral bronchoalveolar lavage, and the concentrations of immunoglobulins in lung washings were compared between normal and involved lungs (33). Increased levels of IgA were present in washings from lungs with cancer. No correlation between local immunoglobulins and cancer chemotherapy was made.

In a recent study carried out at our own institution, the capacity for biosynthesis of complement proteins by normal and diseased alveolar macrophages was evaluated (6). For 8 normal subjects, biosynthetic rates for C2 and factor B fell within a narrow range. For 15 patients, a wide range of synthetic rates was observed. Of interest was 1 patient, receiving prednisone at the time of bronchoscopy, for whom the synthetic rates for C2 and factor B were reduced by 25% (C2) and 30% (factor B) below normal values. These limited observations only serve to highlight the need for a more complete analysis of the impact of immunosuppression on complement function in the human lung.

Finally, the spectrum of pulmonary immunologic abnormalities in patients with AIDS is unknown. Only now are the details of systemic immune dysfunction being described (13,17), and far less information is available regarding pulmonary immunopathology in AIDS. Two preliminary observations are worth noting, however. In one report (64), 5 healthy human volunteers were compared with 11 healthy male homosexuals for the characteristics of bronchoalveolar lavage specimens. There were no significant differences between the groups in numbers of alveolar macrophages, total lymphocytes, or the OKT-4-to-T8 ratio of T lymphocytes in lung lavage fluids. In addition, no differences in immunoglobulin-secreting cells were noted among these subjects. More recently, investigators from the same institution reported their bronchoscopic lavage data for 2 male patients with AIDS (one homosexual, one case of intravenous drug abuse) (51). Each patient had both CMV and *Pneumocystis carinii* pneumonia at the time of lavage. An intense intrabronchial inflammatory response was observed, with increased percentages of polymorphonuclear leukocytes (20 and 60%, respectively), and also increased numbers of immunoglobulin-secreting cells in the lavage fluids. The numbers of lymphocytes in lavages were normal, and the T-lymphocyte subsets in lavage fluids were not examined. These alterations were limited to lung fluids, and the role of the ongoing lung infection versus AIDS itself in producing the local alterations in inflammatory cells could not be determined.

Finally, preliminary work in our own laboratory has examined the capacity of alveolar macrophages from patients with AIDS to develop a respiratory burst. After studying 4 such patients to date (bronchial lavages performed by Dr. Thomas Rossing, Respiratory Division, Brigham and Women's Hospital), we have found 1 patient for whom a respiratory burst did not occur when his alveolar macrophages were stimulated with phorbol myristate acetate.

Thus, it can safely be stated that our current understanding of mechanisms of pulmonary immunopathology in virtually all categories of immunocompromised patients is minimal. For these reasons, considerable work has been carried out in animal models of immunosuppression in an effort to provide insights into this difficult area.

EXPERIMENTAL STUDIES

Animal models of immunosuppression provide a system in which multiple observations, using invasive techniques, over widely differing ranges of immunosuppressing and myelosuppressing treatments can be made. Such models also provide a system in which investigational prophylactic and therapeutic strategies can be evaluated. Although these various animals differ from humans in their responses to immunosuppressives (5), enough information has been accumulated from these models to permit some cautious extrapolations to the clinical setting (1,5).

Alveolar Macrophages

The pulmonary alveolar macrophage is a cell that is critical to pulmonary host defense (16,18). Research in recent years has brought to light an even more complex role for this cell than was originally conceived. Apart from the well-recognized phagocytic and microbicidal activities of the alveolar macrophage, there is now a rapidly expanding list of secretory host defense activities for this cell (6,14, 25,26,35,49). Thus, whereas it remains appropriate to consider the alveolar macrophage as a pivotal component in lung defenses, it is clear that simply examining the effects of immunosuppression on direct antibacterial activities will not be sufficient to fully understand the immunosuppressed alveolar macrophage.

Quantitative Effects of Radiotherapy and Drug Therapy

Numerous studies have described the origin and kinetics of alveolar macrophages. The influences of immunosuppression and myelosuppression on the numbers of these cells both in resting lungs and in infected lungs have also been examined. Despite these multiple studies, a consensus has not been reached on the precise origin and kinetics of these cells. For example, some consider that alveolar macrophages are derived solely from bone marrow (59), whereas others believe that pulmonary interstitial macrophages may replicate and serve as a local means to populate the alveolar spaces with macrophages (20).

In several studies, radiation-induced myelosuppression was employed in an attempt to differentiate between a local origin and bone marrow origin for alveolar macrophages. In one such study (55), beagle dogs were exposed to total-body irradiation and then given bone marrow transplants. Serial blood and bronchial lavage specimens revealed that by 1 week after irradiation, the numbers of blood monocytes were reduced, and by day 21 the numbers of alveolar macrophages were significantly reduced. Furthermore, by day 30, the numbers of blood and alveolar monocyte-macrophages had returned to normal. Sex chromatin studies confirmed that the new alveolar macrophages were of marrow origin. It was concluded (a) that alveolar macrophages are predominantly (or totally) of marrow origin and (b) that myelosuppression reduces the numbers of these cells in alveolar spaces. However, separate studies employing local thoracic irradiation led to a different conclusion. In those studies, only thoracic irradiation was given, and again reduced numbers of alveolar macrophages were described (19,38). It was concluded that suppression of local precursor cells in the lungs accounted for these findings. Unfortunately, neither experimental approach can conclusively solve the dilemma, because total-body irradiation includes lung tissues, and thoracic irradiation includes marrow tissues. Even studies showing greater reduction in alveolar macrophage numbers resulting from total rather than thoracic irradiation (36,60) cannot exclude a local source for macrophages in the lung. Finally, one study employing total-body irradiation of dogs failed to detect any reduction in alveolar macrophage numbers (53). In that study, however, serial lavage was carried out for only 2 weeks following irradiation, a time period that apparently is too short to observe quantitative changes in the lungs (55).

Conflicting data have also been presented regarding drug-induced changes in the alveolar macrophage population. Because experimental designs in these studies have varied in many ways (e.g., animal species, quantitation of lavaged cells only versus total lung cells, dosages and durations of drug therapy), this is not terribly surprising. One example of experimental disagreement is provided by studies of the effects of glucocorticosteroids on alveolar macrophage numbers. It has long been known that steroids decrease the numbers of circulating monocytes. However,

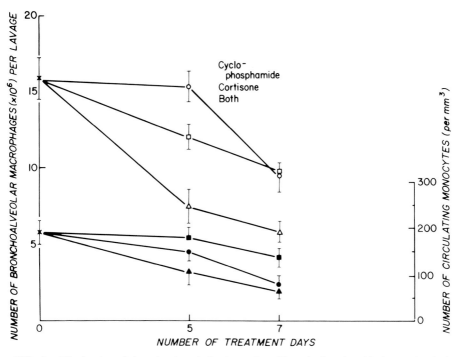

FIG. 1. Effects of week-long treatment of guinea pigs with cyclophosphamide (15 mg/kg/day) or cortisone acetate (100 mg/kg/day), or both, on numbers of circulating monocytes (●,■,▲) and bronchoalveolar macrophages (○,□,△). Only the combined regimen resulted in a statistically significant reduction in numbers of bronchoalveolar macrophages ($p < 0.01$, Student's t test).

Hunninghake and Fauci (23), as well as Lin and associates (31), were unable to detect steroid-induced reductions in numbers of pulmonary macrophages. In contrast, van Oud Alblas and associates found significant reductions in numbers of murine alveolar macrophages using a depot injection of hydrocortisone (58). The methods for collecting cells were different in these studies and included teasing of whole lung tissues (23), lavage only (31), and lavage plus enzyme digestion of lung tissues (58).

The effect of cyclophosphamide, a potent myelosuppressive agent, on the numbers of alveolar macrophages has also been examined. To date, four different groups have been unable to detect cyclophosphamide-induced reductions in numbers of these cells (3,24,41,53).

Studies in our own laboratory have revealed that, in contrast to single-drug therapy with cyclophosphamide or cortisone, combinations of these immunosuppressing and myelosuppressing agents will produce decreases in alveolar macrophage numbers (39–41). When guinea pigs were treated with week-long regimens of cyclophosphamide or cortisone acetate, small reductions (not statistically significant) in lavage-collected macrophages occurred (Fig. 1). However, when a combined regimen was used, a highly significant decrease in cell counts was noted

(Fig. 1). Others have also examined a similar combined regimen in dogs and have not found reduced numbers of alveolar macrophages (53). However, the dosages used in the latter study were far lower than those employed in the guinea pig model. Thus, it appears that high dosages of multiple-drug regimens are most likely to reduce the alveolar macrophage population.

Functional Defects Associated with Immunosuppression

Phagocytic-microbicidal activity

Whereas irradiation does not appear to affect the phagocytic function of alveolar macrophages (55), drug-induced immunosuppression does. However, the influence of drugs on phagocytic and microbicidal macrophage activity is clearly dose-dependent. Furthermore, drug-induced defects may vary according to the type of microorganism. Early studies suggested that unusually high doses of cyclophosphamide altered the capacity of rat alveolar macrophages for ingestion and destruction of *S. aureus* (32). More recently, studies in our own laboratory have used regimens of cortisone and cyclophosphamide designed to provide clinically relevant serum levels of these drugs in guinea pigs. Lower doses of cortisone plus cyclophosphamide had no effect on either the phagocytic or bactericidal capacity of alveolar macrophages when challenged *in vitro* with *Pseudomonas aeruginosa* (40). On raising the dose of cyclophosphamide, however, a reduction in phagocytic (but not bactericidal) capacity occurred (40). Of interest were studies using the lower dose regimen, in which intrapulmonary (44) and intrabronchial (41) killing of *P. aeruginosa* was impaired, despite an intact phagocytic capacity of leukocytes (40). However, dramatic reductions in numbers of intrapulmonary polymorphonuclear leukocytes (PMN) *(vide infra)* and alveolar macrophages occurred in these studies. Taken together, these findings suggest that a reduction in phagocytic numbers alone, without reduced phagocytic-microbicidal functions, is sufficient to significantly impair lung defenses.

In other studies, a dose-related effect of glucocorticosteroid on alveolar macrophage anti-*Listeria* activity was noted (2). In these experiments, alveolar macrophages obtained by lavage were challenged *in vitro* with *Listeria monocytogenes*. Lower dosages of cortisone did not affect macrophage function, but higher dosages resulted in reduced intracellular killing, while phagocytic rates remained intact (Table 2). This contrasts with the findings noted earlier for *P. aeruginosa* and argues that different drugs, dosages, and specific pathogens may all influence the mechanism of pulmonary immunosuppression.

In additional studies, the mechanism for the dose-related decrease in listericidal activity by cortisone-treated alveolar macrophages was sought. It was found that for the higher dosage of cortisone (but not the lower dosage) there was a significant reduction in the respiratory burst (Table 2). Thus, just as previously noted for neutrophils (34), it appears that alveolar macrophage oxidative microbicidal activity may be impaired during steroid treatment.

TABLE 2. *Dosage-dependent effects of cortisone acetate on anti-*Listeria *activity of alveolar macrophages*

Study groups[a]	Phagocytosis[b] (cpm)	Killing index[b] (cpm/CFU)	Superoxide anion production[c]
Normal	732 ± 113	3.06 ± 0.44	11.3 ± 0.6
Low-dosage cortisone	685 ± 94	3.50 ± 0.97	9.9 ± 0.6
High-dosage cortisone	773 ± 78	1.43 ± 0.15[d]	4.0 ± 0.3[d]

[a]Normals treated with subcutaneous (s.c.) saline. Low-dosage: cortisone, 100 mg/kg/day for 1 week (s.c.). High-dosage: cortisone, 200 mg/kg/day for 1 week.
[b]See Blackwood and Pennington (2) for details of assays (^{35}S-labeled *Listeria* used in assays).
[c]Expressed as nanomoles ferricytochrome c reduced for 10^6 cells during 45 min stimulation with phorbol myristate acetate (5 μg/ml).
[d]Different than normal, $p < 0.05$, Student's t test.

Nonspecific cell cytotoxicity

Another effector function of macrophages is direct cytotoxic activity. The effects of immunosuppressing drugs on this function have been assayed for guinea pig alveolar macrophages using a phytohemagglutinin-induced or antibody-dependent assay, employing ^{51}Cr-labeled sheep erythrocyte targets. Both cortisone acetate administration (23) and cyclophosphamide administration (24) resulted in reduced cytotoxic function. For both drugs, a repetitive dosing regimen appeared to be necessary in order to evoke this response.

Alveolar macrophage locomotive capacity and secretion of chemotactic factor

Activated random migration and chemotactic responsiveness to unidirectional stimuli appear to be important components of alveolar macrophage behavior. The specific influence of immunosuppressive agents on this cellular function was sought in guinea pigs treated with week-long regimens of either cyclophosphamide or cortisone acetate (46). A potent chemotactic agent, formyl-methionyl-leucyl-phenylalanine (f-met-leu-phe), was used for these studies. Whereas cyclophosphamide treatment did not impair chemotactic responses, cortisone treatment resulted in a 60% reduction in normal chemotaxis ($p<0.02$). In additional studies, guinea pigs treated with cortisone plus cyclophosphamide demonstrated reduced accumulation of alveolar macrophages in lung tissues during experimental *P. aeruginosa* pneumonia (Fig. 2) (44). Whether or not this defect in mobilization of alveolar macrophages toward chemotactic stimuli is clinically important is unknown. However, past studies have shown that adding cortisone to cyclophosphamide results in mortality from experimental pneumonia exceeding that found with cyclophosphamide treatment alone (44). Thus, it may be that this is one mechanism by which steroids are additive with other agents in depressing lung defenses.

More recently, the immunosuppressive fungal metabolite cyclosporin A has been evaluated in rats for its effect on alveolar macrophage chemotaxis (9). Both *in vitro* exposure and a month-long treatment regimen (5 mg/kg/day) resulted in significant

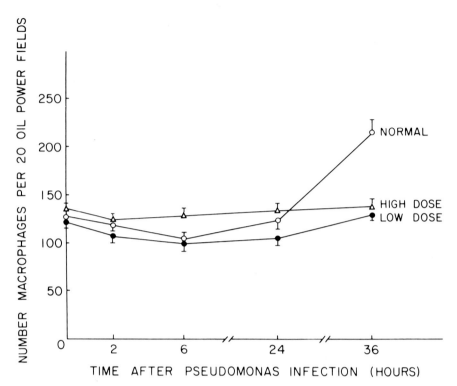

FIG. 2. Quantitation of macrophage inflammatory response in lung tissues of guinea pigs during *Pseudomonas* pneumonia. Values are mean numbers macrophages per 20 oil-power ($\times$ 1,000) fields of lung tissue. Low-dosage group: cortisone acetate, 100 mg/kg/day, for 7 days (subcutaneous) plus cyclophosphamide, 15 mg/kg/day, for 7 days (intraperitoneal). High-dosage group: cortisone (as above) plus cyclophosphamide, 30 mg/kg/day, for 7 days.

impairment of alveolar macrophage chemotactic responses to f-met-leu-phe. In contrast, daily injections of azathioprine did not impair macrophage chemotaxis. Of some interest in this study was the finding that whereas the chemotactic response to f-met-leu-phe was impaired, the response to activated serum (C5a) was not. Furthermore, co-administration of prednisolone during cyclosporin treatment partially abrogated the impairment in chemotactic reactivity. Clearly, more information in this complex area will be useful. In fact, because cyclosporin A is emerging as one of the most valuable agents for transplant patients, there should be considerable incentive to study the spectrum of effects of this agent on lung defenses.

Closely related to these findings, and also appropriate to the discussion of alveolar macrophage secretory functions *(vide infra)*, are studies to determine whether or not immunosuppression reduces the secretion of the previously described alveolar-macrophage-derived neutrophil chemotactic factors (25,35). Guinea pig alveolar macrophages secrete a 5,000-dalton chemotactic factor that has been detected with *in vivo* and *in vitro* techniques (28). Studies in our laboratory have demonstrated

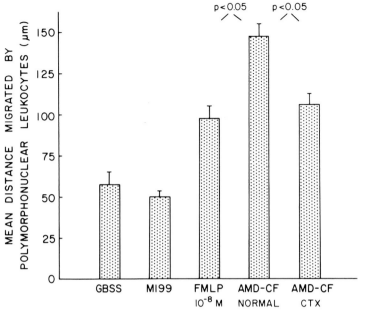

FIG. 3. Chemotactic potency for PMN of alveolar-macrophage-derived chemotactic factor (AMD-CF) from normal versus cyclophosphamide-treated (CTX, 15 mg/kg/day × 7 days) guinea pigs; Gey's balanced salt solution (GBSS) and medium 199 (M199) used as negative controls, and 10^{-8}-M f-met-leu-phe (FMLP) used as a positive control.

that both cortisone treatment and cyclophosphamide treatment of guinea pigs significantly impair the secretion of this chemotactic factor (Fig. 3) (46). Again, the clinical significance of these findings has yet to be determined. However, any adverse effect on the generation of a PMN reaction in infected lungs is well known to reduce survival from infection (7,11,45,47,54).

Secretory functions

The human alveolar macrophage is a potent secretory cell (26), and many of these secretory products have at least potential roles in defense of the lung against infection. Unfortunately, very little information currently exists to describe the effects of immunosuppression on the secretion of these products.

One line of investigation has examined the influence of immunosuppressive drugs on alveolar-macrophage-derived chemotactic factor, as discussed earlier. In a similar study design, guinea pigs were treated with either cyclophosphamide or cortisone acetate, and the effects of these drugs on alveolar macrophage biosynthesis of complement proteins were assessed (48). It was found that both cyclophosphamide and cortisone treatment significantly ($p<0.001$) reduced the synthesis of C2 and C4 by alveolar macrophages (Table 3). For cortisone, this effect was seen as early as 24 hr after a single dose, whereas for cyclophosphamide a week-long

TABLE 3. *Influence of cyclophosphamide and cortisone acetate treatment on biosynthesis of complement by alveolar macrophages in tissue culture*

Study group[a]	Biosynthesis by alveolar macrophages[b]		Serum concentrations[c]	
	C2	C4	C2	C4
Normal	7.8 ± 0.6	12.6 ± 1.2	4.1 ± 0.1	20.6 ± 2.3
Cyclophosphamide	2.9 ± 0.2[d]	2.7 ± 0.5[d]	3.8 ± 0.4	18.5 ± 4.1
Cortisone	2.8 ± 0.2[d]	3.1 ± 0.3[d]	3.2 ± 0.3	17.9 ± 1.6

[a]Normals received saline subcutaneously (s.c.) and intraperitoneally (i.p.); cyclophosphamide group received 15 mg/kg/day (i.p.) for 1 week; cortisone group received 100 mg/kg/day (s.c.) for 1 week.
[b]Values are means (± SEM), expressed as effective molecules of hemolytically active C ($\times 10^{-7}$/μg DNA); see Pennington et al. (48) for details.
[c]Expressed as effective molecules ($\times 10^{-12}$ ml).
[d]Different from normal, $p < 0.001$, Student's t test.

regimen was needed to induce the defect. Furthermore, whereas C2 and C4 production by alveolar macrophages was decreased, serum complement levels in drug-treated animals remained normal (Table 3). The latter finding argues once again for the necessity of studying local lung defense functions rather than attempting to extrapolate from systemic findings to presumed lung functions. Also of interest in this study was the finding that cortisone treatment decreased the spontaneous release by macrophages of lysozyme into tissue culture fluids, whereas cyclophosphamide treatment actually resulted in increased lysozyme release by alveolar macrophages. Neither immunosuppressive agent altered the total protein secreted by alveolar macrophages. Taken together, these data indicate that immunosuppressive agents may selectively impair the biosynthesis of specific secretory products by alveolar macrophages and that in some cases secretory products may actually be increased.

Obviously, the effects of immunosuppressive agents on alveolar macrophage biosynthesis and secretory activities are areas of potential importance. Future studies designed to examine the effects of these agents on secretory products such as neutrophil-activating factor (49), IL-1 (56), complement proteins (6), and leukotriene B_4 (14) warrant high investigative priority.

Oxygen metabolism

A number of past studies have demonstrated that oxygen metabolism plays an integral role in microbicidal activities of neutrophils (30). Studies in recent years have extended these observations to include the alveolar macrophage. In fact, it appears that the same defect in intermediate oxygen metabolism (i.e., production of toxic oxygen radicals such as superoxide anion) that occurs in neutrophils from patients with chronic granulomatous disease also occurs in the alveolar macrophage populations of these patients (21). Although past studies have indicated that glucocorticosteroids impair oxygen metabolism in neutrophils (34), little information exists regarding the effects of immunosuppression on alveolar macrophage oxygen utilization. Work in our own laboratory has recently correlated impaired listericidal activity by cortisone-treated alveolar macrophages with reduced respiratory burst (Table 2). Thus, it is reasonable to assume that during high-dosage regimens of glucocorticosteroids, impairment of oxidative metabolism might result in impaired local defenses against infection. In another recent report, a 52% reduction in superoxide anion release by zymosan-stimulated rat alveolar macrophages after *in vitro* exposure to cyclosporin A was described (9). However, when cyclosporin A was given to rats by intraperitoneal injections over a 1-month period, alveolar macrophages were not affected. Further studies with cyclosporin A given at different dosages may provide insight into this discrepancy.

Alveolar macrophage participation in cell-mediated immunity

A number of studies have illustrated that a lymphocyte-directed, cell-mediated immune system is intact in the lung (see Chapter 4). Alveolar macrophages presumably may function both as initiator cells (e.g., antigen processing, IL-1 secretion) and as effector cells (e.g., activation by lymphokines for cytotoxic or microbicidal activity) in this system. Although few data currently exist to describe the effects of immunosuppressive agents on the interaction of alveolar macrophages with lymphocytes in the lung, a large body of information on the effects of disease states (e.g., sarcoidosis) on this interaction has been accumulating, suggesting disease-related changes in this interaction (27). It should not be long until studies to define drug-induced effects on alveolar macrophage function in this system are available.

Influence of Immunosuppressive and Myelosuppressive Agents on PMN Inflammation in the Lung

It has been fashionable in recent years to emphasize the role of alveolar macrophages as the critical phagocytic cells in defense of the lung (16,18). However, studies in the 1940s (63), as well as recent experimental (7) and clinical (11,45,54) observations, have clearly illustrated the importance of an intact local PMN inflammatory response for optimal lung defense from infection. Accordingly, we have carried out in our laboratory a detailed analysis to describe the influence of two commonly employed immunosuppressive and myelosuppressive agents (cyclophosphamide and a glucocorticosteroid) on the kinetics of PMN inflammtion in acutely infected lungs (40,41,44). For these studies, drug-treated and normal guinea pigs were infected with *P. aeruginosa* by intratracheal instillation. Parameters for evaluation included survival, intrabronchial or intrapulmonary killing of bacteria, and degree of cellular inflammation at timed intervals. Initial studies revealed that a combination regimen of cortisone plus cyclophosphamide, given in doses sufficient to decrease myelopoiesis, resulted in a significant reduction in acute PMN influx to infected airways (Fig. 4 and 5) (40). Specifically, normal animals demonstrated

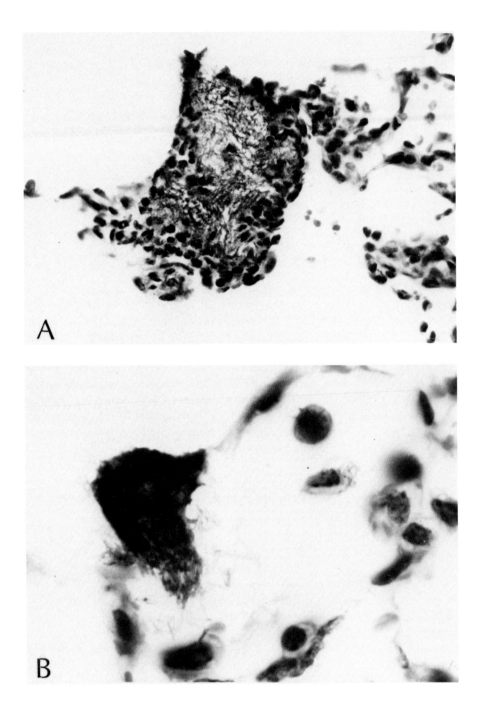

FIG. 4. Guinea pig lung 2 hr after infection with *P. aeruginosa*. **A:** In tissue from a normal animal, a clump of bacteria in an alveolar duct is surrounded predominantly by PMN, with some macrophages. ×400. **B:** In tissue from an animal given immunosuppressive therapy with cortisone acetate and cyclophosphamide, a clump of bacteria in an alveolar duct is seen with no PMN response. Two macrophages are seen phagocytizing bacteria. ×1,000.

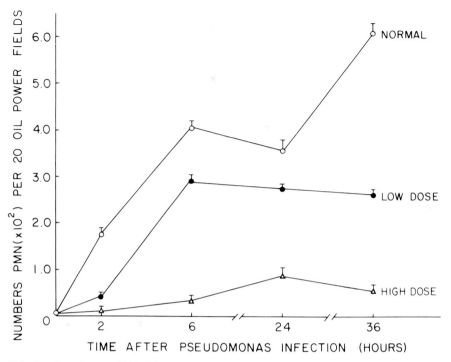

FIG. 5. Quantitation of PMN inflammatory responses in lung tissues of guinea pigs during *Pseudomonas* pneumonia. Values are mean numbers of PMN per 20 oil-power (× 1,000) fields of lung tissue. Low-dosage and high-dosage groups as defined in Fig. 2.

increases in percentages of PMN in bronchial fluids from 5% before infection to 24% 2 hr after infection, whereas drug-treated animals had only 4% PMN in airways 2 hr after infection. By 24 hr after infection, the differences between groups were even more pronounced (Fig. 5 and 6). Next, the differential influence of cyclophosphamide alone versus cortisone alone on PMN lung inflammation was studied (41). It was found that cyclophosphamide alone, but not cortisone alone, impaired local PMN inflammation in bronchial fluids after infection (Fig. 7). Furthermore, adding cortisone to cyclophosphamide did not further impair PMN influx to lungs. These results correlated well with the drug-induced effects on circulating numbers of PMN.

Finally, studies were carried out to determine the effects of decreased PMN inflammatory reactions in the lung on outcome from pneumonia, as well as intrapulmonary killing of bacteria (44). Of interest was a direct relationship between survival and the magnitude of PMN inflammation in lung tissues (44). Furthermore, cortisone alone did not lead to reduced survival or impaired PMN reaction in the lungs. However, adding cortisone to cyclophosphamide did reduce survival, suggesting that a functional deficiency, separate from the impaired PMN inflammation, may have been induced by adding steroids *(vide supra)*. Examination of rates of

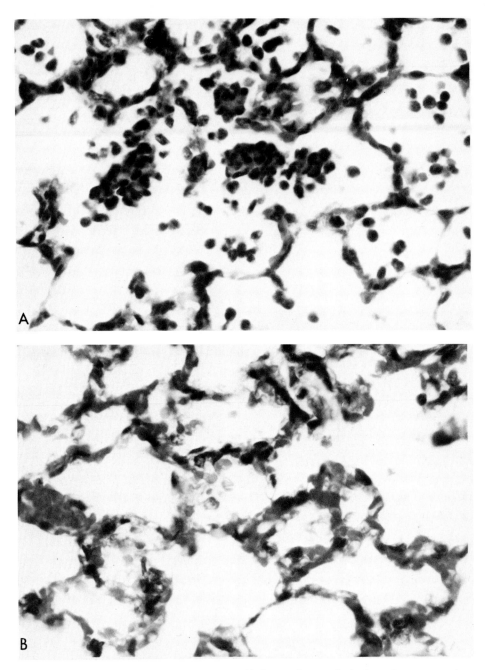

FIG. 6. Guinea pig lung 24 hr after infection with *P. aeruginosa.* **A:** In tissue from a normal animal, severe acute pneumonia, with numerous PMN and macrophages, can be seen. There is minimal thickening of alveolar septae. ×400. **B:** In tissue from an animal given immuno-suppressive therapy with cortisone acetate and cyclophosphamide, there is severe acute pneu-monia, with virtual absence of PMN. Scattered macrophages can be seen. Alveolar thickening is uniformly present, with prominent vasodilation, congestion of capillaries with red blood cells, and focal intraalveolar hemorrhage. ×400.

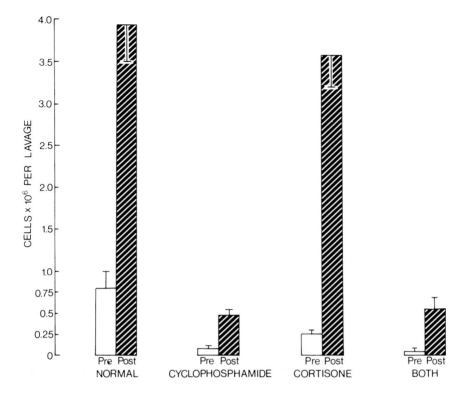

FIG. 7. Numbers of PMN in bronchoalveolar lavage fluid before (Pre) and 2 hr after (Post) lung challenge with *Pseudomonas* organisms. Values are means ± SE for 6 animals.

intrapulmonary killing correlated with the findings in survival and PMN inflammation analyses (Fig. 8). These studies are confirmatory of the clinical suspicion that the degree of PMN influx to infected lung tissues is perhaps the single most important facet of local defense against acute bacterial pneumonia. It has yet to be determined if the reduction in local PMN numbers is simply a result of decreased numbers of circulating PMNs or is at least partially due to the fact that immunosuppressive agents impair alveolar macrophage secretion of neutrophil-directed chemotactic factor (46).

Influence of Immunosuppressive and Myelosuppressive Agents on Lymphocyte Numbers and Function in the Lung

The presence of both T and B lymphocytes in human and animal lungs has been well documented elsewhere in this volume, and these cells may exhibit independent behavior under certain circumstances (4,29). Only a few studies have described the quantitative influence of immunosuppression on pulmonary lymphocyte populations, and even less is known regarding drug effects on intrapulmonary lymphocyte function in host defense.

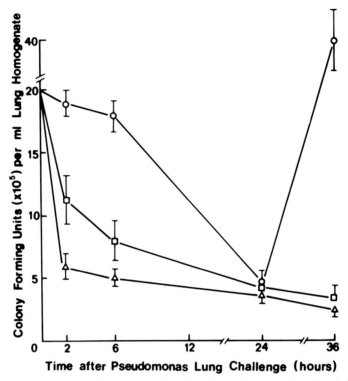

FIG. 8. Clearance of viable *P. aeruginosa* from lung tissue of guinea pigs after challenge. Animals were normal (triangles) or immunosuppressed with cortisone acetate plus low-dosage cyclophosphamide (squares) or with cortisone acetate plus high-dosage cyclophosphamide (circles). Values are means ± SE for a minimum of 6 animals in each group at each interval.

As was noted earlier for alveolar macrophages, there is no guarantee that drug- or radiation-induced quantitative changes in circulating numbers of lymphocytes will be reflected by similar changes in the bronchopulmonary tissues. Reynolds and associates observed profound blood lymphopenia in dogs within 1 week after total-body irradiation (53). However, there were no concomitant decreases in the numbers of lymphocytes recovered from bronchial lavage, with observations made up to 12 days after irradiation. In the same experimental system, dogs were treated with either cyclophosphamide or methylprednisolone, or both agents, and again monitored for circulating and pulmonary lymphopenia. All regimens produced lymphopenia in both compartments. However, when the steroid was given on an alternate-day basis, less notable reductions in lung and blood lymphocytes occurred.

Domby and Whitcomb extended these observations by studying the effects of glucocorticosteroid treatment of guinea pigs on the T-lymphocyte subset in bronchoalveolar spaces (8). They demonstrated that a week-long regimen of cortisone treatment resulted in a 30% reduction in the number of T lymphocytes recovered by lung lavage.

In an attempt to demonstrate the functional consequences of immunosuppression of the pulmonary cell-mediated immune system, we recently carried out experiments in a guinea pig model of experimental *L. monocytogenes* pneumonia (2). We reasoned that because cell-mediated immunity is the principal means of host defense against this facultative intracellular pathogen (4,57), drug-induced defects in local defenses against *Listeria* would be indicative of defective cell-mediated immune function. Guinea pigs were employed because this species most closely resembles humans in its susceptibility to glucocorticosteroids (5). It was clear that cortisone treatment impaired lung defenses to *Listeria* and that this impairment was dose-related. Week-long cortisone regimens of 100 mg/kg/day reduced survival from *Listeria* pneumonia to 67%, whereas control groups routinely survived this same challenge inocula (10^5 colony-forming units). When the cortisone dosage was increased to 200 mg/kg/day, survival was reduced to zero. Deaths in the high-dosage group occurred over the first 5 days, as contrasted with later deaths in the low-dosage group. Sequential cultures of lungs from normal and drug-treated guinea pigs also revealed dose-related impairment in killing of *Listeria* in lungs (Fig. 9). Furthermore, blood cultures were positive in 1 of 23 controls during experimental infection and in 13 of 26 animals receiving the low-dosage regimen of cortisone.

To explore the mechanisms by which lung defenses against *Listeria* were impaired, the influences of cortisone on pulmonary lymphocytes and alveolar macrophages were examined. The low-dosage regimen produced highly significant reductions in numbers of T lymphocytes, both in blood and in bronchoalveolar spaces (Fig. 10). In contrast, the low-dosage regimen did not affect alveolar macrophage number or listericidal activity, when assayed using an *in vitro* technique. At the high dosage, however, a significant reduction in alveolar macrophage listericidal capacity occurred (Table 2). It thus appeared that reduced numbers of T lymphocytes in lungs may have resulted in a modest impairment of lung defense to *Listeria* (low dosage) and that the additional impairment in alveolar macrophage listericidal capacity in the high-dosage group resulted in a profound impairment of lung defenses.

Additional *in vitro* and *in vivo* studies are clearly needed to further explore immunosuppression of cell-mediated immunity in the lung. The potential for enhancing local lung defenses with one or more of the rapidly expanding group of immunostimulants offers a clear incentive to better our understanding of the precise mechanisms by which the immune defects occur in lungs.

Influences of Immunosuppression on Humoral Immunity in the Lung

Studies of humoral immunity in the lung are hindered by the difficulty in performing accurate quantitation of immunoglobulins in the lower respiratory tract. Nevertheless, considerable efforts have been made to quantitate immunoglobulins in bronchial secretions and also to monitor the antibody-forming cells (B lymphocytes) in lungs (see Chapter 5). Unfortunately, almost no information exists to

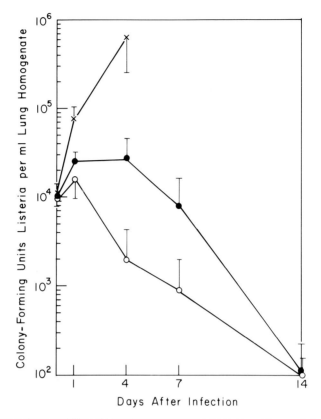

FIG. 9. Intrapulmonary killing of *Listeria* during pneumonia in normal *(open circles)*, low-dosage *(filled circles)*, and high-dosage *(crosses)* cortisone-treated guinea pigs. Values are means ± SEM for 4 to 9 animals for each study group at each time point.

describe the effects of immunosuppressive drugs on these local factors. Unpublished studies in our own laboratory using guinea pigs have revealed that 1-week regimens of cyclophosphamide, but not cortisone, result in significant reductions in bronchoalveolar B lymphocytes. Clearly, much more work remains before we achieve complete understanding of the influence of immunosuppression on humoral immune function in the lung.

CONCLUSION

Taken together, the body of information presented in the section dealing with experimental studies is rather sizable. Nevertheless, compared with the detailed understanding of the systemic immune system, both in normal and in immunosuppressed settings, our understanding of pulmonary immunopathology is limited. The rapid expansion of information dealing with biological response modifiers (e.g., interleukins, interferons) and the advanced technologies to produce these materials

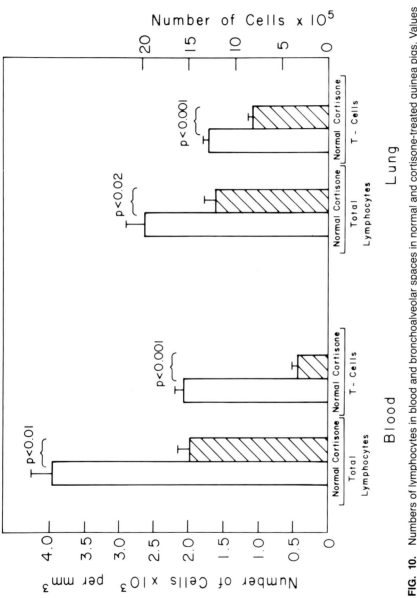

FIG. 10. Numbers of lymphocytes in blood and bronchoalveolar spaces in normal and cortisone-treated guinea pigs. Values are means ± SEM, with 4 to 12 animals per group.

in meaningful quantities offer a compelling reason for further studies to define precise mechanisms of pulmonary immunosuppression. Only with full awareness of these mechanisms can there be a rational means for selecting appropriate new therapeutic or prophylactic interventions in these high-risk patients.

ACKNOWLEDGMENTS

This work was supported in part by USPHS grant HL-21997. I want to thank Ms. Sahira Ansari for preparing the manuscript.

REFERENCES

1. Balow, J. E., Hurley, D. L., and Fauci, A. S. (1975): Immunosuppressive effects of glucocorticosteroids: Differential effect of acute vs. chronic administration on cell-mediated immunity. *J. Immunol.*, 114:1072–1076.
2. Blackwood, L. L., and Pennington, J. E. (1982): Dose-dependent effect of glucocorticosteroids on pulmonary defenses in a steroid-resistant host. *Am. Rev. Respir. Dis.*, 126:1045–1049.
3. Buhles, W. C., and Shifrine, M. (1977): Effects of cyclophosphamide on macrophage numbers, functions and progenitor cells. *J. Reticuloendothel. Soc.*, 5:285–297.
4. Cantey, J. R., Hand, W. L., Hughes, C. G., Lund, M. E., and King, N. L. (1974): Cell-mediated immunity after bacterial infection of the lower respiratory tract. *J. Clin. Invest.*, 54:1125–1134.
5. Claman, H. N. (1972): Corticosteroids and lymphoid cells. *N. Engl. J. Med.*, 287:388–397.
6. Cole, F. S., Matthews, W. J., Rossing, T. H., Gash, D. J., Lichtenberg, N. A., and Pennington, J. E. (1983): Complement biosynthesis by human bronchoalveolar macrophages. *Clin. Immunol. Immunopathol.*, 27:153–159.
7. Dale, D. C., Reynolds, H. Y., Pennington, J. E., Elin, R. J., Pitts, T. W., and Graw, R. G. (1975): Granulocyte transfusion therapy of experimental *Pseudomonas* pneumonia. *J. Clin. Invest.*, 54:664–671.
8. Domby, W. R., and Whitcomb, M. E. (1978): The effects of corticosteroid administration on the bronchoalveolar cells obtained from guinea pigs by lung lavage. *Am. Rev. Respir. Dis.*, 117:893–896.
9. Drath, D. B., and Kahan, B. D. (1983): Alterations in rat pulmonary macrophage function by the immunosuppressive agents cyclosporin, azathioprine, and prednisolone. *Transplantation*, 35:588–592.
10. Eickhoff, T. C., Olin, D. B:, Anderson, R. J., and Shaffer, L. A. (1972): Current problems and approaches to diagnosis of infection in renal transplant recipients. *Transplant. Proc.*, 4:693–697.
11. Fanta, C. H., and Pennington, J. E. (1981): Fever and new lung infiltrates in the immunocompromised host. *Clin. Chest Med.*, 2:19–39.
12. Fanta, C. H., and Pennington, J. E. (1983): Pneumonia in the immunocompromised host. In: *Respiratory Infections: Diagnosis and Management*, edited by J.E. Pennington, pp. 171–185. Raven Press, New York.
13. Fauci, A. S., Macher, A. M., Longo, D. L., Lane, H. C., Rook, A. H., Masur, H., and Gelman, E. P. (1984): Acquired immunodeficiency syndrome: Epidemiologic, clinical, immunologic, and therapeutic considerations. *Ann. Intern. Med.*, 100:92–106.
14. Fels, A. O. S., Pawlowski, N. A., Cramer, E. B., King, T. K. C., Cohn, Z. A., and Scott, W. A. (1982): Human alveolar macrophages produce leukotriene B_4. *Proc. Natl. Acad. Sci. U.S.A.*, 79:7866–7870.
15. Golde, D. W., Finley, T. N., and Cline, M. J. (1974): The pulmonary macrophage in acute leukemia. *N. Engl. J. Med.*, 290:875–878.
16. Goldstein, E., Lipperts, W., and Warshauer, D. (1974): Pulmonary alveolar macrophage: Defender against bacterial infection of the lung. *J. Clin. Invest.*, 54:519–526.
17. Gottlieb, M. S., Groopman, J. E., Weinstein, W. M., Fahey, J. L., and Detels, R. (1983): The acquired immunodeficiency syndrome. *Ann. Intern. Med.*, 99:208–220.
18. Green, G. M., and Kass, E. H. (1964): The role of the alveolar macrophage in the clearance of bacteria from the lung. *J. Exp. Med.*, 119:167–175.

19. Gross, N. J. (1977): Alveolar macrophage number: An index of the effect of radiation on the lungs. *Radiat. Res.*, 72:325–332.
20. Hocking, W. G., and Golde, D. W. (1979): The pulmonary-alveolar macrophage. *N. Engl. J. Med.*, 301:580–587, 639–645.
21. Hoidal, R. J., Fox, R. B., and Repine, J. E. (1979): Defective oxidative metabolic responses in vitro of alveolar macrophages in chronic granulomatous disease. *Am. Rev. Respir. Dis.*, 120:613–618.
22. Huertas, V. E., Port, F. K., Rozas, V. V., and Niederhuber, J. E. (1976): Pneumonia in recipients of renal allografts. *Arch. Surg.*, 111:162–166.
23. Hunninghake, G. W., and Fauci, A. S. (1977): Immunological reactivity of the lung. III. Effects of corticosteroids on alveolar macrophage cytotoxic effector function. *J. Immunol.*, 118:146–150.
24. Hunninghake, G. W., and Fauci, A. S. (1977): Immunological reactivity of the lung. IV. Effect of cyclophosphamide on alveolar macrophage cytotoxic effector function. *Clin. Exp. Immunol.*, 27:555–559.
25. Hunninghake, G. W., Gadek, J. E., Fales, H. M., and Crystal, R. G. (1980): Human alveolar macrophage-derived chemotactic factor for neutrophils. *J. Clin. Invest.*, 66:473–483.
26. Hunninghake, G. W., Gadek, J. E., Kawanami, O., Ferrans, V. J., and Crystal, R. G. (1979): Inflammatory and immune processes in the human lung in health and disease. Evaluation by bronchoalveolar lavage. *Am. J. Pathol.*, 97:149–206.
27. Hunninghake, G. W., Gadek, J. E., Young, R. C., Kawanami, O., Ferrans, V. J., and Crystal, R. G. (1980): Maintenance of granuloma formation in pulmonary sarcoidosis by T lymphocytes within the lung. *N. Engl. J. Med.*, 302:594–598.
28. Hunninghake, G. W., Gallin, J. I., and Fauci, A. S. (1978): Immunologic reactivity of the lung: The in vivo and in vitro generation of a neutrophil chemotactic factor by alveolar macrophages. *Am. Rev. Respir. Dis.*, 117:15–23.
29. Kaltreider, H. B. (1976): Expression of immune mechanisms in the lung. *Am. Rev. Respir. Dis.*, 113:347–379.
30. Klebanoff, S. J. (1980): Oxygen metabolism and the toxic properties of phagocytes. *Ann. Intern. Med.*, 93:480–489.
31. Lin, H.-S., Kuhn, C., and Chen, D.-M. (1982): Effects of hydrocortisone acetate on pulmonary alveolar macrophage colony-forming cells. *Am. Rev. Respir. Dis.*, 125:712–715.
32. Lockard, V. G., Sharbaugh, R. J., Arhelger, R. B., and Grogan, J. B. (1971): Ultrastructural alterations in phagocytic functions of alveolar macrophages after cyclophosphamide administration. *J. Reticuloendothel. Soc.*, 9:97–107.
33. Mandel, M. A., Dvorak, K. J., Worman, L. W., and Decross, J. J. (1976): Immunoglobulin content in the bronchial washings of patients with benign and malignant pulmonary disease. *N. Engl. J. Med.*, 295:694–698.
34. Mandell, G. L. (1973): Interaction of intraleukocytic bacteria and antibiotics. *J. Clin. Invest.*, 120:613–618.
35. Merrill, W. W., Jaegel, G. P., Matthay, R. A., and Reynolds, H. Y. (1980): Alveolar macrophage-derived chemotactic factor: Kinetics of *in vitro* production and partial characterization. *J. Clin. Invest.*, 65:268–276.
36. Moyer, R. F., and Riley, R. F. (1969): Effect of whole-body and partial-body x-irradiation on the extractable cellular components of the lung with special consideration to the alveolar macrophage. *Radiat. Res.*, 39:716–730.
37. Neiman, P. E., Thomas, E. D., Reeves, W. C., Ray, C. F., Sale, G., Lernerk, K. G., Buckner, C. D., Clift, R. A., Storb, R., Weiden, P. L., and Fefer, A. (1976): Opportunistic infection and interstitial pneumonia following marrow transplantation for aplastic anemia and hematologic malignancy. *Transplant. Proc.*, 8:663–667.
38. Peel, D. M., and Coggle, J. E. (1980): The effect of X irradiation on alveolar macrophages in mice. *Radiat. Res.*, 81:10–19.
39. Pennington, J. E. (1977): Quantitative effects of immunosuppression on bronchoalveolar cells. *J. Infect. Dis.*, 136:127–131.
40. Pennington, J. E. (1977): Bronchoalveolar cell response to bacterial challenge in the immunosuppressed lung. *Am. Rev. Respir. Dis.*, 116:885–893.
41. Pennington, J. E. (1978): Differential effects of cyclophosphamide and cortisone acetate on bronchoalveolar phagocytic cell populations. *Am. Rev. Respir. Dis.*, 118:319–324.

42. Pennington, J. E. (1978): Infection in the compromised host: Recent advances and future directions. *Semin. Infect. Dis.*, 1:142–202.
43. Pennington, J. E. (1983): Pneumonia in the acquired immune deficiency syndrome. In: *Respiratory Infections: Diagnosis and Management*, edited by J. E. Pennington, pp. 187–190. Raver Press, New York.
44. Pennington, J. E., and Ehrie, M. G. (1978): Pathogenesis of *Pseudomonas aeruginosa* pneumonia during immunosuppression. *J. Infect. Dis.*, 137:764–774.
45. Pennington, J. E., and Feldman, N. T. (1977): Pulmonary infiltrates and fever in patients with hematologic malignancy: Assessment of transbronchial biopsy. *Am. J. Med.*, 62:581–587.
46. Pennington, J. E., and Harris, E. A. (1981): Influence of immunosuppression on alveolar macrophage chemotactic activities in guinea pigs. *Am. Rev. Respir. Dis.*, 123:299–304.
47. Pennington, J. E., and Herman, P. G. (1983): Pneumonia in the immunocompromised host. In: *Iatrogenic Thoracic Complications*, edited by P. G. Herman, pp. 35–47. Springer-Verlag, New York.
48. Pennington, J. E., Matthews, W. J., Marino, J. T., and Colten, H. R. (1979): Cyclophosphamide and cortisone acetate inhibit complement biosynthesis by guinea pig bronchoalveolar macrophages. *J. Immunol.*, 123:1318–1321.
49. Pennington, J. E., Rossing, T. H., and Boerth, L. W. (1983): The effect of human alveolar macrophages on the bactericidal capacity of neutrophils. *J. Infect. Dis.*, 148:101–109.
50. Ramsey, P. G., Rubin, R. H., Tolkoff-Rubin, N. E., Cosimi, A. B., Russell, P. S., and Greene, R. (1980): The renal transplant patient with fever and pulmonary infiltrates: Etiology, clinical manifestations, and management. *Medicine (Baltimore)*, 59:206–222.
51. Rankin, J. A., Walzer, P. D., Dwyer, J. M., Schrader, C. E., Enriquez, R. E., and Merrill, W. W. (1983): Immunologic alterations in bronchoalveolar lavage fluid in the acquired immunodeficiency syndrome (AIDS). *Am. Rev. Respir. Dis.*, 128:189–194.
52. Reynolds, H. Y. (1983): Normal and defective respiratory host defenses. In: *Respiratory Infections: Diagnosis and Management*, edited by J. E. Pennington, pp. 1–23. Raven Press, New York.
53. Reynolds, H. Y., Kazmierowski, J. A., and Dale, D. C. (1976): Changes in the composition of canine respiratory cells obtained by bronchial lavage following irradiation or drug immunosuppression. *Proc. Soc. Exp. Biol. Med.*, 151:756–761.
54. Sickles, E. A., Young, V. M., Greene, W. H., Wiernik, P. H. (1973): Pneumonia in acute leukemia. *Ann. Intern. Med.*, 79:528–534.
55. Springmeyer, S. C., Altman, L. C., Kopecky, K. J., Deeg, H. J., and Storb, R. (1982): Alveolar macrophage kinetics and function after interruption of canine marrow function. *Am. Rev. Respir. Dis.*, 125:347–351.
56. Toews, G. B., Vial, W. C., Dunn, M. M., and Lipscomb, M. F. (1983): Human alveolar macrophages produce interleukin-1. *Am. Rev. Respir. Dis.*, 127:60.
57. Truitt, G. L., and Mackaness, G. (1971): Cell-mediated resistance to aerogenic infection of the lung. *Am. Rev. Respir. Dis.*, 104:829–842.
58. van Oud Alblas, A. B., van der Linden-Schrever, B., Mattie, H., and van Furth, R. (1981): The effect of glucocorticosteroids on the kinetics of pulmonary macrophages. *J. Reticuloendothel. Soc.*, 30:1–14.
59. van Oud Alblas, A. B., and van Furth, R. (1979): Origin, kinetics, and characteristics of pulmonary macrophages in the normal steady state. *J. Exp. Med.*, 149:1504–1518.
60. Velo, G. P., and Spector, W. G. (1973): The origin and turnover of alveolar macrophages in experimental pneumonia. *J. Pathol.*, 109:7–19.
61. Winston, D. J., Gale, R. P., Meyer, D. V., and Young, L. S. (1979): Infectious complications in human bone marrow transplantation. *Medicine (Baltimore)*, 58:1–31.
62. Winston, D. J., Territo, M. C., Winston, G. H., Miller, M. J., Gale, R. P., and Golde, D. W. (1982): Alveolar macrophage dysfunction in human bone marrow transplant recipients. *Am. J. Med.*, 73:859–866.
63. Wood, W. B., Jr. (1941): Studies on the mechanism of recovery in pneumococcal pneumonia. I. The action of type specific antibody upon the pulmonary lesion of experimental pneumonia. *J. Exp. Med.*, 73:201–222.
64. Young, K. R., Rankin, J. A., Paul, E. S., Matthay, R. A., Merrill, W. W., and Reynolds, H. Y. (1983): Pulmonary and systemic immunologic analysis in asymptomatic homosexual males. *Am. Rev. Respir. Dis.*, 127:55 (abstract).

Advances in Host Defense Mechanisms, Vol. 4,
edited by J. I. Gallin and A. S. Fauci.
Raven Press, New York © 1985.

Infectious Diseases of the Gastrointestinal Tract

*Claire B. Panosian and **Sherwood L. Gorbach

*Division of Infectious Diseases, UCLA–Olive View Memorial Medical Center, Van Nuys,
California 91405, and Department of Medicine, UCLA School of Medicine, University of
California at Los Angeles, Los Angeles, California 90024; and **Division of Infectious
Diseases, Tufts University School of Medicine, Tufts–New England Medical Center
Hospital, Boston, Massachusetts 02111

The human gastrointestinal tract is an ecosystem that is remarkable both for its complexity and its homeostasis. Indigenous mechanisms that contribute to the regulation of a healthy bowel environment include the native gut flora, gastric acidity, small-intestine motility, and mucosal immune systems. Some pathogenic organisms directly circumvent these innate defenses. The establishment of an intestinal infection may also reflect primary failure of one or more host systems. This chapter will begin with a brief summary of normal gut bacteriology and physiology as they relate to prevention of gastroenteritis, followed by a review of current concepts of pathogenesis and host defense in the common bacterial and viral intestinal infections of humans.

GENERAL PRINCIPLES OF HOST DEFENSE IN THE GASTROINTESTINAL TRACT

The human gastrointestinal tract is characterized by a series of ecologic environments, and the normal resident flora that inhabit these regions demonstrate impressive quantitative and qualitative variations (1). Because few microorganisms can survive the acid environment of the stomach, bacterial counts exceeding 10^3 colony-forming units (CFU) are rarely found in this organ. The predominant organisms (*Streptococcus, Lactobacillus*, and fungi) in the stomach reflect a saliva-borne inoculum from the oral cavity. The small intestine constitutes a zone of transition: Although they are more numerous, the organisms present in the duodenum, jejunum, and proximal ileum are qualitatively similar to those of the stomach. In the distal ileum, however, Gram-negative bacteria begin to outnumber Gram-positive species. The progressively lower redox potential of this region also permits the growth of anaerobic microorganisms such as *Bacteroides, Bifidobacterium, Fusobacterium*, and *Clostridium*. Once past the ileocecal sphincter, bacterial concentrations in the cecum increase to 10^{11} to 10^{12} CFU/ml, and anaerobes outnumber coliforms in the large intestine by a factor of 10^2 to 10^4.

Although the average human colon harbors more than 400 bacterial species, fecal organisms are remarkably constant over prolonged periods of time (2). This stability is in part determined by microbial interactions. Facultative organisms help to maintain the reduced environment of the colon by consuming available oxygen that might otherwise jeopardize the survival of more oxygen-sensitive anaerobic species. Other bacterial factors that serve to inhibit overgrowth of native or exogenous bacteria include antibiotic-like substances such as those elaborated by *Bacillus subtilis* and various strains of *Escherichia coli*. Anaerobes and some facultative bacteria also produce short-chain fatty acids that are inhibitory to microbial growth at the pH and Eh (oxidation–reduction potential) of the colon. Whether as a consequence of the foregoing or other control mechanisms, bacterial generation time in the intestinal tract is generally limited to one to four divisions per day (3).

In view of the stabilizing influences exerted by the normal intestinal flora on its own constituency, antibiotic therapy can serve as a very real risk factor for the development of intestinal infection. For example, pretreatment of mice with streptomycin has been shown to lower the disease-producing inoculum of *Salmonella* from 10^6 to fewer than 10 organisms (4). Antimicrobial therapy can also convert asymptomatic human carriage of *Salmonella* into acute enteritis (5). More recently, the use of a variety of oral and parenteral antibiotics has been linked to overgrowth of *C. difficile* in the human gut, resulting in an entity termed "antibiotic-associated" or "pseudomembranous" colitis. The resulting disease includes both necrotizing and secretory features mediated by two separate toxin activities of *C. difficile* (6).

In the absence of mitigating circumstances, the prevention of small-bowel overgrowth with resident organisms is largely accomplished by normal intestinal peristalsis. This process facilitates the transit of ingested bacteria into the colon. In clinical situations such as the blind-loop syndrome, in which intestinal motility is impaired, a dense bacterial overgrowth of the small bowel results. In addition, intestinal infections with *Shigella flexneri* and *Salmonella typhimurium* are more readily established in experimental animals when gut motility is inhibited (7,8). In human volunteers, prolonged fecal excretion of *S. flexneri* was observed in subjects who received the antiperistaltic regimen of diphenoxylate hydrochloride and atropine (Lomotil) during their acute diarrheal illness (9).

Another physiologic mechanism that influences the stability of gut ecology is gastric acid. Patients who are achlorhydric or who have undergone gastrectomy demonstrate significantly higher counts of aerobic and anaerobic bacteria in the stomach and small intestine (1). Clinical infections due to pathogenic organisms such as *Vibrio cholerae, Giardia lamblia*, and *Salmonella* also occur with greater frequency in this setting (10). Neutralization of gastric acidity with sodium bicarbonate has been shown to reduce the dose of *V. cholerae* needed to infect normal volunteers from 10^8 to 10^4 organisms (11); similarly, concomitant administration of an antacid compound increases the attack rate of experimentally induced shigellosis and *E. coli* diarrhea (12). In contrast to the situation with gastric acid, the influence of enteric secretions on resident or pathogenic intestinal flora is unresolved. Succus entericus, pancreatic juice, and unconjugated bile acids do not appear to exhibit *in vivo* antibacterial activity (1).

The frequent clinical observation that breast-fed infants exhibit fewer intestinal infections than do bottle-fed babies has recently led to heightened interest in human milk as a mediator of intestinal host defense. In developing countries, many mothers have demonstrable antibody (primarily secretory IgA) in their breast milk with specificity directed against such common diarrheal pathogens as enterotoxigenic *E. coli, V. cholerae*, and rotavirus (13,14). In one study of Bangladeshi infants, ingestion of cholera-specific breast milk antibody did not prevent intestinal infection with *V. cholerae* O1, but it did appear to protect colonized infants from overt clinical disease (15). The ability of human milk to avert intestinal disease in infants may also be related to components other than antibody. Breast milk from Swedish women has been found to contain nonimmunoglobulin substances, characterized as high-molecular-weight glycoproteins, that inhibit both the pili-mediated adherence of *E. coli* and the binding of enterotoxins of *E. coli* and *V. cholerae* (16). In studies of breast milk from American lactating women, Cleary et al. (17) described another protective factor that is a nonlactose carbohydrate; this substance prevented lethal intestinal fluid loss in suckling mice exposed to the heat-stable toxin (ST) of *E. coli*. Yet another immunoglobulin-independent, possibly lipase-mediated, phenomenon was reported recently whereby the intestinal protozoal pathogens *G. lamblia* and *Entamoeba histolytica* were directly killed by exposure to normal human milk (18).

EPIDEMIOLOGY AND ETIOLOGY

The worldwide impact of acute gastrointestinal infection is enormous. The vast majority of victims are infants and children in the developing countries of Asia, Africa, and Latin America. Between 1977 and 1978, an estimated 3 to 5 billion cases of diarrhea occurred in these areas, accounting for 5 to 10 million deaths (19). Although these same stark morbidity and mortality figures do not apply to North American populations, acute gastroenteritis is still second only to the common cold as a cause of illness in U.S. families (20).

Many factors influence the incidence and etiologic spectrum reported for intestinal infection worldwide. Important parameters include the geographic locale, the vehicle of transmission, the season of the year, the age of subjects studied, and, often, the investigator's bias to seek a specific causative agent. Epidemiologic surveys must always be interpreted with these considerations in mind. Nonetheless, the ability to implicate a specific enteropathogen in patients with diarrhea has improved greatly during the past decade. Earlier diagnostic yields of 20 to 25% have now increased to a range of 50 to 80% (21). This accomplishment can be attributed both to the availability and use of better diagnostic techniques and to the recognition of previously unappreciated etiologic agents. Specifically, bacteria such as enterotoxigenic *E. coli*, noncholera vibrios, *Campylobacter jejuni*, and *Yersinia enterocolitica*, as well as the rotavirus and the Norwalk-agent virus, have now been added to the list of more traditional pathogens causing gastrointestinal infection. With this broader knowledge of etiology and pathogenesis has come hope for application of directed strategies for prevention and treatment of these ubiquitous agents of disease.

BACTERIAL INFECTIONS OF THE GASTROINTESTINAL TRACT

The human gut is an organ with a limited repertoire of responses to various disease states. Consequently, diarrhea (conventionally defined as a twofold or greater increase in the wet weight of stool relative to habitual output) often becomes the final common clinical pathway for acute gastrointestinal infections due to a variety of agents. From a pathophysiologic perspective, however, intestinal pathogens utilize several mechanisms in order to overcome normal host defenses and cause disease. These mechanisms have been best studied in bacteria, but similar principles of virulence may also apply to viruses and protozoa that infect the human gastrointestinal tract.

With the proviso that some organisms exhibit multiple virulence factors, three pathogenetic properties have been described that allow for initial characterization of most bacterial intestinal pathogens:

1. Adherence to the mucosal surface by specialized structures and receptors, permitting colonization (prototype species: enterotoxigenic *E. coli*)

2. Elaboration of enterotoxins, altering intestinal fluid and electrolyte transport (prototype species: *V. cholerae,*), or cytotoxins, which directly injure the host cell (prototype species: *C. difficile*)

3. Direct invasion, producing necrosis and inflammation of mucosal epithelium (prototype species: *Shigella* sp.)

For some bacteria, these specialized functions are encoded by chromosomal genes. Other properties such as mucosal adherence and enterotoxin production by various pathogenic strains of *E. coli* are determined by extrachromosomal elements (plasmids) transmissible to related organisms. There are, in addition, other less well studied mechanisms by which intestinal microorganisms display pathogenicity. Representative examples include (a) unusual bacterial motility *(V. cholerae)* (22), (b) intracellular survival and replication (*Salmonella* sp.) (23), (c) elaboration of lytic enzymes that aid in mucosal penetration *(E. histolytica, V. cholerae)* (24,25), and elaboration of substances that mimic the actions of intestinal hormones *(E. histolytica)* (26) or interfere with the autonomic motor function of the intestine *(E. coli)* (27).

In the following sections, specific representative bacterial infections of the human gastrointestinal tract will be presented, with relatively brief clinical description and a major emphasis on recent concepts of pathogenesis and host defense.

Cholera and Other Vibrios

Cholera is a severe diarrheal disorder that can produce dehydration and death within hours of onset. As the prototype of toxin-mediated secretory diarrheas, no disease has contributed more to our current knowledge of intestinal physiology. The causative agent, *V. cholerae*, is a curved, motile Gram-negative rod existing as two biotypes (classical and El Tor). Both biotypes have produced worldwide pandemics of disease. The current El Tor pandemic, thought to have begun in Indonesia in 1961, has now progressed throughout Asia, Africa, and pockets of southern Europe.

V. cholerae is an exclusive pathogen of humans, and fecally contaminated food or water is its usual vehicle of transmission. Consequently, the disease is concentrated in areas where modern sanitation and water purification are lacking. The inoculum of organisms required to produce symptomatic infection in normal hosts is very large, on the order of 10^9. Following acute disease, up to 5% of patients become transient asymptomatic carriers and thus provide a reservoir in which the pathogen can "overwinter."

As with all infectious diseases, there is a spectrum of clinical manifestations due to *V. cholerae*. The typical syndrome associated with the organism consists of overwhelming isotonic diarrhea and dehydration. The fecal effluent contains minimal protein and no inflammatory cells. Because *V. cholerae* itself is neither invasive nor otherwise capable of histologic injury, this dramatic secretory process entirely reflects the action of cholera toxin on the small-intestine epithelium. The actual enterotoxin produced by all wild strains of *V. cholerae* is a protein of molecular weight 84,000 constructed of A and B subunits at a ratio of 1:5. The B subunit is responsible for binding to a receptor on the mucosal cell membrane (identified as the GM_1 ganglioside), whereas the A subunit binds and activates adenyl cyclase located on the inner cellular membrane of the intestinal epithelial cell. According to current data, the resulting increased levels of cyclic AMP (cAMP) both stimulate direct secretion of chloride by intestinal crypt cells and inhibit absorption of neutral sodium chloride by intestinal villous cells (28).

Following an attack of acute cholera, specific serum antibodies of two types can be demonstrated: a vibriocidal antibody directed against bacterial somatic antigen, and an antitoxin antibody. In areas of high endemicity such as the Indian subcontinent, the level of vibriocidal antibody rises with age and correlates with significant protection against recurrent disease; consequently, acute cholera in endemic areas is largely a disease of young children. Nonetheless, the critical defense against cholera is probably mediated by mucosal immune systems involving intestinal antibodies. Antibodies retrieved from small-intestine fluid or feces of experimental animals recovering from cholera infection appear to inhibit both the mucosal binding of *V. cholerae* organisms and the specific binding of cholera toxin to its GM_1 ganglioside receptor (21). In addition, oral immunization of experimental animals with cholera toxin confers protection against subsequent challenge with either live *V. cholerae* organisms (29) or cholera toxin (30). Because the commercial parenteral whole-cell cholera vaccine that is currently available provides only limited protection (50% efficacy lasting 3–6 months), these findings have fostered interest in a cholera toxoid vaccine. Ongoing trials thus far indicate that 80% of volunteers in

Bangladesh given a single oral or intramuscular immunization with B-subunit cholera toxoid developed a rise in local intestinal secretory antitoxin (31).

Acute diarrheal disease due to a noncholera marine vibrio, *V. parahemolyticus*, was first recognized in 1951. This agent is now estimated to cause almost 50% of cases of food-borne gastroenteritis in the summer months in Japan (32), presumably linked to the consumption of raw or undercooked seafood. In contrast to *V. cholerae*, the pathogenicity of *V. parahemolyticus* has been attributed to adherence, colonization, and invasion of the human ileum; the production of a thermostable hemolysin by the organism may also contribute to its virulence (33).

Other halophilic vibrios that are pathogenic for humans include *V. mimicus, V. vulnificus*, and *V. alginolyticus*. The first of these agents was recently recovered during the course of acute gastroenteritis from 19 patients who shared a penchant for raw oysters; however, only two of the isolated strains elaborated choleralike enterotoxin in conventional assays, again implying that other pathogenetic mechanisms were operative (34). *V. alginolyticus* and *V. vulnificus* are primarily associated with soft-tissue and/or otic infection following marine exposure, although some patients infected with *V. vulnificus* also present with septicemia. In this setting, bacteremia may reflect dissemination from a gastrointestinal portal of entry (33). *Aeromonas hydrophila* is a final member of the Vibrionaceae family recently appreciated as a significant cause of childhood gastroenteritis. In one series, enterotoxin-positive *A. hydrophila* was isolated from the stools of 127 of 975 Australian children with diarrhea during a 12-month prospective study (35).

Escherichia coli

E. coli is the most common facultative bacteria in the normal fecal flora, and until recently it commanded little notice as an important diarrheal pathogen. Over the past decade, however, this picture has radically changed. It is now known that certain strains of *E. coli* can produce gastroenteritis by several different mechanisms, leading to the following designations: enterotoxigenic (ETEC), enteropathogenic (EPEC), and enteroinvasive (EIEC). These agents are found worldwide. In particular, ETEC is responsible for the majority of cases of adult traveler's diarrhea and also causes dehydrating gastroenteritis in small children throughout the developing world.

ETEC

It was not long after the pathophysiology of cholera was elucidated that certain plasmid-bearing strains of *E. coli* were found to produce a similar clinical picture of secretory diarrhea without associated mucosal damage or bacteremia. Two toxins were subsequently found in these isolates. The heat-labile toxin of *E. coli* (LT) is physiologically and antigenically similar to cholera toxin: It has a high molecular weight (80,000), is immunogenic, and stimulates the adenylate cyclase/AMP system in small-intestine epithelium by binding to the GM_1 ganglioside. The kinetics and clinical effects of LT are similar to those of cholera toxin, because LT produces a delayed secretion of isotonic fluid that persists for hours after the binding event. LT is detected *in vitro* by morphologic changes in tissue culture (Y-1 adrenal cells or Chinese hamster ovary cells) or by enzyme-linked immunosorbent assay.

The second, heat-stable, toxin of *E. coli* (ST) is distinctly different from LT. It has a low molecular weight ($\sim 4,500$), acts on mucosal receptors of both the small bowel and large bowel, and probably mediates its secretory effects through activation of guanylate cyclase. These effects dissipate rapidly when ST is washed out of the gut lumen of experimental animals. Although ST has classically been detected by its ability to elicit fluid secretion in the infant mouse intestine, new evidence indicates that a second group of ST molecules may exhibit secretory effects only in ligated intestinal loops from rabbits or pigs (36). In addition, techniques such as molecular cloning, nucleotide sequence analysis, and nucleic acid hybridization now suggest that at least two genes encode for ST molecules in human isolates of ETEC (37). One of these gene products (STIa) has previously been seen in human, bovine, and porcine ETEC, but the second toxin (STIb) may be confined solely to ETEC strains of human origin (37).

Following the ingestion of contaminated food or water, colonization of the small intestine by ETEC precedes the development of diarrhea. The actual process of colonization is related to specific protein antigens on the bacterial cell surface in the form of pili, or fimbriae. Some of these pili have been termed colonization factor antigens (CFA-I and CFA-II); they are characterized in part by a pattern of mannose-resistant hemagglutination when reacted with human group A or bovine erythrocytes (38). Pili from human ETEC isolates have also been found to bind to human buccal cells, and the inhibition of this event by specific pili antisera has provided experimental support for at least three additional adherence factors (39). In general, isolates of ETEC recovered from human patients with diarrhea are both fimbriated and enterotoxigenic (containing LT or ST or both). However, a porcine strain possessing the K88 surface antigen was no longer capable of causing diarrhea in piglets when this bacteria selectively lost its genetic ability to synthesize pili while retaining toxin production (40).

Antibodies against the enterotoxins and colonization factors of ETEC have been demonstrated in infected patients. Epidemiologic studies indicate that individuals who reside in areas endemic for ETEC have a lowered risk of acquiring traveler's diarrhea due to these organisms (41). Such observations suggest that immunization with some component of ETEC is a plausible control strategy. Fimbrial antigens have been used to stimulate colostral antibody in pregnant pigs, cows, and sheep; however, the resulting protection of neonatal animals extended only to rechallenge with a homologous fimbriated strain and merely limited the disease severity (42). More recently, extensive work by Klipstein et al. (42) has led to the production of a cross-linked toxoid vaccine containing both synthetic ST (coupled to a protein carrier) and the B unit of purified porcine LT. Immunization with this preparation gave significant increases in mucosal IgA antitoxin titers in rats and protected the animals against viable strains of human and porcine ETEC containing both ST and LT.

EPEC

Since the first recognition over 50 years ago of sporadic epidemics of diarrhea in nurseries, *E. coli* has been associated with gastroenteritis in this setting. The subsequent development by Kauffman of a serotyping system based on O, H, and K antigens of Enterobacteriaceae helped to elucidate the epidemiology of such outbreaks, linking approximately 15 O serotypes of *E. coli* (especially O55 and O111) with this clinical syndrome. These strains are now conventionally designated as enteropathogenic. Although they consistently lack enterotoxic activity, some EPEC serotypes elaborate a cytotoxin that produces distinctive changes in Vero-cell tissue cultures (43). This toxin is also immunologically similar to the toxin of *Shigella dysenteriae* type 1 (44) and may be carried on a bacteriophage (45).

Another unusual form of EPEC diarrhea is characterized by widespread entero-adherence, leading to a syndrome of jejunal overgrowth and mucosal injury in infants (46). Investigation of this clinical entity has been aided by study of RDEC-1, an enteroadherent strain of *E. coli* that causes diarrhea in rabbits by an apparently similar mechanism. In the rabbit model, RDEC-1 binds to membranous (M) cells of the lymphoid follicle epithelium of Peyer's patches soon after inoculation, and widespread ileal, cecal, and colonic epithelial colonization is apparent only 3 days later (47). If these animal data can be extrapolated to human disease, antigenic processing by lymphocytes of the gastrointestinal tract may be an early event in this form of *E. coli* diarrhea.

EIEC

The earliest evidence that certain serotypes of *E. coli* could display frankly in-vasive behavior was published in 1967, when investigators in Japan and Brazil simultaneously reported an association between *E. coli* and an illness resembling bacillary dysentery. In many respects these strains of *E. coli* are similar to *Shigella* organisms: They express common somatic antigens, and they also share the capacity to penetrate colonic intestinal epithelial cells. In addition, EIEC are often nonmotile and may not ferment lactose as rapidly as do other *E. coli* strains, thus causing confusion with *Shigella* organisms during primary isolation from stool.

In order to confirm the invasive property of a suspected EIEC strain, the Sereny test is performed. This procedure entails inoculation of a fresh suspension of organisms into the conjunctival sac of a guinea pig; the result is judged positive if purulent inflammation develops within 1 to 7 days. The presence of a high-molecular-weight plasmid (120–140 megadaltons) in all Sereny-positive EIEC (48), as well as in some virulent *Shigella* species (49), further suggests that acquired genetic homology may partly explain the similar *in vivo* features of these two bacterial enteropathogens.

Other E. coli

In early 1982, a domestic outbreak of hemorrhagic colitis occurred that was ultimately traced to consumption of undercooked hamburger meat. A rare *E. coli* serotype (O157:H7) was isolated from stools of affected patients (50). This isolate was notable because it lacked both toxigenic and invasive characteristics and was not known to be among the previously recognized group of EPEC strains. The primary pathogenic mechanism of *E. coli* O157 awaits further verification, but preliminary studies have shown that this serotype produces a cytotoxin similar to that of *S. dysenteriae* type 1 (51). Bacterial extracts and culture supernatants of three U.S. clinical isolates were cytotoxic for cultured HeLa cells, an effect that could be neutralized by rabbit antiserum to purified Shiga toxin (51).

Campylobacter

C. jejuni is a newly recognized enteric pathogen with a vast reservoir in animals. Because the agent is fastidious and its optimal culture conditions have been defined only in the past decade, an appreciation of its significance is just now emerging. In North America and Europe, *C. jejuni* is estimated to cause 3 to 14% of unselected cases of gastroenteritis (52). Epidemiologic evidence has linked infection to consumption of contaminated products (especially poultry, unpasteurized milk, and water), contact with domestic animals, and travel abroad. In such reports, fecal isolation of *C. jejuni* has been almost universally associated with symptomatic disease. In contrast, fecal isolation of *C. jejuni* in developing countries is most common in infants and young children and does not necessarily correlate with acute diarrheal illness (53).

The clinical presentation of *Campylobacter* enteritis ranges from a dysenteric form of illness associated with fecal leukocytes and blood to intermittent watery diarrhea. Associated pathological changes include widespread mucosal injury that may involve the entire jejunum, ileum, and colon. Although cellular infiltration on biopsy specimens and the occasional detection of bacteremia strongly suggest primary tissue invasion by the organism, the actual pathogenesis of human campylobacteriosis is still debated. The observation that culture supernatants of *C. jejuni* induce a secretory response in jejunal segments of adult rats implies that enterotoxin activity may contribute to the development of diarrhea (54). In addition, other workers have recently reported cytopathic changes and increased cAMP levels in Chinese hamster ovary cells exposed to supernatants of *C. jejuni* (55). Although serum antibodies can be detected following both symptomatic and asymptomatic *Campylobacter* infections (56,53), the precise mechanisms whereby clinical immunity may develop to this agent have not yet been studied.

Shigella

Shigella is an invasive pathogen of the human gastrointestinal tract that produces the disease syndrome known as bacillary dysentery. Strains of *Shigella* are characterized by specific cell wall antigens and are subdivided into the following four species: *S. dysenteriae* (10 serotypes), *S. flexneri* (6 serotypes), *S. boydii* (15 serotypes), and *S. sonnei* (1 serotype). Although *S. flexneri* is the most common isolate in developing countries, *S. dysenteriae* 1, also known as the Shiga bacillus, produces the most virulent clinical disease. In Central America, a five-country pandemic of the latter strain caused over 10,000 deaths in 1968–72, primarily in young children (57). In recent years, *S. sonnei* has replaced *S. flexneri* as the most common domestic species, accounting for the representative figure of 66% of all reported cases of shigellosis in the United States in 1981 (58).

Shigellae are highly host-adapted bacteria, natural pathogens only of humans and a few higher primates. As a consequence, one human infection is always theoretically traceable to another human source, although the route may deviate through contaminated food or liquid. Volunteer studies indicate that an oral dose of 10^5 *Shigella* organisms produces an attack rate of 75%, but experimental infection has been established in humans with as few as 10 to 200 viable bacilli of the virulent *S. dysenteriae* 1 or *S. flexneri* 2a strains (59,60).

Although patients with shigellosis may manifest a spectrum of symptomatic disease, the classic clinical presentation of bacillary dysentery is characterized by fever, abdominal cramps, tenesmus, and the passage of multiple small-volume stools containing blood, mucus, and inflammatory cells. Pathologically, these symptoms and signs reflect direct bacterial invasion of colonic epithelial cells to the level of the submucosa. On the basis of the work of Formal et al. (61,62), it is now believed that multiple chromosomal genes encode for the ability of *Shigella* to invade and proliferate within epithelial cells. In addition, certain strains of *S. flexneri* also possess large 120- to 140-megadalton plasmids containing genetic determinants that contribute to virulence (49).

Elaboration of a unique and potent exotoxin is another important pathogenetic property of all *Shigella* species. In 1960, Vicari et al. (63) reported that a product of *S. dysenteriae* 1 was cytotoxic for cells in tissue culture. The inhibition of protein synthesis by this toxin may be the intracellular event that results in death of infected epithelial cells. Keusch and associates subsequently studied a clinical epidemic strain of *S. dysenteriae* and found that the cytotoxic Shiga toxin also mediated heat-labile enterotoxic activity (demonstrated in isolated segments of rabbit ileum) (64). This finding was consistent with the clinical observation of a secretory diarrheal prodrome in a selected subset of patients with shigellosis. Nonetheless, because live oral challenge with nonpenetrating, enterotoxin-positive mutants of *S. dysenteriae* does not produce overt illness in humans or monkeys (65), mucosal invasion is still the critical event leading to clinical shigellosis.

As further evidence that all *Shigella* species are toxigenic, neutralizing antitoxin has been detected in the sera of patients recovering from *S. dysenteriae, S. flexneri,* and *S. sonnei* infections (66,67). However, serum antitoxin is present in only the IgM antibody fraction and does not appear to confer protection against reinfection (68). Nonetheless, epidemiologic evidence and data from human volunteers who were rechallenged after experimental dysentery do suggest the development of serotype-specific immunity to *Shigella*. Although the precise nature of this protective mechanism is not known, recent work in a rabbit model demonstrated that a vigorous IgA memory response was present in intestinal secretions after oral immunization with multiple doses of a live hybrid *S. flexneri* vaccine strain (69).

The continuing challenge in developing a live oral vaccine for human shigellosis is to retain effective colonization while inhibiting invasive behavior in a stable hybrid strain (70).

Salmonella

The three species of *Salmonella*, *S. typhi*, *S. cholera-suis*, and *S. enteritidis*, are worldwide pathogens responsible for a spectrum of human disease that encompasses typhoid fever, septicemia with or without focal suppuration, acute gastroenteritis, and asymptomatic carrier states. *S. typhi* is remarkably host-adapted to humans, who represent the only natural reservoir of infection. In contrast, the almost 2,000 serotypes of *S. enteritidis* that cause the majority of cases of *Salmonella* gastroenteritis are widely prevalent in domestic and natural animal populations, as well as sewage, river, and sea water. Food and fluid vehicles such as poultry, eggs, milk, and drinking water are most commonly implicated in the transmission of *S. enteritidis*, although infection may be traced to another human host.

The minimum inoculum necessary to establish infection with *S. typhi* is 10^5 organisms, as determined by volunteer studies with the virulent Quailes strain (71). In contrast, the infectivity of *S. enteritidis* varies with serotype and inoculum size; for example, 10^5 *S. enteritidis* serotype *newport* produced illness in some subjects, whereas 10^9 *S. enteritidis* serotype *pullorum*, a strain that is highly adapted to chickens, were unable to produce human disease (72,73). Age, gastric acidity, and the composition of the normal bacterial flora are additional host factors that influence the infectious dose for all *Salmonella* organisms. The relative frequency of hospital outbreaks of *Salmonella* gastroenteritis implies that altered hosts may have enhanced susceptibility to this infection. Some specific disease states with which salmonellosis has been directly associated include malignancy, liver disease, malaria, bartonellosis, schistosomiasis, and hemoglobinopathies such as sickle cell disease (74).

Although the clinical features of typhoid fever will not be comprehensively reviewed here, they essentially reflect the remarkable ability of *S. typhi* to invade bowel mucosa and disseminate to lymphatic foci throughout the body. Following several days of intracellular replication in reticuloendothelial tissue, sequential waves of bacteremia then establish more distant sites of *S. typhi* infection. Nontyphoidal salmonellosis is a more purely gastrointestinal disease, marked by short incubation (6–48 hr), nausea, vomiting, abdominal cramps, diarrhea, and variable fever in up to 50% of patients. Despite the abbreviated clinical course, histologic abnormalities and occasional bacteremia bespeak primary tissue invasion even in the gastroenteritis syndrome. The ileal mucosa and Peyer's patches lymphoid tissue are thought to be the tissue portals of entry for both *S. typhi* and invasive *S. enteritidis*, and the stools of patients acutely infected with either of these pathogens typically contain inflammatory cells.

There are several biologic characteristics that make salmonellae virulent for humans and animals. For nontyphoidal strains, one determinant of virulence is the

O (somatic) antigen contained within the lipopolysaccharide (LPS) capsule of the organism. Organisms that lack the O-specific side chains of the LPS are called "rough" mutants and are unable to cause disease in experimental animals (75). As with other Enterobacteriaceae, circulating LPS may itself mediate a variety of physiologic effects such as fever, complement activation, clotting abnormalities, and hypotension through the action of its endotoxin component.

Because some invasive strains of *Salmonella* also cause intestinal secretory effects in animal models, investigators have sought evidence for enterotoxin production by these organisms. Studies have shown that *Salmonella* infection may initiate the synthesis of prostaglandins, which in turn stimulate adenylate cyclase/cAMP synthesis and attendant fluid accumulation (76). The detection of a *Salmonella* "enterotoxin" in cell-free bacterial filtrates applied in the suckling mouse assay has been less reproducible, and considerable controversy therefore persists regarding the relative contributions of bacterial invasion and pure enterotoxin activity to fluid secretory effects in salmonellosis (77). There is also conflicting evidence regarding the cross-immunogenicity of the putative *Salmonella* enterotoxin with cholera toxin and *E. coli* heat-labile enterotoxin (78).

Another fundamental property that enhances the pathogenicity of *Salmonella* species is their ability to replicate intracellularly within macrophages and thus to resist opsonization and phagocytosis. This mode of infection suggests that the host defense in salmonellosis, as with many other intracellular pathogens, ultimately depends on mechanisms of cellular immunity. Such a theory is supported by early experiments in mice correlating the susceptibility to infection with *S. typhimurium* with the ability to mount a delayed hypersensitivity response to an extract of the organism (23). Subsequent studies in mice demonstrated that natural resistance to *S. typhimurium* (which correlates with the development of delayed hypersensitivity) is genetically determined by products of the Ir gene complex (79). Most recently, both peripheral and intestinal lymphoid cells of C3H/HeN mice were shown to exhibit natural and antibody-mediated cytotoxicity for *S. typhimurium*, whereas macrophages alone were devoid of this spontaneous activity (80).

Paradoxically, the apparent pathogenicity of salmonellae is also increased when host phagocytosis of these organisms is impaired. An increased incidence of salmonellosis is therefore seen in certain disorders such as sickle cell anemia, malaria, bartonellosis, and louse-borne relapsing fever, all of which are characterized by reticuloendothelial blockade. Corroborating animal studies have demonstrated that multiplication of *S. typhimurium* is enhanced during acute experimental hemolysis (81); presumably, as macrophages ingest breakdown products of red blood cells, their ability to phagocytize organisms is reduced. A second phagocytic alteration in patients with sickle cell anemia is related to decreased opsonization of salmonellae due to defective activation of the alternate complement pathway in these individuals (82).

Although humoral immunity may be important in salmonellosis, serologic testing has not been found particularly helpful, for the following reasons: (a) gastroenteritis and carrier states may not elicit a measurable serum antibody response; (b) cross-reacting antibodies from nonrelated salmonellae or coliforms can falsely elevate the typhoid O antigen titer; (c) nonspecific elevations are seen in various inflammatory states and in liver disease; (d) the use of killed typhoid vaccine often results in persistently elevated levels of antibody to the H (flagellar) antigen. As a consequence, there have been few data from humans supporting serum antibody as a defense mechanism against *Salmonella* infection. Nonetheless, some studies do indicate at least partial protection from reinfection mediated by local intestinal immunity. One line of evidence is derived from the finding that women who have recovered from *Salmonella* gastroenteritis secrete specific IgA in their colostrum (83). In another recent series, 6 of 8 patients studied 1 year after documented *Salmonella* enteritis still had significant concentrations of intestinal IgA, whereas serum antibody (IgG) had fallen to levels only marginally higher than those in controls (84). Some degree of clinical immunity has also been observed in volunteers refed the same strain of *Salmonella* with which they were previously infected. Only 50% of subjects thus tested developed a second illness, and the subset that did exhibit recurrent disease required up to six times the original inoculum and still experienced milder symptoms than on initial exposure (85).

The ongoing debate on the respective contributions of cellular immunity and humoral immunity to host defense in salmonellosis bears directly on the design of new vaccines for this disease. Although a killed parenteral vaccine for typhoid fever has been in use for many years, the partial immunity achieved with this preparation can clearly be overcome by an increase in the bacterial inoculum. Some laboratories have therefore investigated newer killed vaccines (whole organisms or subcellular fractions) and reported that the antibodies raised against the O antigen of *S. typhimurium* may be protective in mice, depending on their immunogenetic constitution (86). The alternate school holds that live mutant organisms orally administered are more likely to elicit effective intestinal and cellular defense mechanisms, although concern persists regarding the potential for reversion to virulence in these attenuated bacteria. However, initial results from a clinical field trial of live *S. typhi* strain Ty 21a (a galactose-epimerase-negative, Vi-negative mutant) are promising. This preparation appeared to be safe, stable, and effective (0.2 case per 10,000 children treated in a three-dose regimen versus 4.9 cases per 10,000 control subjects) over a 3-year period of evaluation (87).

Yersinia

Y. enterocolitica is a bacterial pathogen with a wide zoonotic reservoir and diverse clinical manifestations. In some areas of the world, such as Scandinavia and Canada, this agent is a common cause of pediatric gastroenteritis. In adults, it also produces a pseudoappendicitis syndrome, mesenteric adenitis, arthritis, erythema nodosum, and sepsis. Although the incidences of yersiniosis are almost equal for male and female subjects, clinical symptoms may vary with sex; some series have indicated that men infected with *Y. enterocolitica* are likely to develop gastroenteritis, whereas erythema nodosum is more often seen in adult female patients (88). Another interesting epidemiologic observation is the apparent decreased incidence of acute yersiniosis in warm climates or summer months. This finding may be related to the selective ability to grow at cold temperatures (4°C or 25°C) that the organism exhibits in culture.

The actual pathogenesis of disease due to *Y. enterocolitica* is unclear, despite the demonstration of several virulent properties: (a) elaboration of heat-stable enterotoxin (89); (b) penetration of epithelial cells in tissue culture (90); (c) production of keratoconjunctivitis in guinea pigs (Sereny test) (91). The specific serotypes O3, O8, and O9 (prevalent in Canada, the United States, and Scandinavia, respectively) are also markers for clinical pathogenicity. Because these isolates share the ability to produce exudative diarrhea with inflammatory cells, as well as a common potential for extraintestinal sequelae, tissue invasion is probably their primary pathogenetic mechanism. The presence of a 42- to 44-megadalton plasmid in a variety of enteroinvasive serotypes of *Y. enterocolitica* (92) suggests that this genetic mechanism may underlie the acquisition of virulence.

Although clinical diarrhea due to *Y. enterocolitica* usually subsides within 1 to 3 weeks, prolonged fecal excretion of the pathogen is often observed over several months (93). *Y. enterocolitica* is a facultative intracellular bacterium, and cellular immune mechanisms may ultimately be required for resolution of infection. In a recent comparative study of patients suspected of having yersiniosis and asymptomatic controls, the correlation of clinical disease with monospecific antibody titers was inconsistent; in addition, serologic testing proved to be insensitive in infants and immunosuppressed patients with culture-proven infection (94). In contrast, preliminary work suggests that specific lymphocyte transformation responses to *Yersinia* antigen provide a more accurate reflection of acquired host defense during acute disease (95).

VIRAL INFECTIONS OF THE GASTROINTESTINAL TRACT

For many years it has been traditional to ascribe viral causes to those cases of acute gastroenteritis in which bacterial pathogens are not demonstrated. Initial indirect evidence for the role of viruses in human diarrhea was obtained in the 1940s, when human volunteers developed intestinal symptoms following oral administration of bacteria-free filtrates prepared from the stools of patients involved in diarrheal outbreaks (96). Although some outbreaks in the 1950s and 1960s were directly linked to infection with known enteroviruses (echovirus types 11, 14, and 18; Coxsackie B-3) (97), subsequent worldwide epidemiologic studies have failed to support the notion that these agents are common causes of acute intestinal illness (98). Similar early attempts to link adenovirus and human gastroenteritis were confounded by the finding that these viruses were often detected as frequently in the stools of normal persons as in fecal specimens from symptomatic patients (99).

In 1968, an outbreak of diarrhea in Norwalk, Ohio, spurred renewed interest in viral gastroenteritis. Subsequent application of electron microscopy, immune electron microscopy, and other techniques that quantitate viral antigens in stool specimens has greatly advanced our knowledge of viral pathogens of the gastrointestinal tract. Two major classes of viral agents are now considered principally responsible for the majority of cases of viral diarrhea: (a) the Norwalk-like viruses, which characteristically produce explosive family and communitywide epidemics affecting school-age children and adults, and (b) the rotaviruses, agents that are commonly associated with sporadic infantile diarrhea throughout the world. Although astroviruses, calciviruses, and adenoviruses have also been implicated as likely etiologic organisms in some other recent, carefully studied outbreaks, the epidemiologic significance of these agents appears to be of lesser magnitude (98).

Norwalk-like Viruses

In the winter of 1968, 50% of the children attending an elementary school in Norwalk, Ohio, developed an illness lasting 24 to 48 hr, consisting of diarrhea, nausea, vomiting, fever, malaise, myalgias, and abdominal cramps (100). A high attack rate also occurred among family contacts, which enabled investigators to estimate an incubation period of 48 hr preceding the onset of clinical symptoms. Bacteria- and toxin-free stool filtrates from the affected patients did not induce illness in experimental animals and did not yield detectable virus when cell culture was attempted. Nonetheless, intestinal passage of the putative agent through several generations of human volunteers resulted in reproducible clinical disease in 50% of all subjects thus exposed (101). In 1972, a small (27-nm diameter), nonenveloped, round particle of unclear structure was ultimately identified in fecal specimens from these symptomatic volunteers (102). A subsequent CDC survey of 74 outbreaks of nonbacterial gastroenteritis occurring between 1976 and 1980 confirmed the epidemiologic importance of this organism by utilizing both serologic testing and clinical features to link Norwalk-like agents to 42% of these outbreaks (103).

When a stool containing the Norwalk agent is combined with convalescent serum from a recently recovered patient, an aggregation of viral particles occurs that can be identified by electron microscopic examination. This technique provided the initial means for diagnosis of Norwalk disease. By use of the same procedure, other noncultivatable fecal strains have been discovered that are similar to the Norwalk agent in their physical properties but are antigenically distinct and associated with geographically disparate clusters of acute gastrointestinal disease. More recently, radioimmunoassay has facilitated measurement of serum antibody as well as identification of Norwalk-related viruses in stool. At present, at least three serogroups, designated as the Norwalk agent, the Hawaii agent, and the Ditchling agent, are conventionally recognized, and a fourth possible serogroup, known as the Marin agent, has also been described.

The current inability to propagate Norwalk virus in cell culture and the lack of experimental animal models have clearly hindered efforts to understand the pathophysiology of this infection. However, histologic observations in human volunteers do provide some insight. While lacking distinct evidence for viral particles in intestinal tissue, biopsy specimens have revealed characteristic lesions in the proximal small intestine in all symptomatic subjects (104). These histologic abnormalities, which may persist up to 1 week, include shortening of jejunal villi, hyperplastic crypts, vacuolated and cuboidal columnar epithelium, and polymorphonuclear and mononuclear cell infiltration in the lamina propria (104). In addition, fat, lactose, and xylose malabsorptions have been documented in many infected patients. This clinical observation supports the concept that a dysfunction of enterocyte absorption results from the apparent cellular injury. Conversely, the maintenance of normal brush-border adenylate cyclase levels during the disease course (105) implies that Norwalk disease does not produce a classic secretory defect mediated by alterations in cAMP. Because symptomatic volunteers do not demonstrate fecal leukocytes and rectal histology remains normal, infection appears to be limited to the small intestine (106).

Prospective serologic evaluation of human volunteers exposed to the Norwalk agent indicates that many of the subjects who developed gastroenteritis had experienced prior exposure to the virus, as manifested by detectable serum antibodies (107). On the other hand, two studies have demonstrated that the subset of volunteers who remained well after ingestion of infectious stool filtrate had low levels of preexisting antibody or no antibody in their sera and intestinal secretions (107,108). The absence of immunologic recognition of the virus may indicate an effective, nonimmunologic, but currently unknown, mechanism of host defense directed against this agent. One could speculate that susceptibility to the virus is genetically determined and is mediated by receptors on the intestinal cell surface; such an explanation is consistent with the finding of familial clusters of susceptibility and resistance observed during a recent water-borne outbreak of Norwalk disease (109). As an alternative theory, Blacklow and Cukor have suggested that seropositivity and clinical illness may not develop until repetitive exposures to the virus have occurred (98). Nonetheless, following symptomatic infection with the Norwalk virus, serologic titers do rise, correlating with a period of protection against reinfection that lasts for weeks to months. The finding that rechallenge with virus after 27 to 42 months produced recurrent illness in all volunteers previously symptomatic (107) substantiates the conclusion that acquired immunity to Norwalk disease in susceptible hosts is relatively short-lived. In the same study, previously nonsusceptible volunteers did not experience any clinical illness on reexposure to the agent.

Rotavirus

Although rotaviruses have been found in almost every animal species examined, human rotavirus was not identified until 1973, when 9 Australian infants with acute gastroenteritis were studied by intestinal biopsy. Thin-section electron microscopy revealed 65-nm-diameter viral particles in duodenal epithelial cells of 6 of these children (110). Similar structures were subsequently detected in negatively stained stools of many children with acute diarrheal illness (98). In early reports, these viral particles were variously referred to as orbivirus, reovirus-like agent (HRVL), infantile gastroenteritis virus, and duovirus. Although closely related to these other agents, rotaviruses were subsequently differentiated as a unique class of RNA viruses and were named for their distinctive wheel-like appearance. In 1980, Wyatt et al. (111) were able to adapt a strain of human rotavirus to high-titer propagation after multiple passages through gnotobiotic piglets, representing the first successful *in vitro* tissue culture of the human agent. This accomplishment has raised hopes that a mutant human rotavirus or a recombinant strain of animal and human rotavirus may ultimately be used in the development of an oral vaccine.

Rotavirus infection is found throughout the world, with a peak occurrence in 6-month-old to 2-year-old children. In developed countries, it has emerged as the single most important cause of diarrhea in infants and young children who enter hospitals for treatment of acute gastroenteritis, accounting for 39 to 63% of such admissions (97). Although the incidence of rotavirus-related illness in tropical areas is less well documented, it is also believed to be a frequent enteropathogen in the developing world. Recent surveillance has been facilitated by the vast array of diagnostic techniques that have been adapted to detect either the antigen or antibody of rotavirus in human sera and stool. Such methods (which include radioimmunoassay, enzyme-linked immunosorbent assay, immunofluorescence, counterimmunoelectrophoresis, immune-adherence hemagglutination, and complement fixation) have yielded evidence for as many as five clinical serotypes of the agent (112).

Disease due to rotavirus is usually sporadic, and it tends to occur in the cooler months of the year. Severe watery diarrhea is the dominant presentation, with a mean duration of 7 days. Associated clinical findings include low-grade fever (63–100%), vomiting (63–100%), and upper respiratory symptoms (26–75%) (98). The risk of isotonic dehydration is greatest in the most susceptible population: infants under the age of 2 years. Although children in more developed settings are unlikely to have life-threatening sequelae, a recent study in Bangladesh determined that dehydration following rotavirus infection was responsible for a mortality of 6.5 per 1,000 (113). In any given region, adult patients experience active symptoms from the agent much less frequently than do children; however, two series that studied adults who had visited either Honduras or Mexico implicated rotavirus infection in up to one-third of cases of traveler's diarrhea acquired in those countries (114).

Histologic evidence suggests that rotavirus selectively infects the villi of the small-intestine epithelium. Virus particles can actually be visualized in tissue by transmission electron microscopy, localizing in the distended cisternae of the endoplasmic reticulum within epithelial cells (112). In contrast, examination by light microscopy of small-intestine biopsies of 17 infected patients revealed severe injury in only two specimens; a spectrum of nonspecific abnormalities and inflammation was seen in the remainder (115). All of these changes resolved by 3 to 8 weeks after infection. In the same group of patients, depression of disaccharidase activities (maltase, sucrase, or lactase) was found in 14 of 16 studied. Isolated jejunal villus enterocytes from pigs infected with human rotavirus showed no decreases in the expected levels of cAMP (116), a finding similar to that observed in humans with Norwalk virus infection.

An attempt has been made to correlate a state of protection from rotavirus with the presence of specific serum and intestinal antibodies. By routine screening, it appears that 60 to 75% of neonates have serum antibody to rotavirus (probably maternally acquired); these values progressively increase to reach 80 to 95% in children older than 2 years (112). Despite seropositivity, however, up to 50% of newborns surveyed excreted rotavirus, and this neonatal infection did not appear to confer immunity against reinfection later in infancy or early childhood (117).

The apparent dissociation between serum antibody levels and intestinal colonization with rotavirus has naturally stimulated an investigation of specific mucosal immunity that may be mediated by secretory IgA. As supportive evidence, the incidence of clinical rotavirus disease is significantly decreased in breast-fed infants over bottle-fed control babies (118), and the level of rotavirus-specific IgA in human breast milk correlates with this acquired protection (119). Similarly, lambs fed colostrum containing antirotavirus immunoglobulin are protected from infection with the agent (120). Most interesting, there is evidence in a small group of adult volunteers orally inoculated with type 2 rotavirus that the level of type-2-specific IgA in jejunal fluid is a better marker for resistance to infection than is serum IgG (121). Type-1-specific IgA in the intestinal secretions of these subjects did not appear to confer protection against type 2 challenge. Questions yet unanswered include the immunologic cross-reactivity of other rotavirus serotypes, the duration and mechanism of the intestinal immune response, and the validity of serum markers as a reflection of gut antibody-mediated host defense against rotavirus after repeat exposures to the agent.

REFERENCES

1. Simon, G. L., and Gorbach, S. L. (1984): Intestinal flora in health and disease. *Gastroenterology*, 86:174–193.
2. Gorbach, S. L., Nahas, L., Lerner, P. I., and Weinstein, L. (1967): Studies of intestinal microflora. I. Effects of diet, age and periodic sampling on numbers of fecal microorganisms in man. *Gastroenterology*, 53:845–855.
3. Gibbons, R. J., and Kapsimalis, B. (1967): Estimates of the overall role of growth of the intestinal microflora of hamsters, guinea pigs and mice. *J. Bacteriol.*, 93:510–512.
4. Bohnhoff, M., Drake, B. L., and Miller, C. P. (1954): Effect of streptomycin on susceptibility of intestinal tract to experimental *Salmonella* infection. *Proc. Soc. Exp. Biol. Med.*, 86:133–137.
5. Rosenthal, S. L. (1969): Exacerbation of *Salmonella* enteritis due to ampicillin. *N. Engl. J. Med.*, 280:147–148.
6. Tedesco, F. J. (1982): Pseudomembranous colitis: Pathogenesis and therapy. *Med. Clin. North Am.*, 66:655–664.
7. Formal, S. B., Abrams, G. D., Schneider, H., and Sprinz, H. (1963): Experimental *Shigella* infections. VI. Role of the small intestine in an experimental infection of guinea pigs. *J. Bacteriol.*, 85:119–125.
8. Kent, T. H., Formal, S. B., and LaBrec, E. H. (1966): Acute enteritis due to *Salmonella typhimurium* in opium-treated guinea pigs. *Arch. Pathol.*, 81:501–508.
9. Dupont, H. L., and Hornick, R. B. (1973): Adverse effect of therapy in shigellosis. *J.A.M.A.*, 226:1525–1528.
10. Giannella, R. A., Broitman, S. A., and Zamcheck, N. (1973): Influence of gastric acidity on bacterial and parasitic enteric infections. *Ann. Intern. Med.*, 78:271–276.

11. Cash, R. I., Music, S., Libonati, J., Snyder, M. J., Wenzel, R. P., and Hornick, R. B. (1974): Response of man to infection with *V. cholerae*: I. Clinical, serologic and bacteriologic response to a known inoculum. *J. Infect. Dis.*, 129:45–52.

12. Plotkin, G. R., Kluge, R. M., and Waldman, R. H. (1979): Gastroenteritis: Etiology, pathophysiology and clinical manifestations. *Medicine (Baltimore)*, 58:95–114.

13. Holmgren, J., Hanson, L. A., and Carlson, B. (1975): Neutralizing antibodies against *Escherichia coli* and *Vibrio cholerae* enterotoxins in human milk from a developing country. *Scand. J. Immunol.*, 5:867–871.

14. Yolken, R. H., Wyatt, R. G., Mata, L., Urrutia, J. J., Garcia, B., Chanock, R. B., and Kapikian, A. Z. (1978): Secretory antibody directed against rotavirus in human milk—measurement by means of enzyme-linked immunosorbent assay. *J. Pediatr.*, 93:916–921.

15. Glass, R. I., Svennerholm, A. M., Stoll, B. J., Khan, M. R., Hossain, K. M. B., Huq, M. I., and Holmgren, J. (1983): Protection against cholera in breast-fed children by antibodies in breast milk. *N. Engl. J. Med.*, 308:1389–1392.

16. Holmgren, J., Svennerholm, A. M., and Ahren, C. (1981): Non-immunoglobulin fraction of human milk inhibits bacterial adhesion (hemagglutination) and enterotoxin binding of *Escherichia coli* and *Vibrio cholerae*. *Infect. Immun.*, 33:136–141.

17. Cleary, T. G., Chambers, J. P., and Pickering, L. K. (1983): Protection of suckling mice from the heat-stable enterotoxin of *Escherichia coli* by human milk. *J. Infect. Dis.*, 148:1114–1119.

18. Gillin, F. D., Reiner, D. S., and Wang, C. S. (1983): Human milk kills parasitic intestinal protozoa. *Science*, 221:1290–1292.

19. Walsh, J. A., and Warren, K. A. (1979): Selective primary health care: An interim strategy for disease control in developing countries. *N. Engl. J. Med.*, 301:967–974.

20. Dingle, J. H., Badger, G. F., Feller, A. E., Hodges, R. G., Jordan, W. S., and Rammelkamp, C. H. (1953): A study of illness in a group of Cleveland families. I. Plan of study and certain general observations. *Am. J. Hyg.*, 58:16–30.

21. Giannella, R. A. (1981): Pathogenesis of acute bacterial diarrheal disorders. *Annu. Rev. Med.*, 32:341–357.

22. Guentzel, M. D., and Berry, L. J. (1975): Motility as a virulence factor for *Vibrio cholerae*. *Infect. Immun.*, 11:890–897.

23. Mitsuhashi, S., Sata, I., and Tanaka, T. (1961): Experimental salmonellosis: Intracellular growth of *Salmonella enteritidis* ingested in mononuclear phagocytes of mice and cellular basis of immunity. *J. Bacteriol.*, 81:863–868.

24. Neal, R. A. (1960): Enzymic proteolysis by *Entamoeba histolytica*: Biochemical characteristics and relationship with invasiveness. *Parasitology*, 50:531–550.

25. Schneider, D. R., and Parker, C. D. (1982): Purification and characterization of the mucinase of *Vibrio cholerae*. *J. Infect. Dis.*, 145:474–482.

26. McGowan, K., Kane, A., Asarkof, N., Wicks, J., Guerina, V., Kellum, J., Baron, S., Gintzler, A. R., and Donowitz, M. (1983): *Entamoeba histolytica* causes intestinal secretion: Role of serotonin. *Science*, 221:762–764.

27. Mathias, J. R., Nogueira, J., Martin, J. L., Carlson, G. M., and Giannella, R. A. (1982): *Escherichia coli* heat stable toxin: Its effect on motility of the small intestine. *Am. J. Physiol.*, 242:G360–363.

28. Carpenter, C. C. J. (1982): The pathophysiology of secretory diarrheas. *Med. Clin. North Am.*, 66:597–610.

29. Pierce, N. F., Cray, W. C., and Engel, P. F. (1980): Antitoxic immunity to cholera in dogs immunized with cholera toxin. *Infect. Immun.*, 27:632–637.

30. Holmgren, J., Svennerholm, A. M., Ouchterlony, O., Andersson, A., Wallerstrom, G., and Westerberg-Berndtsson, U. (1975): Antitoxic immunity in experimental cholera: Protection and serum and local antibody responses in rabbits after enteral and parenteral immunization. *Infect. Immun.*, 12:1331–1340.

31. Svennerholm, A. M., Sack, D. A., Holmgren, J., and Bardhan, P. K. (1982): Intestinal antibody responses after immunization with cholera B subunit. *Lancet*, 1:305–307.

32. Blake, P. A., Weaver, R. E., and Hollis, D. G. (1980): Diseases of humans (other than cholera) caused by vibrios. *Annu. Rev. Microbiol.*, 34:341–367.

33. Rodrick, G. E., Hood, M. A., and Blake, N. J. (1982): Human vibrio gastroenteritis. *Med. Clin. North Am.*, 66:665–671.

34. Shandera, W. X., Johnston, J. M., Davis, B. R., and Blake, P. A. (1983): Disease from infection with *Vibrio mimicus*, a newly recognized *Vibrio* species. *Ann. Intern. Med.*, 99:169–171.

35. Burke, V., Gracey, M., Robinson, J., Peck, D., Beaman, J., and Bundell, C. (1983): The microbiology of childhood gastroenteritis: *Aeromonas* species and other infective agents. *J. Infect. Dis.*, 148:68–74.

36. Gyles, C. L. (1979): Limitations of the infant mouse test for *Escherichia coli* heat stable enterotoxin. *Can. J. Comp. Med.*, 43:371–379.

37. Mosely, S. L., Samadpour-Motalebi, M., and Falkow, S. (1983): Plasmid association and nucleotide sequence relationships of two genes encoding heat stable enterotoxin production in *Escherichia coli*. *J. Bacteriol.*, 156:441–443.

38. Evans, D. G., Evans, D. J., and Dupont, H. L. (1977): Virulence factors of enterotoxigenic *E. coli*. *J. Infect. Dis.*, 136:S118–S123.

39. Deneke, C. F., Thorne, G. M., and Gorbach, S. L. (1981): Serotypes of attachment pili of enterotoxigenic *Escherichia coli* isolated from humans. *Infect. Immun.*, 32:1254–1260.

40. Smith, H. W., and Linggood, M. A. (1971): Observations on the pathogenic properties of the K88, Hly and Ent plasmids of *Escherichia coli* with particular reference to porcine diarrhea. *J. Med. Microbiol.*, 4:467–485.

41. Evans, J. J., Ruiz-Palacios, G., Evans, D. G., Dupont, H. L., Pickering, L. K. and Olarte, J. (1977): Humoral immune response to the heat-labile enterotoxin of *Escherichia coli* in naturally acquired diarrhea and antitoxin determination by passive immune hemolysis. *Infect. Immun.*, 16:781–788.

42. Klipstein, F. A., Engert, R. A., Clements, J. D., and Houghten, R. A. (1983): Protection against human and porcine enterotoxigenic strains of *Escherichia coli* in rats immunized with a cross-linked toxoid vaccine. *Infect. Immun.*, 40:924–929.

43. Konowalchuk, J., Speirs, J. I., and Stavric, S. (1977): Vero response to a cytotoxin of *Escherichia coli*. *Infect. Immun.*, 18:775–779.

44. O'Brien, A. D., LaVeck, G. D., Thompson, M. R., and Formal, S. B. (1982): Production of *Shigella dysenteriae* type 1-like cytotoxin by *Escherichia coli*. *J. Infect. Dis.*, 146:763–769.

45. Scotland, S. M., Smith, H. R., Willshaw, Q. A., and Rowe, B. (1983): Vero cytotoxin production in strain of *Escherichia coli* is determined by genes carried on bacteriophage. *Lancet*, 2:216.

46. Rothbaum, R., McAdams, J., Giannella, R., and Partin, J. C. (1982): A clinicopathologic study of enterocyte-adherent *Escherichia coli*; a cause of protracted diarrhea in infants. *Gastroenterology*, 83:441–454.

47. Inman, L. R., and Cantey, J. R. (1983): Specific adherence of *Escherichia coli* (strain RDEC-1) to membranous (M) cells of the Peyer's patch in *Escherichia coli* diarrhea in the rabbit. *J. Clin. Invest.*, 71:1–8.

48. Silva, R. M., Toledo, M. R. F., and Trabulsi, L. R. (1982): Correlation of invasiveness with plasmid in enteroinvasive strains of *Escherichia coli*. *J. Infect. Dis.*, 146:706.

49. Sansonetti, P. J., Hale, T. L., Dammin, G. J., Kapfer, C., Collins, H. H., Jr., and Formal, S. B. (1983): Alterations in the pathogenicity of *Escherichia coli* K-12 after transfer of plasmid and chromosomal genes from *Shigella flexneri*. *Infect. Immun.*, 39:1392–1402.

50. Riley, L. W., Remis, R. S., Helgerson, S. D., McGee, H. B., Wells, J. G., Davis, B. R., Hebert, R. J., Olcott, E. S., Johnson, L. M., Hargrett, N. T., Blake, P. A., and Cohen, M. L. (1983): Hemorrhagic colitis associated with a rare *Escherichia coli* serotype. *N. Engl. J. Med.*, 308:681–685.

51. O'Brien, A. D., Lively, T. A., Chen, M. E., Rothman, S. W., and Formal, S. B. (1983): *Escherichia coli* O157:H7 strains associated with hemorrhagic colitis in the United States produce a *Shigella dysenteriae* 1 (Shiga) like cytotoxin. *Lancet*, 1:702.

52. Blaser, M. J., and Reller, L. B. (1981): *Campylobacter* enteritis. *N. Engl. J. Med.*, 305:1444–1452.

53. Glass, R. I., Stoll, B. J., Huq, M. I., Struelens, M. J., Blaser, M., and Kibriya, A. K. M. G. (1983): Epidemiologic and clinical features of endemic *Campylobacter jejuni* infection in Bangladesh. *J. Infect. Dis.*, 148:292–296.

54. Fernandez, H., Neto, U. F., Fernandes, F., Pedra, M. A., and Trabulsi, L. R. (1983): Culture supernatants of *Campylbacter jejuni* induce a secretory response in jejunal segments of adult rats. *Infect. Immun.*, 40:429–431.

55. Ruiz-Palacios, G. M., Torres, J., Torres, N. I., Escamilla, E., Ruiz-Palacios, B. R., and Tamayo, J. (1983): Cholera-like enterotoxin produced by *Campylobacter jejuni*. Characterization and clinical significance. *Lancet*, 2:250–252.

56. Blaser, M. J., Berkowitz, I. D., LaForce, F. M., Cravens, J. S., Reller, L. B., and Wang, W. L. (1979): *Campylobacter* enteritis: Clinical and epidemiologic features. *Ann. Intern. Med.*, 91:179–185.

57. Mata, L. J., Gangarosa, E. J., Caceres, A., Perera, D. R., and Mejicanos, M. L. (1970): Epidemic Shiga bacillus dysentery in Central America: I. Etiologic investigations in Guatemala, 1969. *J. Infect. Dis.*, 122:170–180.

58. (1982): Shigellosis—United States, 1981. *Morbid. Mortal. Weekly Rep.*, 31:681–682.

59. Levine, M. M., Dupont, H. L., Formal, S. B., Hornick, R. B., Takeuchi, A., Gangarosa, E. J., Snyder, M. J., and Libonati, J. P. (1973): Pathogenesis of *Shigella dysenteriae* 1 (Shiga) dysentery. *J. Infect. Dis.*, 127:261–270.

60. Dupont, H. L., Hornick, R. B., and Snyder, M. J. (1972): Immunity in shigellosis. II. Protection induced by oral live vaccine or primary infection. *J. Infect. Dis.*, 125:12–16.

61. Formal, S. B., Gemski, P., Baron, L. S., and LaBrec, E. H. (1971): A chromosomal locus which controls the ability of *Shigella flexneri* to evoke keratoconjunctivitis. *Infect. Immun.*, 3:73–79.

62. Formal, S. B., LaBrec, E. H., Kent, T. H., and Falkow, S. (1965): Abortive intestinal infection with an *Escherichia coli-Shigella flexneri* hybrid strain. *J. Bacteriol.*, 89:1374–1382.

63. Vicari, G., Olitzki, A. L., and Olitzki, Z. (1960): The action of thermolabile toxin of *Shigella dysenteriae* on cells cultivated *in vitro*. *Br. J. Exp. Pathol.*, 41:179–189.

64. Keusch, G. T., Grady, G. F., Mata, L. J., and McIver, J. (1972): The pathogenesis of *Shigella* diarrhea. I. Enterotoxin production by *Shigella dysenteriae* 1. *J. Clin. Invest.*, 51:1212–1218.

65. Gemski, P. A., Takeuchi, A., Washington, O., and Formal, S. B. (1972): Shigellosis due to *S. dysenteriae*. Relative importance of mucosal invasion versus toxin production in pathogenesis. *J. Infect. Dis.*, 126:523–530.

66. Keusch, G. T., Jacewicz, M., Levine, M. M., Hornick, R. B., and Kochwa, S. (1976): Pathogenesis of *Shigella* diarrhea. Serum anticytotoxin antibody response produced by toxigenic and nontoxigenic *Shigella dysenteriae* 1. *J. Clin. Invest.*, 57:194–202.

67. Keusch, G. T., and Jacewicz, M. (1977): The pathogenesis of *Shigella* diarrhea. VI. Toxin and antitoxin in *Shigella flexneri* and *Shigella sonnei* infections in humans. *J. Infect. Dis.*, 135:552–556.

68. Keusch, G. T. (1982): Shigellosis. In: *Bacterial Infections in Humans*, edited by A. S. Evans and H. A. Feldman, pp. 487–509. Plenum, New York.

69. Keren, D. J., Kern, S. E., Bauer, D. H., Scott, P. J., and Porter, P. (1982): Direct demonstration in intestinal secretions of an IgA memory response to orally administered *Shigella flexneri* antigens. *J. Immunol.*, 128:475–479.

70. Thorne, G. A., and Gorbach, S. L. (1977): *Shigella* vaccines, *Shigella* pathogens—Dr. Jekyll and Mr. Hyde. *J. Infect. Dis.*, 136:601–604.

71. Hornick, R. B., Greiseman, S. E., Woodward, T. E., DuPont, H. L., Dawkins, A. T., and Snyder, M. J. (1970): Typhoid fever: Pathogenesis and immunological control. *N. Engl. J. Med.*, 283:686–691, 736–746.

72. McCullough, N. B., and Eisele, C. W. (1951): Experimental human salmonellosis. III. Pathogenicity of strains of *Salmonella newport*, *Salmonella derby* and *Salmonella bareilly* obtained from spray-dried whole egg. *J. Infect. Dis.*, 89:209–213.

73. McCullough, N. B., and Eisele, C. W. (1951): Experimental human salmonellosis. IV. Pathogenicity of strains of *Salmonella pullorum* obtained from spray-dried whole egg. *J. Infect. Dis.*, 89:259–265.

74. Bennett, I. L., and Hook, E. W. (1959): Infectious diseases (some aspects of salmonellosis). *Annu. Rev. Med.*, 10:1–20.

75. Makela, P. H., Valtonen, V. V., and Valtman, M. (1973): Role of O-antigen (lipopolysaccharide) factors in the virulence of *Salmonella*. *J. Infect. Dis.*, 128S:581–585.

76. Giannella, R. A., Gots, R. E., Charney, A. N., Greenough, W. B., and Formal, S. B. (1975): Pathogenesis of *Salmonella*-mediated intestinal fluid secretion: Activation of adenyl cyclase and inhibition by indomethacin. *Gastroenterology*, 69:1238–1245.

77. Peterson, J. W. (1980): *Salmonella* toxin. *Pharmacol. Ther.*, 11:719–724.

78. Baloda, S. B., Faris, A., Krovacek, K., and Wadstrom, T. (1983): Cytotonic enterotoxins and cytotoxic factors produced by *Salmonella enteritidis* and *Salmonella typhimurium. Toxicon*, 21:785–796.

79. Plant, J., and Glynn, A. A. (1974): Natural resistance to *Salmonella* infection, delayed hypersensitivity and Ir genes in different strains of mice. *Nature*, 248:345–347.

80. Nencioni, L., Villa, L., Boraschi, D., Berti, B., and Tagliabue, A. (1983): Natural and antibody-dependent cell-mediated activity against *Salmonella typhimurium* by peripheral and intestinal lymphoid cells in mice. *J. Immunol.*, 130:903–907.

81. Kaye, D., and Hook, E. W. (1963): The influence of hemolysis on susceptibility to *Salmonella* infection: Additional observations. *J. Exp. Med.*, 91:518–527.

82. Hand, W. L., and King, N. L. (1977): Serum opsonization of *Salmonella* in sickle cell anemia. *Am. J. Med.*, 64:388–395.

83. Allardyce, R. A., Shearman, D. J. C., McClelland, D. B. L., Marwick, K., Simpson, A. J., and Laidlaw, R. B. (1974): Appearance of specific colostral antibodies after clinical infection with *Salmonella typhimurium. Br. Med. J.*, 3:307–309.

84. LaBrooy, J. T., Shearman, D. J. C., and Rowley, D. (1982): Antibodies in serum and secretions one year after *Salmonella* gastroenteritis. *Clin. Exp. Immunol.*, 48:551–554.

85. McCullough, N. B., and Eisele, C. W. (1951): Experimental human salmonellosis. II. Immunity studies following experimental illness with *Salmonella melaeagridis* and *Salmonella anatum. J. Immunol.*, 66:595–608.

86. Eisenstein, T. K., and Sultzer, B. M. (1983): Immunity to *Salmonella* infection. *Adv. Exp. Med. Biol.*, 162:261–296.

87. Wahdan, M. H., Serie, C., Cerisier, Y., Sallam, S., and Germanier, R. (1982): A controlled field trial of live *Salmonella typhi* strain Ty 21a oral vaccine against typhoid: Three-year results. *J. Infect. Dis.*, 145:292–295.

88. Vantrappen, G, Geboes, K., and Ponette, E. (1982): *Yersinia* enteritis. *Med. Clin. North Am.*, 66:639–654.

89. Pai, C. H., Mors, V., and Toma, S. (1978): Prevalence of enterotoxigenicity in human and nonhuman isolates of *Yersinia enterocolitica. Infect. Immun.*, 22:334–338.

90. Maki, M., Gronroos, P., and Vesikari, T. (1978): *In vitro* invasiveness of *Yersinia enterocolitica* isolated from children with diarrhea. *J. Infect. Dis.*, 138:677–680.

91. Zink, D. L., Feeley, J. C., Wells, J. G., Vanderzant, C., Vickery, J. C., Roof, W. D., and O'Donovan, G. A. (1980): Plasmid-mediated tissue invasiveness in *Yersinia enterocolitica. Nature*, 283:224–226.

92. Aulisio, C. C. G., Hill, W. E., Stanfield, J. T., and Sellers, R. L. (1983): Evaluation of virulence factor testing and characteristics of pathogenicity in *Yersinia enterocolitica. Infect. Immun.*, 40:300–335.

93. Marks, M. I., Pai, C. H., and LaFleur, L. (1981): *Yersinia enterocolitica* gastroenteritis in children and their families. In: *Yersinia enterocolitica*, edited by E. J. Bottone, pp. 95–104. CRC Press, Boca Raton, Fla.

94. Bottone, E. J., and Sheehan, D. J. (1983): *Yersinia enterocolitica*: Guidelines for serologic diagnosis of human infection. *J. Infect. Dis.*, 5:898–906.

95. Vuento, R. (1983): Antigen-specific lymphocyte transformation in patients with recent yersiniosis. *Acta Pathol. Microbiol. Immunol. Scand.*, 91C:89–93.

96. Gordon, I., Ingraham, H. S., and Kerns, R. F. (1947): Transmission of epidemic gastroenteritis to human volunteers by oral administration of fecal filtrates. *J. Exp. Med.*, 86:409–422.

97. San Joaquin, V. H., and Marks, M. I. (1982): New agents in diarrhea. *Ped. Infect. Dis.*, 1:53–65.

98. Blacklow, N. R., and Cukor, G. (1981): Viral gastroenteritis. *N. Engl. J. Med.*, 304:397–406.

99. Yow, M. D., Melnick, J. L., Blattner, R. J., Stephenson, W. B., Robinson, N. M., and Burkhardt, M. A. (1970): The association of viruses and bacteria with infantile diarrhea. *Am. J. Epidemiol.*, 92:33–39.

100. Adler, J., and Zickl, R. (1969): Winter vomiting disease. *J. Infect. Dis.*, 119:668–673.

101. Blacklow, N. R., Dolin, R., and Fedson, D. S. (1972): Acute infectious non-bacterial gastroenteritis: Etiology and pathogenesis. *Ann. Intern. Med.*, 76:993–1008.

102. Kapikian, A. Z., Wyatt, R. G., and Dolin, R. (1972): Visualization by immune electron microscopy of a 27-nm particle associated with acute infectious nonbacterial gastroenteritis. *J. Virol.*, 10:1075–1081.

103. Kaplan, J. E., Gary, G. W., Baron, R. C., Singh, N., Schonberger, L. B., Feldman, R., and Greenberg, H. B. (1982): Epidemiology of Norwalk gastroenteritis and the role of Norwalk virus in outbreaks of acute nonbacterial gastroenteritis. *Ann. Intern. Med.*, 96:756–761.

104. Schreiber, D. S., Blacklow, N. R., and Trier, J. S. (1973): The mucosal lesion of the proximal small intestine in acute infectious nonbacterial gastroenteritis. *N. Engl. J. Med.*, 288:1318–1323.

105. Levy, A. G., Widerlite, L., Schwartz, C. J., Dolin, R., Blacklow, N. R., Gardner, J. D., Kimberg, D. V., and Trier, J. S. (1976): Jejunal adenylate cyclase activity in human subjects during viral gastroenteritis. *Gastroenterology*, 70:321–325.

106. Schreiber, D. S., Trier, J. S., and Blacklow, N. R. (1977): Recent advances in viral gastroenteritis. *Gastroenterology*, 73:174–183.

107. Parrino, T. A., Schreiber, D. S., Trier, J. S., Kapikian, A. Z., and Blacklow, N. R. (1977): Clinical immunity in acute gastroenteritis caused by the Norwalk agent. *N. Engl. J. Med.*, 297:86–89.

108. Blacklow, N. R., Cukor, G., Bedigian, M. K., Echeverria, P., Greenberg, H. B., Schreiber, D. S., and Trier, J. S. (1979): Immune response and prevalence of antibody to Norwalk enteritis virus as determined by radioimmunoassay. *J. Clin. Microbiol.*, 10:903–909.

109. Koopman, J. S., Eckert, E. A., Greenberg, H. B., Strohm, B. C., Isaacson, R. E., and Monto, A. S. (1982): Norwalk virus enteric illness acquired by swimming exposure. *Am. J. Epidemiol.*, 115:173–177.

110. Bishop, R. F., Davidson, G. P., Holmes, I. H., and Ruck, B. J. (1973): Virus particles in epithelial cells of duodenal mucosa from children with acute nonbacterial gastroenteritis. *Lancet*, 2:1281–1283.

111. Wyatt, R. G., James, W. D., Bohl, E. H., Theil, K. W., Saif, L. J., Kalica, A. R., Greenberg, H. B., Kapikian, A. Z., and Chanock, R. M. (1980): Human rotavirus type 2: Cultivation *in vitro*. *Science*, 207:189–191.

112. Wolf, J. L., and Schreiber, D. S. (1982): Viral gastroenteritis. *Med. Clin. North Am.*, 66:575–595.

113. Black, R. E., Merson, M. H., Huq, I., Alim, A. R. M. A., and Yunus, M. (1981): Incidence and severity of rotavirus and *Escherichia coli* diarrhea in rural Bangladesh. Implication for vaccine development. *Lancet*, 1:141–143.

114. Smith, C. C., Aurelian, L., and Santosham, M. (1983): Rotavirus-associated travellers diarrhea: Neutralizing antibody in asymptomatic infections. *Infect. Immun.*, 41:829–833.

115. Davidson, G. P., and Barnes, G. L. (1979): Structural and functional abnormalities of the small intestine in infants and young children with rotavirus enteritis. *Acta Pediatr. Scand.*, 68:181–186.

116. Davidson, G. P., Gall, D. G., Petric, M., Butler, D. G., and Hamilton, J. R. (1977): Human rotavirus enteritis induced in conventional piglets. Intestinal structure and transport. *J. Clin. Invest.*, 60:1402–1409.

117. Bishop, R. F., Barnes, G. L., Cipriani, E., and Lund, J. S. (1983): Clinical immunity after neonatal rotavirus infection. *N. Engl. J. Med.*, 309:72–76.

118. Bishop, R. F., Cameron, D. J. S., Veenstra, A. A., and Barnes, G. L. (1979): Diarrhea and rotavirus infection associated with differing regimens of post-natal care of newborn babies. *J. Clin. Microbiol.*, 9:525–529.

119. McLean, B. S., and Holmes, I. H. (1981): Effects of antibodies, trypsin and trypsin inhibitors on susceptibility of neonates to rotavirus infection. *J. Clin. Microbiol.*, 13:22–29.

120. Snodgrass, D. R., and Wells, P. W. (1976): Rotavirus infections in lambs: Studies on passive protection. *Arch. Virol.*, 52:201–205.

121. Kapikian, A. Z., Wyatt, R. G., Greenberg, H. B., Kalica, A. R., Kim, H. W., Brandt, C. W., Rodriguez, W. J., Parrott, R. H., and Chanock, R. M. (1980): Approaches to immunization of infants and young children against gastroenteritis due to rotavirus. *Rev. Infect. Dis.*, 2:459–469.

Subject Index